CLINICAL REASONING

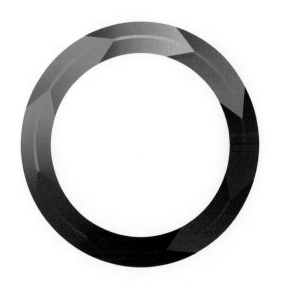

Dedication

This book is dedicated to my son Tyler and my daughter Madeline—inspirational healthcare professionals who make a difference in people's lives every day.

Tracy Levett-Jones

SECOND EDITION

CLINICAL REASONING

Learning to think like a nurse

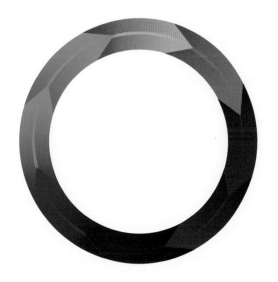

EDITED BY
TRACY LEVETT-JONES

Copyright © Pearson Australia (a division of Pearson Australia Group Pty Ltd) 2018

Pearson Australia
707 Collins Street
Melbourne VIC 3008

www.pearson.com.au

Senior Portfolio Manager: Mandy Sheppard
Development Editor: Judith Bamber
Project Manager: Bronwyn Smith
Production Manager: Abhishek Agarwal, iEnergizer Aptara®, Ltd
Content Developer: Stephen Razos
Rights and Permissions Editor: Emma Gaulton
Production Controller: Bradley Smith
Lead Editor/Copy Editor: Sandra Goodall
Proofreader: iEnergizer Aptara®, Ltd
Indexer: iEnergizer Aptara®, Ltd
Cover and internal design by Natalie Bowra
Typeset by iEnergizer Aptara®, Ltd

Printed in Malaysia (CTP-PJB)

1 2 3 4 5 22 21 20 19 18

National Library of Australia
Cataloguing-in-Publication Data

Title:	Clinical reasoning : learning to think like a nurse / edited by Tracy Levett-Jones.
Edition:	2nd edition
ISBN:	9781488616396 (paperback)
Notes:	Includes index.
Subjects:	Nursing—Textbooks.
	Nursing—Study and teaching.
	Medical logic.
Other Creators/Contributors:	Levett-Jones, Tracy, editor.

Pearson Australia Group Pty Ltd   ABN 40 004 245 943

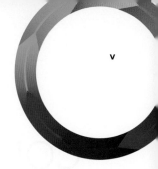

BRIEF CONTENTS

CONTENTS

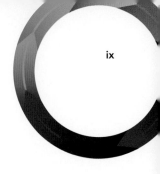

CHAPTER 12

Caring for a person with a complex and chronic health condition   216

Rachel Rossiter and Teresa Stone

CHAPTER 13

Caring for a person experiencing an acute psychotic episode   236

Anna Treloar and Peter Ross

CHAPTER 14

Caring for an older person with altered cognition   254

Sharyn Hunter, Frances Dumont and Jacqui Culver

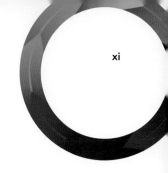

ABOUT THE EDITOR

Tracy Levett-Jones, PHD, RN, MED & WORK, BN, DIPAPPSC (NURSING), is Professor of Nursing Education at the University of Technology, Sydney. She has been the recipient of multiple teaching and research awards, and has led a number of funded research projects designed to improve the quality of teaching and learning for healthcare students, and ultimately improve patient outcomes. Tracy has also authored numerous books, book chapters, journal articles and blogs. Her research interests include clinical reasoning, interprofessional communication, patient safety, cultural competence, belongingness, empathy and simulation. Tracy's doctoral research explored the clinical placement experiences of students in Australia and the United Kingdom.

CONTRIBUTORS

Ms Jacqui Culver RN, BN, MMP
Nurse Practitioner Aged Care (Palliative & Dementia), Hunter New England Health

Ms Frances Dumont RN, MSN, BN, BED
Former Dementia Delirium Clinical Nurse Consultant, Hunter New England Health

Ms Natalie Govind RN, BN (HON), GRAD CERT ICU, PHD CANDIDATE
Lecturer, Faculty of Health, University of Technology Sydney

Dr Stephen Guinea BN, GRAD DIP VOC ED TRAIN, PHD
Senior Lecturer, Coordinator of Health Simulation, Faculty of Health Sciences, Australian Catholic University

Mr Nathan Haining RN, BN, GRAD CERT CRIT CARE
Clinical Nurse Educator, Neuroscience, Westmead Hospital

Dr Kerry Hoffman RN, BSC, GRAD DIP ED, DIP HEALTH SCI, MN, PHD
Lecturer, School of Nursing and Midwifery, University of Newcastle

Dr Sharyn Hunter PHD, RN, BSC (HONS), GRAD CERT (AGED CARE), GRAD CERT TERTIARY TEACHING
Senior Lecturer, School of Nursing and Midwifery, University of Newcastle

Professor Christine Imms BAPPSC (OT), MSC, PHD
National Head of School, Allied Health, Australian Catholic University

Ms Marcia Ingles RN
Clinical Nurse Specialist, Emergency Department, Belmont Hospital

Professor Tracy Levett-Jones PHD, RN, MED & WORK, BN, DIPAPPSC (NURSING)
Professor of Nursing Education, Faculty of Health, University of Technology Sydney

Professor Vanessa McDonald PHD, BN, RN, DIP HEALTH SCI
Professor, School of Nursing and Midwifery, University of Newcastle

Ms Jessica McKirkle BN, GRAD DIP CHILDREN, ADOLESCENT AND FAMILY HEALTH
Lecturer, School of Nursing, Midwifery & Paramedicine, Australian Catholic University

Ms Veronica Mills RN, BN, MHLTH SC
Casual Academic, School of Nursing and Midwifery, CQ University, Diabetic Educator

Associate Professor David Newby PHD, GRAD DIP EPI, BPHARM
Acting Discipline Lead, Clinical Pharmacology, School of Medicine and Public Health, University of Newcastle

Ms Elizabeth Newman RN, GRAD CERT NURS. SCIENCE (APHERESIS), MASTER OF NURSING (NURSE PRACTITIONER)
Nurse Practitioner Bone Marrow Transplant & Apheresis, Concord Repatriation General Hospital, Conjoint Lecturer, School of Nursing and Midwifery, University of Newcastle

Ms Lorinda Palmer MN, RN, BSC, DIP ED, GRAD DIP (NURSING), PHD CANDIDATE
Lecturer, School of Nursing and Midwifery, University of Newcastle

Ms Caroline Phelan RN, MPH, BN, PHD CANDIDATE
Clinical Nurse Consultant Pain Management, Hunter Integrated Pain service

Dr Victoria Pitt RN, PHD, MNUR (RESEARCH), GRAD DIP NURS (PAL. CARE), GRAD CERT TERTIARY TEACHING, DIP APSC (NURSING)
Bachelor of Nursing Program Convenor, School of Nursing and Midwifery, University of Newcastle

Ms Loretto Quinney RN, RM, CCRN, BAAPPSC, GRAD CERT MNG, PHD CANDIDATE
Lecturer, School of Nursing and Midwifery, Australian Catholic University

Professor Kerry Reid-Searl PHD, RN, RM, BHLTHSC, MCLINED
 Professor of Nursing, School of Nursing and Midwifery,
 CQ University

Mr Peter Ross RN
 Mental Health Nurse, Mid North Coast Correctional Centre

Dr Rachel Rossiter D.HSC, RN, MN (NP), MCOUNSELLING, BCOUNSELLING, BHLTHSC
 Associate Professor of Nursing (Nurse Practitioner),
 Charles Sturt University

Mr Peter Sinclair RN, BN, RENAL CERT, MPHIL, PHD CANDIDATE
 Lecturer, School of Nursing and Midwifery, University of
 Newcastle

Professor Teresa Stone PHD, RN, RMN, BA, M HEALTH MANAGEMENT, GRAD
 CERT TERTIARY TEACHING
 Professor, International Nursing, Faculty of Health
 Sciences, Yamaguchi University

Dr Anna Treloar RN, CMHN, MA, MPHC, PHD
 Lecturer, School of Nursing and Midwifery, University of
 Newcastle

Associate Professor Pamela van der Riet PHD, RN, MED, BA, DIP ED
 (NURSING), ICU/CCU CERT
 Associate Professor, School of Nursing and Midwifery,
 University of Newcastle

Ms Bree Walker RN, BN
 Nurse Educator, Paediatrics, Rockhampton Hospital

Dr Amanda Wilson RN, BA (HONS), MCA, PHD
 Senior Lecturer, School of Nursing and Midwifery,
 University of Newcastle

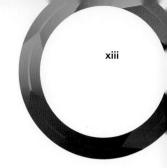

PREFACE

FOR STUDENTS

Having sufficient 'cue sensitivity' to detect potential errors only applies to the interested, engaged nurse. The indifferent detached nurse . . . would not be alert to subtle patient changes that may occur with deterioration in their health or medical errors . . .

(Benner, 2001, p. 136)

Competent nursing practice requires not only knowledge and skills but also sophisticated thinking abilities. Safe and effective nurses use disciplined, systematic and logical thought processes to guide their practice and inform their decision making. Their clinical reasoning ability is a key factor in the provision of quality care and the prevention of adverse patient outcomes.

In order to become a competent nurse, it is essential to learn the process and steps of clinical reasoning. Students need to understand the rules that determine how cues influence clinical decisions and the connections between cues, decisions and outcomes (Benner, 2001). Becoming skilled in clinical reasoning does not happen serendipitously. It requires practice, determination and active engagement in deliberate learning activities; it also requires reflection on activities designed to improve performance.

This second edition of *Clinical Reasoning* includes 17 authentic, engaging and meaningful chapters that will guide you through the clinical reasoning process while challenging you to think critically and creatively about the nursing care you provide. Three new chapters have been added to the collection: Chapters 10, 13 and 15. Like the others, these new chapters each promote deep learning and provide opportunities for you to rehearse how you will respond to emergent clinical situations in ways that are both person-centred and clinically astute.

The scenarios included in each chapter have been adapted from real clinical situations that occurred in healthcare and community settings. The clinical conditions that feature in this book are framed by Australia's National Health Priorities, and the patients/clients profiled are of different ages and from different cultural backgrounds. Each chapter emphasises patient safety and quality care; and there are references to the National Safety and Quality Health Service (NSQHS) Standards (2017) as well as the Nursing and Midwifery Board of Australia (NMBA) *Registered Nurse Standards for Practice* (2016).

We hope you enjoy learning about clinical reasoning and that this book helps you on your journey to becoming a safe, person-centred and competent nurse.

HOW TO USE THIS BOOK

While there is no one way to read this book, here are some suggested approaches. Start with Chapter 1; it will help you to understand the importance of clinical reasoning and introduce you to the process. Chapter 2 then takes you through the clinical reasoning process by juxtaposing two scenarios: the first demonstrates what can happen when clinical reasoning is not used and the second 'rewinds' and illustrates how effective clinical reasoning skills can make a significant difference to patient outcomes. With the foundation skills from Chapter 1 and the application skills from Chapter 2, you will be prepared for the other chapters. Scan the list of contents and select the topics that interest you the most, that you are currently studying or that you have encountered in your clinical practice. Your lecturers may also prescribe certain chapters as part of your required course work. While many of the chapters illustrate how effective clinical reasoning skills can help you recognise and manage patient deterioration early and, in effect, 'rescue' the patient, Chapter 17 considers the ethical implications of withholding potentially life-saving treatments when an attempt to 'rescue' may not be in the person's best interests or in accord with their wishes. These are some of the most difficult clinical decisions that can be made, and require effective clinical and moral reasoning skills.

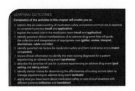

Learning outcomes are listed at the beginning of the chapter, and a sequential, step-through approach is used to tell an 'unfolding story'.

Key concepts integrated throughout the book include person-centred care, holistic practice, empathy, therapeutic communication, intra- and interprofessional communication, cultural competence, pathophysiology and safe medication practices.

Advanced organisers are provided to enhance understanding and recall of the clinical reasoning cycle.

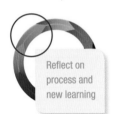

Reflect on process and new learning

Questions (multiple-choice, true or false, rank and sort, and short-answer) provide multiple opportunities to test your knowledge, make mistakes and learn from the process.

Answers to the questions are provided on the *Clinical Reasoning* website (www.pearson.com.au/9781488616396).

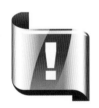

Something to think about boxes highlight important points within each chapter.

Reflective thinking is the final stage of the clinical reasoning cycle and, in order for you to maximise your learning, guided reflection questions are provided at the end of each scenario. Answers to these questions are not provided, as their purpose is to help you think critically and creatively about what you have learned and, most importantly, how your learning will inform and translate to your future practice.

Margin notes provide helpful hints, advice and links to relevant resources.

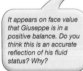

It appears on face value that Giuseppe is in a positive balance. Do you think this is an accurate reflection of his fluid status? Why?

Suggested readings are provided at the beginning of each chapter to enable preparation for the learning activities.

Further reading lists are provided at the end of each chapter to build on and extend your knowledge about topics of interest.

A **glossary** of terms is provided on page 330.

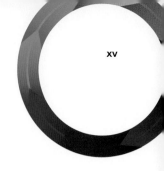

FOR EDUCATORS

Nursing or Midwifery programs must enable the development of clinical reasoning, problem solving and critical thinking.

(World Health Organization, 2008)

This book is premised on the understanding that a requisite level of clinical reasoning skills is imperative for safe and effective nursing practice. This requires educators to model, teach and assess students' developing clinical reasoning skills, in both academic and clinical settings. The scenarios in this book have been developed to encourage the acquisition of both content knowledge (domain-specific) and process knowledge (clinical reasoning ability). The constructivist approach adopted will allow both undergraduate and postgraduate students to construct knowledge by being actively engaged in learning that is situated, experiential and authentic. The unfolding stories provide meaningful opportunities for reiterative learning which leads to deeper levels of processing, thus improving retention and recall of information. The consistent structure of the scenarios allows for cognitive rehearsal of the clinical reasoning process to enable students to integrate these cognitive skills into their repertoire of clinical behaviours.

The scenarios can be used in multiple ways: as stimulus materials prior to or during tutorial activities or online learning; for self-directed learning, assignments and exam preparation; or for continuing professional development. Additionally, the scenarios can be used as a framework for the development of simulation scenarios using manikins, standardised patients/actors or a range of other modalities.

The reflective thinking activities can be used to design assignment and exam questions, for tutorial discussion or to structure debriefing following simulation sessions. They can also be extended and contextualised by adding specific questions that align with your course objectives.

Feedback from students about the first edition of this book has been consistently positive. For example:

- *Each chapter made me feel like an investigator trying to put all the clues together to solve the patient problem.*
- *The scenarios showed me how I jump to conclusions before considering the information given; I learnt that some things aren't always what they seem.*
- *The scenarios involved constant thinking and decision making and I found them to be a great tool for learning what could go wrong when a patient's nursing diagnosis is incorrect.*
- *Going step by step through the clinical reasoning cycle was a good way to learn. I found it made me research a lot of things I didn't know and look into conditions I was unfamiliar with.*

In writing this book for nursing students, our aim has been to have a positive impact on patient safety and quality care. We hope that you find the scenarios engaging, meaningful and beneficial in your teaching of clinical reasoning.

The most important practical lesson that can be given to nurses is to teach them what to observe – how to observe – what symptoms indicate improvement – what the reverse – which are of importance – which are none – which are the evidence of neglect – and of what kind of neglect.

(Florence Nightingale, 1860, p. 105)

Tracy Levett-Jones and the 'Thinking like a nurse' writing team

REFERENCES

Benner, P. (2001). *From Novice to Expert: Excellence and Power in Clinical Nursing Practice.* Upper Saddle River, NJ: Prentice Hall.

Florence Nightingale. (1860). *Notes on Nursing: What It Is and What It Is Not.* New York: D. Appleton and Co. Reprint 1969. New York: Dover Publications, Inc.

World Health Organization. (2008). *Global Standards for the Initial Education of Professional Nurses and Midwives.* Geneva: WHO.

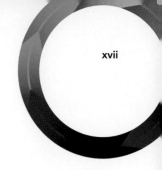

ACKNOWLEDGEMENTS

First, I would like to acknowledge and offer sincere thanks to my wonderful writing team. Their commitment to student learning, patient safety and person-centred care informs every chapter and has resulted in a book that will inspire, motivate and engage nursing students. Next, I would like to thank the expert clinicians and academics who reviewed the book for accuracy, authenticity and relevance. Finally, thank you to the editorial and production team at Pearson, including Mandy Sheppard, Senior Portfolio Manager; Judith Bamber, Development Editor; Bronwyn Smith, Project Manager; Bernadette Chang, Editorial Design and Production Manager; Emma Gaulton, Senior Rights and Permissions Editor; and Sandra Goodall, Lead Editor/Copy Editor.

REVIEWERS

Ms Shannon Barnes, Lecturer, Australian Catholic University

Mrs Rhonda Beggs, Lecturer, Griffith University

Miss Nicole Blakey, Senior Lecturer & National Professional Practice Lead (Nursing), Australian Catholic University

Dr Denise Blanchard, Senior Lecturer, Charles Sturt University

Mr Adam Burston, Lecturer, Australian Catholic University

Ms Tara Flemington, The University of Sydney

Ms Jacqueline Fong, Lecturer/Nursing Practitioner, The University of Sydney

Dr Julie Hanson, Lecturer, University of the Sunshine Coast

Mrs Peta Harbour, Lecturer, Charles Darwin University

Dr Debbie Massey, Senior Lecturer, University of the Sunshine Coast

Mr Thomas K. Mathew, Lecturer, The University of Melbourne

Ms Peta Reid, Lecturer, Australian Catholic University

Ms Annette Saunders, Lecturer, University of Tasmania

Mrs Rosemary Saunders, Senior Lecturer, Edith Cowan University

FIRST EDITION

The publisher would like to thank and acknowledge the valuable work of the following previous contributors to the first edition of this text:

Chapter 1 Clinical reasoning: What it is and why it matters
Dr Kerry Hoffman, *The University of Newcastle*

Chapter 3 Caring for a person with fluid and electrolyte imbalance
Dr Kerry Hoffman, *The University of Newcastle*
Dr Jennifer Dempsey, *The University of Newcastle*

Chapter 5 Caring for a child with type 1 diabetes
Ms Lea Vieth, *Rockhampton Hospital*

Chapter 6 Caring for a person experiencing respiratory distress and hypoxia
Mrs Raelene Kenny, *Port Macquarie Base Hospital and The University of Newcastle*
Dr Jennifer Dempsey, *The University of Newcastle*

Chapter 7 Caring for a person with a cardiac condition
Dr Jennifer Dempsey, *The University of Newcastle*
Mrs Raelene Kenny, *Port Macquarie Base Hospital and The University of Newcastle*

Chapter 9 Caring for a person receiving blood component therapies
Dr Jennifer Dempsey, *The University of Newcastle*

CHAPTER 1

CLINICAL REASONING: WHAT IT IS AND WHY IT MATTERS

TRACY LEVETT-JONES

LEARNING OUTCOMES

Completion of the activities in this chapter will enable you to:

○ explain what it means to 'think like a nurse'

○ define and explain the process of clinical reasoning

○ justify why nursing students need to learn about clinical reasoning

○ discuss how clinical reasoning errors can adversely affect patient outcomes

○ explain the relationship between clinical reasoning and critical thinking

○ explain how stigmatising, stereotyping, preconceptions and assumptions can negatively impact clinical reasoning

○ explore and discuss different types of clinical reasoning errors.

Nurses are the caregivers most directly involved with patients 24/7, responsible for monitoring and assessing clinical changes in patients, intervening when necessary, and communicating changes in status to ensure appropriate intervention and coordination of care. (Duffield et al., 2007)

INTRODUCTION

In this chapter, we begin to explore what it means to 'think like a nurse'. We define and discuss the importance of clinical reasoning, outline the clinical reasoning process and illustrate how clinical errors are linked to poor reasoning skills. This chapter creates a foundation for the ones that follow and a backdrop to a series of authentic and clinically relevant clinical scenarios.

Learning to 'think like a nurse' is challenging and requires commitment, practice and multiple opportunities for application of learning. However, the benefits are significant for you, as a curious, competent and intelligent nurse, and also for the people who will be the recipients of your care. Simply stated, effective clinical reasoning skills improve the quality of patient care, prevent adverse patient outcomes and enhance nurses' work satisfaction.

WHAT DOES IT MEAN TO 'THINK LIKE A NURSE'?

While there are a number of similarities in the way nurses and other health professionals think, there are also significant differences. Unlike many health professionals who 'treat' and 'retreat', therapeutic relationships between nurses and their patients can extend over hours, days or even longer. During this time, nurses maintain constant vigilance and engage in multiple episodes of clinical reasoning for each person in their care, responding to the complex nature of the illness experience in ways that are authentic, holistic and person-centred.

> *'Thinking like a nurse' is a form of engaged moral reasoning. Educational practices must help students engage with patients with a deep concern for their well being. Clinical reasoning must arise from this engaged, concerned stance, always in relation to a particular patient and situation and informed by generalised knowledge and rational processes, but never as an objective, detached exercise. (Tanner, 2006, p. 209)*

WHY IS CLINICAL REASONING IMPORTANT?

Nurses are required to care for and make decisions about complex patients with diverse health needs. As they are responsible for a significant proportion of the clinical judgments in healthcare, their ability to respond to challenging and dynamic situations requires not only psychomotor skills and knowledge, but also sophisticated thinking abilities.

A body of evidence has identified that clinical reasoning skills have a positive impact on patient outcomes while, conversely, nurses with poor clinical reasoning skills often fail to detect patient deterioration, resulting in a failure to rescue (Cooper et al., 2011). Clinical reasoning errors have been implicated as a key factor in the majority of adverse patient outcomes (Institute of Medicine, 2010). The reasons for this are multidimensional and include the tendency to make errors in time-sensitive situations where there is a large amount of complex data to process, and difficulties in distinguishing between a clinical problem that needs immediate attention and one that is less acute (Hoffman, 2007).

WHAT IS CLINICAL REASONING?

Clinical reasoning is a systematic and cyclical process that guides clinical decision making, particularly in unpredictable, emergent and non-routine situations, and leads to accurate and informed clinical judgments. Clinical reasoning is defined as 'the process by which nurses (and other clinicians) collect cues, process the information, come to an understanding of a patient problem or situation, plan and implement interventions, evaluate outcomes, and reflect on and learn from the process' (Levett-Jones et al., 2010, p. 516). The clinical reasoning cycle (Figure 1.1) is informed by a body of research undertaken by Hoffman (2007) and Levett-Jones et al. (2010).

THE CLINICAL REASONING PROCESS

A diagram showing the clinical reasoning cycle and describing the nursing actions that occur during each stage is provided in Figure 1.2. The cycle begins at 1200 hours and moves in a clockwise direction through eight stages: *look, collect, process, diagnose, plan, act, evaluate* and *reflect*. Although each stage is presented as a separate and distinct element in this diagram, in reality clinical reasoning is a dynamic process and nurses often combine one or more stages or move back and forth between them before reaching a diagnosis, taking action and evaluating outcomes. Table 1.1 provides an example of a nurse's clinical reasoning while caring for a man following surgery for an abdominal aortic aneurysm.

Stages of the clinical reasoning cycle

1. Consider the patient situation

During the first stage of the clinical reasoning cycle, the nurse begins to gain an initial impression of the patient and identifies salient features of the situation. This first impression, which Tanner (2006) refers to as 'noticing', is critical but can be negatively influenced by the nurse's preconceptions, assumptions and biases.

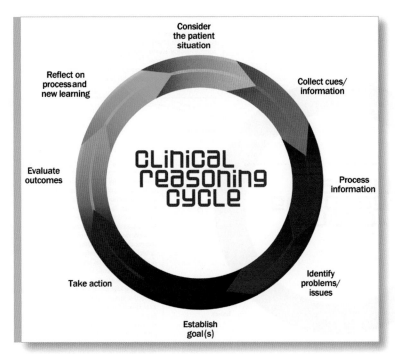

Figure 1.1
The clinical reasoning cycle

Source: T. Levett-Jones, K. Hoffman, Y. Dempsey, S. Jeong, D. Noble, C. Norton, J. Roche & N. Hickey (2010). The 'five rights' of clinical reasoning: An educational model to enhance nursing students' ability to identify and manage clinically 'at risk' patients. *Nurse Education Today, 30*(6), 515–20.

2. Collect cues/information

The importance of the cue collection stage of the clinical reasoning cycle cannot be underestimated, as early subtle cues when missed can lead to adverse patient outcomes (Levett-Jones et al., 2010). During the second stage, the nurse begins to collect relevant information about the patient. He/she reviews the information that is currently available, including the handover report, the patient's medical and social history, clinical documentation, electronic medical records and other available information.

The nurse then identifies additional information that is required, such as vital signs and/or a focused health assessment. Importantly, the nurse focuses on collecting specific cues relevant to the person's condition at this point in time. When appropriate, the nurse also seeks to elicit the patient's understanding of the situation and the family's or carer's concerns.

Lastly, the nurse recalls knowledge related to the patient's particular situation. A breath and depth of knowledge is therefore imperative for accurate clinical reasoning. Unless a nurse has a deep understanding of the applied sciences, especially pathophysiology, the ability to make sense of and correctly interpret cues will be impacted.

3. Process information

In the third stage of the clinical reasoning cycle, the nurse interprets the cues that have been collected and identifies significant aberrations from normal. Cues are grouped into meaningful clusters; clinical patterns are identified, inferences are made and hypotheses are generated. During this stage, experienced nurses call upon their wide repertoire of previous clinical experiences matching the features of patient's presentation with other similar situations. They are also able to 'think ahead' anticipating potential outcomes and complications depending on the particular course of action (or inaction).

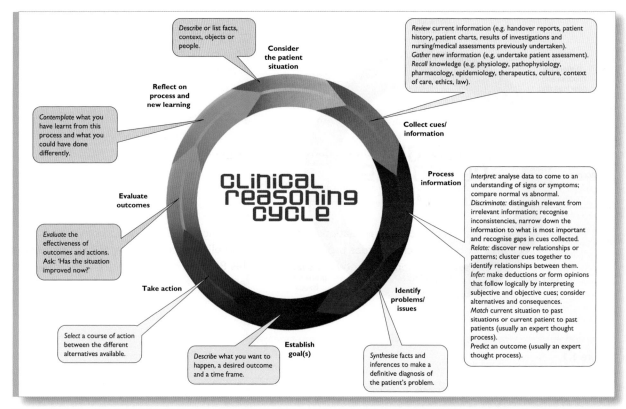

Figure 1.2
The clinical reasoning process with descriptors

Source: Adapted from T. Levett-Jones, K. Hoffman, Y. Dempsey, S. Jeong, D. Noble, C. Norton, J. Roche & N. Hickey (2010). The 'five rights' of clinical reasoning: An educational model to enhance nursing students' ability to identify and manage clinically 'at risk' patients. *Nurse Education Today*, *30*(6), 515–20.

Table 1.1 *Phases of the clinical reasoning cycle with examples*

Process	Description	Example of a nurse's thinking
Consider the patient situation	**Describe** person and context.	Mr Smith is a 60-year-old man admitted to ICU yesterday following surgery for an abdominal aortic aneurysm (AAA).
Collect cues/ information	**Review** current information (e.g. handover reports, patient history, patient charts, results of investigations and nursing/medical assessments previously undertaken)	Mr Smith has a history of hypertension and he takes beta-blockers. His BP was 140/80 mmHg an hour ago.
	Gather new information (e.g. undertake patient assessment).	Mr Smith's vital signs are: T 37.6°C, PR 116, RR 20, BP 110/60 mmHg. His urine output is averaging 20 mL/hr. He has an epidural running @ 10 mL/hr.
	Recall knowledge (e.g. physiology, pathophysiology, pharmacology, epidemiology, therapeutics, culture, context of care, ethics, law).	BP and PR are influenced by fluid status. Epidurals can lower the BP because they can cause vasodilation.

Table 1.1 *Phases of the clinical reasoning cycle with examples (continued)*

Process information	**Interpret:** analyse cues to come to an understanding of signs or symptoms. Compare normal vs abnormal.	Mr Smith's BP is low, especially for a person with a history of hypertension. He is tachycardic and oliguric.
	Discriminate: distinguish relevant from irrelevant information; recognise inconsistencies; narrow down information to what is most important; recognise gaps in cues collected.	Although Mr Smith is slightly febrile, I'm more concerned about his hypotension, tachycardia and oliguria.
	Relate: discover new relationships or patterns; cluster cues together to identify relationships between them.	Although Mr Smith's hypotension, tachycardia and oliguria could be signs of impending shock, his BP decreased soon after we increased his epidural rate.
	Infer: make deductions or form opinions that follow logically by interpreting subjective and objective cues; consider alternatives and consequences.	Mr Smith's BP is probably low because of his epidural and blood loss during surgery.
	Match current situation to past situations or current patient to past patients (usually an expert thought process).	AAAs are often hypotensive post-op.
	Predict an outcome (usually an expert thought process).	If we don't give Mr Smith a fluid challenge, he could develop acute kidney injury or go into shock.
Identify the problem/issue	**Synthesise** facts and inferences to make a definitive nursing diagnosis.	Mr Smith has reduced cardiac output related to decreased intravascular volume and vasodilation evidenced by hypotension, tachycardia and oliguria.
Establish goals	**Describe** what you want to happen, a desired outcome and a time frame.	To improve Mr Smith's cardiac output, haemodynamic status and urine output over the next 1–2 hours.
Take action	**Select** a course of action between the different alternatives available.	I will phone the medical officer (using ISBAR) to request an order for a fluid challenge, increased IV rate and aramine if needed.
Evaluate	**Evaluate** the effectiveness of outcomes and actions. Ask: 'Has the situation improved now?'	Mr Smith's BP has improved and his urine output is now averaging > 30 mL/hr. I'll continue to monitor him as he may need another fluid challenge or aramine later.
Reflect on process and new learning	**Contemplate** what you have learnt from this process and what you could have done differently.	I now understand … I should have … Next time I will …

Source: K. Hoffman (2007). A comparison of decision-making by 'expert' and 'novice' nurses in the clinical setting, monitoring patient haemodynamic status post abdominal aortic aneurysm surgery. Unpublished PhD thesis, University of Technology, Sydney; and T. Levett-Jones, K. Hoffman, Y. Dempsey, S. Jeong, D. Noble, C. Norton, J. Roche & N. Hickey (2010). The 'five rights' of clinical reasoning: An educational model to enhance nursing students' ability to identify and manage clinically 'at risk' patients. *Nurse Education Today, 30*(6), 515–20.

4. Identify problems/issues

Improving the diagnostic process is not only possible, but it also represents a moral, professional, and public health imperative. **(Institute of Medicine, 2010)**

The fourth stage of the cycle is where the nurse synthesises all of the information that has been collected and processed in order to identify the most appropriate nursing diagnoses. A three-part 'actual' diagnosis or a two-part 'risk' diagnosis may be formulated. The accuracy of this step is critical as the nursing diagnosis is used to determine appropriate goals of care and subsequent nursing actions. The following examples are adapted from Berman et al. (2017).

Nursing diagnosis

1. A nursing **diagnosis** is a problem that becomes apparent following a thorough and systematic interpretation of subjective and objective data. An actual nursing diagnosis consists of the person's **problem**, the related **aetiology** (causal relationship between a problem and its related or risk factors), and supporting **evidence**/cues.

   For example: *Dehydration* related to *post-operative nausea* and *vomiting* evidenced by *dry mucous membranes, oliguria, poor skin turgor, hypotension* and *tachycardia.*

2. A **risk nursing diagnosis** is a clinical judgment about a potential problem where the presence of **risk factors** indicates that a problem may develop unless nurses intervene appropriately. A risk diagnosis is written in two parts and does not include signs and symptoms.

   For example: *Risk of infection* related to *skin tear* and *type 2 diabetes.*

5. Establish goals

The fifth stage of the cycle is where the nurse clarifies and prioritises the goals of care depending on urgency. Goals must be SMART (**S**pecific, **M**easureable, **A**chievable, **R**ealistic and **T**imely) and designed to address the nursing diagnoses previously identified. Without SMART goals, the nurse cannot determine the efficacy of their actions.

6. Take action

In this stage the nurse selects the most appropriate course of action to achieve the goals of care and address the nursing diagnoses. The nurse also decides who is best placed to undertake the interventions, and who should be notified and when.

7. Evaluate outcomes

This stage requires the nurse to re-examine objective and subjective data (patient cues) in order to evaluate how effective the nursing interventions have been, and whether the patient's problem has improved. If the evaluation identifies that the patient's condition has not improved, the nurse reconsiders the patient's situation and seeks to identify a more appropriate course of action. There may be a need to engage in a new cycle of clinical reasoning at this stage.

8. Reflect on process and new learning

Effective clinical reasoning requires both cognitive and metacognitive (thinking about one's thinking) skills in order to develop the ability to 'think like a nurse' (Mezirow, 1990). Thus, the final step of the clinical reasoning cycle involves reflection. This requires nurses to critically review their practice with a view to refinement, improvement or change. Reflection is intrinsic to learning. It is a deliberate, orderly and structured intellectual activity that allows nurses to process their experience, and explore their understanding of what they did, why they did it, and the impact it had on themselves and others (Boud, 2015).

Nurses reflect *in* and *on* practice by asking themselves questions such as:

- What happened and why?
- What was done well and what should be improved?
- What should be done differently if presented with the same or similar situation?
- What has been learnt that can be used when caring for other patients?
- What is needed to improve future practice, for example more knowledge about a specific condition or more practice in particular skills?

CLINICAL REASONING AND CRITICAL THINKING

As a client's status changes, the nurse must recognise, interpret, and integrate new information and make decisions about the course of action to follow. For satisfactory client outcomes clinical reasoning goes hand in hand with critical thinking. (Martin, 2002, p. 245)

Clinical reasoning is dependent on a critical thinking 'disposition' (Scheffer & Rubenfeld, 2000). Critical thinking is a complex collection of cognitive skills and affective habits of the mind and has been described as the process of analysing and assessing thinking with a view to improving it (Paul & Elder, 2007). To think like a nurse requires you to learn the knowledge, ideas, skills, concepts and theories of nursing, and develop your intellectual capacities to become a disciplined, self-directed, critical thinker capable of clinical reasoning (Paul & Elder, 2007).

Nurses who are critical thinkers strive to be clear, accurate, precise, logical and fair when they listen, speak, read and write (Paul & Elder, 2007). Critical thinkers think deeply and broadly, eliminating irrelevant, inconsistent and illogical thoughts as they reason about patient care. The quality of their thinking improves over time and through reflection (Norris & Ennis, 1989). Below is a list of attributes nurses need to develop their critical thinking and clinical reasoning skills (Scheffer & Rubenfeld, 2000, p. 358; Rubenfeld & Scheffer, 2006, pp. 16–24):

- **A holistic and contextual perspective**—consideration of the whole person, taking into account the entire situation, including relationships, background and environment
- **Creativity**—the ability and desire to generate, discover or restructure ideas; and the ability to imagine alternatives
- **Inquisitiveness**—a thoughtful, questioning and curious approach; and an eagerness to explore possibilities and alternatives
- **Perseverance**—a dedication to the pursuit of knowledge despite any obstacles that are encountered
- **Intuition**—insightful patterns of knowing brought about by previous experiences and pattern recognition
- **Flexibility**—the capacity to adapt, modify or change thoughts, ideas and behaviours
- **Academic integrity**—seeking the truth through sincere, honest processes, even if the results are contrary to one's assumptions or beliefs
- **Reflexivity**—contemplation of assumptions, thinking and behaviours for the purpose of deeper understanding and self-evaluation
- **Confidence**—a firm belief in one's reasoning abilities
- **Open-mindedness**—receptiveness to different views and sensitivity to one's biases, prejudices, preconceptions and assumptions.

QUESTIONING ASSUMPTIONS AND UNDERSTANDING ERRORS

Nurses are human and we make the same kinds of thinking errors in our practice as we do in our day-to-day lives. Sometimes we overlook or misinterpret the significance of an important cue, or we jump to conclusions or fail to take into account alternative possibilities or options. Additionally, preconceptions, assumptions, biases, stereotypes and stigmatism can negatively influence our clinical reasoning and in some cases even prevent clinical reasoning from occurring. We may be unaware of the assumptions and prejudices that we hold as they are often long-standing and deeply embedded. For this reason nurses must develop insight and self-awareness by deliberately reflecting on their biases and preconceptions. Failure to do so can undermine the accuracy of clinical reasoning and consequently patient safety. Nurses can help avoid clinical reasoning errors by being mindful and reflective, and by using the multitude of decision support resources available to help them make a decision. They can also maintain a healthy skepticism and make it a habit to ask: 'What is influencing my thinking about this patient?', 'Could my interpretation be flawed?' and 'What other nursing diagnosis is possible in this situation?'.

Table 1.2 provides a list of clinical reasoning errors, many of which arise because of flawed assumptions and beliefs. Some of these errors are then illustrated in the narratives that follow.

Table 1.2   *Clinical reasoning errors*

Error	Definition
Anchoring	The tendency to lock onto salient features in the patient's presentation too early in the clinical reasoning process, and failing to adjust this initial impression in the light of later information. This error is compounded by confirmation bias.
Ascertainment bias	When a nurse's thinking is shaped by prior assumptions and preconceptions, for example ageism, stigmatism and stereotyping.
Confirmation bias	The tendency to look for confirming evidence to support a nursing diagnosis rather than look for disconfirming evidence to refute it, despite the latter often being more persuasive and definitive.
Diagnostic momentum	Once labels are attached to patients, they tend to become stickier and stickier. What started as a possibility gathers increasing momentum until it becomes definite and other possibilities are excluded.
Fundamental attribution error	The tendency to be judgmental and to blame patients for their illnesses (dispositional causes) rather than examine the circumstances (situational factors) that may have been responsible. Patients with a mental illness and from minority or marginalised groups are at particular risk of this error.
Overconfidence bias	A tendency to believe we know more than we do. Overconfidence bias reflects a tendency to act on incomplete information, intuition or hunches. Too much faith is placed on opinion instead of carefully collected cues. This error may be augmented by anchoring.
Premature closure	The tendency to accept a nursing diagnosis without sufficient evidence and before it has been fully verified. This error accounts for a high proportion of inaccurate or incomplete nursing diagnoses.
Psych-out error	People with a mental illness are particularly vulnerable to clinical reasoning errors, and co-morbid conditions may be overlooked or minimalised. A variant of this error occurs when medical conditions (such as hypoxia, delirium, electrolyte imbalance and head injuries) are misdiagnosed as psychiatric conditions.
Unpacking principle	Failure to collect and unpack all of the relevant cues, and consider differential diagnoses may result in significant possibilities being missed.

Source: Adapted from P. Croskerry (2003). The importance of cognitive errors in diagnosis and strategies to minimize them. *Academic Medicine, 78*(8), 1–6.

Examples of clinical reasoning errors

Some of the clinical reasoning errors listed in Table 1.2 are illustrated here with authentic clinical experiences. As you read these narratives, it will become evident that even experienced, committed and well-intentioned health professionals can make errors if they allow their thinking process to be clouded by assumptions, preconceptions and stereotypes. Environmental and situational factors such as noise, fatigue, stress, multitasking and interruptions can also impede thinking processes. As you read these examples, it is important to reflect on your own biases and prejudices, and any personal or contextual factors that negatively influence your thinking, as this will enhance your self-awareness, emotional intelligence and clinical reasoning ability.

Fundamental attribution error

This incident occurred when I was a newly registered nurse working on a medical ward. The patient was an elderly man (70+ years) who was admitted for a stroke. During his admission the man had some degree of hemiparesis from his stroke; however, this subsided to a large degree. The man appeared to be extremely resistive to our efforts to make him as independent as possible. He wanted a great deal of assistance with his activities of daily living and more than required for his level of disability. He required constant encouragement to participate in any sort of physical activity, no matter how minimal. The man was eventually transferred to a rehabilitation unit. Some weeks later he returned to our ward as he would 'not participate' in his rehabilitation program. The handover reported that he had 'failed rehab'. I judged him on his previous behaviour and I assumed he was just lazy (based on the information from the rehab staff). On his return to my ward he continued to constantly want assistance and seemed to be determined to become dependent. I insisted (often strenuously and on reflection harshly) that he walk and participate in his own care. Around this time he also started to mention pain which hadn't really featured till then. He was investigated and was found to have widespread bony metastasis from an unknown primary cancer. He died three weeks later. I was astounded and felt very guilty as I had judged this man, making assumptions that were proven to be erroneous. I did, however, ensure that this man received the very best care for the last three weeks of his life.

Doctor Jennifer Dempsey
University of Newcastle

Ascertainment bias

While employed as a mental health nurse in a GP practice I assessed a 65-year-old woman, Alice,[1] who was referred by her GP as he was concerned about her mental state. Upon assessment I found Alice had been diagnosed three years prior with the degenerative neurological condition, amyotrophic lateral sclerosis (ALS). She was divorced, lived alone in a council flat in a small seaside village and had limited contact with her daughter and grandchildren who lived six hours drive away. She had a prior history that included childhood sexual abuse, a previous suicide attempt (in the context of domestic violence) and two episodes of major depression which had responded well to psychotropic medication and supportive psychotherapy.

Although Alice had significant physical symptoms that affected her mobility at times, she described having managed well until four months ago when her relationship with her daughter had deteriorated severely. The abandonment had increased her sense of isolation and this estrangement appeared to have been a trigger for a relapse into major depression, with severe depressive symptoms, including increased loss of motivation, tearfulness, disordered sleep, loss of appetite and a heightened sense of hopelessness and suicidal ideation. Further discussion revealed that her GP had initiated a neurological review, which revealed minimal deterioration in physical functioning, and an aged care assessment (ACAT), with a view to increasing the level of support services available to Alice.

After consultation with Alice's GP, it was agreed that a psychiatrist review was warranted and I prepared a comprehensive referral to the mental health services. At the time I was working part-time with the Community Mental Health Team and thus was present at the intake meeting where all referrals were reviewed as part of a

---

1 **Pseudonym**

multi-disciplinary team process. The nurse from the Acute Care Service responsible for presenting the referrals to the team commenced reading the referral. Before he had finished, he commented, 'This is a waste of time; of course the woman's depressed, who wouldn't be with a degenerative illness; besides, she's old.' Another team member responded, 'Tell the GP to refer her to palliative care.'

Sadly for Alice, the mental health service declined a psychiatrist review; the Mental Health Service for Older Persons likewise declined a review and recommended instead that the application process for placement in an aged care facility be started. Alice's 'real' issues were not addressed because of the ageism and preconceptions of the mental health team.

Associate Professor Rachel Rossiter
Charles Sturt University

Anchoring

Working as a nurse educator, I had been paged to come to recovery. Two RNs were seeking advice about the management of a patient (Mrs L) who had had a left hip replacement and was in severe pain, very distressed and calling out loudly and incoherently. The anaesthetist had been notified but was in theatre with another patient. Mrs L had been given morphine by the anaesthetist before being transferred to recovery. As ordered, she was given three further bolus doses of morphine at 3-minute intervals but with minimal effect. The nurses were encouraging her to use her PCA button but she was not coherent enough to comply. I tried to do a thorough pain assessment but was hampered in my attempts as the patient was unable to reply to my questions. I did an assessment of the wound … the dressing was dry and intact and the bellovac draining a small amount. There was a small amount of urine in the catheter bag. I examined the area surrounding the wound convinced that there must be a surgical problem. It appeared normal and I could see no obvious reason for the pain.

Time was passing without any improvement and we were all becoming anxious and concerned about Mrs L's distress and pain. I was about to phone the anaesthetist again but decided to check her wound one more time. In the process I briefly noticed that Mrs L's catheter had not been taped to her leg and was actually lying under her thigh. Lifting it over her leg I saw that it had also been kinked. As I untwisted it, urine began to quickly flow. Within minutes there was close to 1600 mL in the catheter bag and Mrs L had drifted off into a morphine-induced state. Her resps were now 6 and oxygen sats 85 per cent. We increased the oxygen to 10 L per minute with little effect and phoned the anaesthetist for an order of naloxone as she had become narcotised. Had I not anchored onto the belief that Mrs L's pain must be coming from the surgical site I would have done a more comprehensive assessment, identified the cause of her pain, not administered as much morphine, and prevented respiratory depression from occurring. Checking that catheters are draining properly and not kinked or blocked became part of my routine post-operative patient assessment following this experience.

Professor Tracy Levett-Jones
University of Technology, Sydney

REFERENCES

Berman, A., Synder, S., Levett-Jones, T., Dwyer, T., Hales, M., Harvey, N., … Stanley, D. (2017). *Kozier and Erb's Fundamentals of Nursing* (4th edn). Sydney: Pearson.

Boud, D. (2015). Feedback: Ensuring that it leads to enhanced learning. *The Clinical Teacher, 12*(1), 3–7.

Cooper, S., Buykx, P., McConnell-Henry, T., Kinsman, L. & McDermott, S. (2011). Simulation: Can it eliminate failure to rescue? *Nursing Times, 107*(3).

Croskerry, P. (2003). The importance of cognitive errors in diagnosis and strategies to minimize them. *Academic Medicine, 78*(8), 1–6.

Duffield, C., Roche, M., O'Brien-Pallas, L., Diers, D., Alsbett, C., King, M., … Hall, J. (2007). *Gluing It Together: Nurses, Their Work Environment and Patient Safety*. University of Sydney, NSW.

Hoffman, K. (2007). A comparison of decision-making by 'expert' and 'novice' nurses in the clinical setting, monitoring patient haemodynamic status post abdominal aortic aneurysm surgery. Unpublished PhD thesis, University of Technology, Sydney.

Institute of Medicine. (2010). *The Future of Nursing: Focus on Education*. Accessed March 2017 at <www.nursingworld.org/MainMenuCategories/ThePracticeofProfessionalNursing/workforce/IOM-Future-of-Nursing-Report-1>.

Levett-Jones, T., Hoffman, K., Dempsey, Y., Jeong, S., Noble, D., Norton, C., … Hickey, N. (2010). The 'five rights' of clinical reasoning: An educational model to enhance nursing students' ability to identify and manage clinically 'at risk' patients. *Nurse Education Today, 30*(6), 515–20.

Martin, C. (2002). The theory of critical thinking. *Nursing Education Perspectives, 23*(5), 241–47.

Mezirow, J. (1990). *Fostering Critical Reflection in Adulthood: A Guide to Transformative and Emancipatory Learning*. San Francisco: Jossey Bass.

Norris, S. P. & Ennis, R. H. (1989). *Evaluating Critical Thinking*. Pacific Grove, CA: Midwest Publications, Critical Thinking Press.

Paul, R. & Elder, L. (2007). *The Thinker's Guide for Students on How to Study and Learn a Discipline*. Dillon Beach, USA: Foundation for Critical Thinking Press.

Rubenfeld, M. & Scheffer, B. (2006). *Critical Thinking Tactics for Nurses*. Boston: Jones and Bartlett.

Scheffer, B. & Rubenfeld, M. (2000). A consensus statement on critical thinking in nursing. *Journal of Nursing Education, 39*, 352–59.

Tanner, C. (2006). Thinking like a nurse: A research-based model of clinical judgement in nursing. *Journal of Nursing Education, 45*(6), 204–11.

CHAPTER 2

CARING FOR A PERSON EXPERIENCING AN ADVERSE DRUG EVENT

TRACY LEVETT-JONES AND DAVID NEWBY

LEARNING OUTCOMES

Completion of the activities in this chapter will enable you to:

O explain why an understanding of medication safety and person-centred care is essential to competent practice (**recall** and **application**)

O explain the nurse's role in the medication team (**recall** and **application**)

O identify potential clinical manifestations of an adverse drug event that will guide the collection and interpretation of appropriate cues (**gather**, **review**, **interpret**, **discriminate**, **relate** and **infer**)

O identify potential risk factors for medication safety and from medication errors (**match** and **predict**)

O review clinical information to identify the main nursing diagnoses for a patient experiencing an adverse drug event (**synthesise**)

O describe the priorities of care for a patient experiencing an adverse drug event (**goal setting** and **taking action**)

O identify clinical criteria for determining the effectiveness of nursing actions taken to manage experiencing an adverse drug event (**evaluate**)

O apply what you have learnt about medication safety to new clinical situations with different patients (**reflection** and **translation**).

There are two types of healthcare practitioner—one who has made a mistake and one who will make a mistake. (www.nicpld.org/online/gov/module2/default.asp)

INTRODUCTION

Medication errors result from multiple factors; they include knowledge and skill deficits, ineffective teamwork, poor communication between health professionals and between health professionals and the people they care for, and medication calculation errors (World Health Organization, 2012). However, nursing students (and sometimes more senior nurses) often assume that if they learn about pharmacology and the 'six rights', and practise the technical aspects of medication administration, medication safety will be assured. In reality, there are many contextual and interpersonal factors that impact on safe medication practices. Additionally, each person who is the recipient of care will respond in individual ways to the medications prescribed and will need to be monitored for these responses. Clinical reasoning skills allow nurses to manage the many interconnected and complex factors that influence medication safety.

In this chapter, two scenarios related to medication safety are juxtaposed. The first scenario describes what actually occurred in the care of Mr Giuseppe Esposito. In the second scenario, we 'rewind' and illustrate what might have happened had the nursing student caring for Mr Esposito demonstrated effective clinical reasoning skills. These scenarios are typical of those played out in Australian hospitals every day. They illustrate how clinical reasoning can make a difference in promoting patient safety and managing an adverse drug event; and how health assessment and effective communication skills are key components of medication safety. Importantly, these scenarios will help you to understand your role and the difference you can make, even as a nursing student or graduate nurse, to your patients' clinical outcomes.

KEY CONCEPTS

adverse drug event
medication error
medication safety

SUGGESTED READINGS

A. Berman, S. Synder, T. Levett-Jones, T. Burton & N. Harvey (Eds). (2017). *Skills in Clinical Nursing* (1st Australian edn). Sydney: Pearson.
Unit 6: Medication administration

T. Levett-Jones (Ed.) (2014). *Critical Conversations for Patient Safety: An Essential Guide for Health Professionals*. Sydney: Pearson.
Chapter 9: Communicating to promote medication safety

SCENARIO 2.1   What did happen …

SETTING THE SCENE

One of the causes of medication errors is inconsistent and inaccurate use of medication abbreviations. Which of these medication prescriptions is incorrect? Access this link for the approved terms for use in Australian hospitals: <www.safetyandquality.gov.au/wp-content/uploads/2012/01/32060v2.pdf>.

Reid-Searl et al. (2008) refer to this practice as 'being near'. Although a commonly used form of supervision during medication administration, it is neither legal nor professional.

Do you know the laws that control the administration of medications in your state or territory?

Would these results be considered 'normal' for Mr Esposito?

Mr Giuseppe Esposito, 81 years, was admitted to the medical ward of Griffith Community Hospital with dehydration as a result of suspected gastroenteritis. He'd had vomiting and diarrhoea for two days prior to admission. Intravenous (IV) fluids were commenced and his diarrhoea and vomiting began to improve the following day, although some nausea persisted. Mr Esposito's IV was not resited when it 'tissued' later that evening.

On the second day following Mr Esposito's admission, Madeline Rose, a first-year student nurse, was to administer his usual oral medications (frusemide 80 mg, digoxin 125 mcg and enalapril 20 mg) at 0800.

At first she was supervised by a registered nurse (RN), but when another nurse called for assistance the RN left to attend to a patient in a nearby bed saying to Madeline, 'Keep going—I'll watch what you are doing from over here.'

Madeline was new to the ward, and felt quite intimidated by the RN who was mentoring her, so she continued to administer the medications following the 'six rights' of medication administration (right patient, right drug, right dose, right time, right route and right documentation) as she had been taught at university. Madeline had heard of each of the medications but did not know very much about them. She did not refer to a drug reference, as she was conscious that the RN was busy and wanted to get on with the medication round for her other patients.

Later that morning, the RN told Madeline that the bed was needed and asked her to quickly shower Mr Esposito, take his vital signs and get him ready for discharge. Madeline entered Mr Esposito's room and explained that his daughter would be in to pick him up soon but that she was going to take him to have a shower first. As Mr Esposito got out of bed he staggered a little and said, 'I'm a bit wobbly today' but quickly regained his balance. Madeline reassured him that she would put a shower chair in the bathroom for him. She was concerned as time was getting away, so she settled Mr Esposito in the shower then left to pack up his belongings. When Madeline returned, she found him leaning forward in the chair with his head down. Mr Esposito reassured her by saying, 'Don't you worry, love, it's just the hot water … it made me a bit giddy.' So she helped him dress, then walked with him back to his room and sat him in the chair next to his bed to wait for his daughter. Mr Esposito asked Madeline to pass him his glasses saying, 'My eyes are bad today.'

Madeline returned a few minutes later with an electronic blood pressure machine and took Mr Esposito's temperature, pulse, respiration and blood pressure, as she had been instructed. His vital signs were: T 36.6°C, PR 64, RR 20, BP 120/70 mmHg. Madeline then documented the observations in Mr Esposito's chart.

The RN was busy when Mr Esposito's daughter arrived, so she asked Madeline to give him his discharge papers and take him to the car in a wheelchair.

Mr Esposito's daughter took her father home. She would have preferred that he spent a few days in town with her but he refused, saying that he wanted to get back to the farm and that his dog would be fretting without him. She made him a sandwich and a cup of tea, ensured he was comfortable, and left saying she would be back in a couple of hours after she had finished with some things at work. Mr Esposito, relieved to be home and feeling very tired, fell asleep in his recliner chair. He woke up an hour later needing to go to the bathroom. He began to walk to the bathroom but felt very dizzy. Later he couldn't recall whether he lost his footing or fainted, but when he regained consciousness he had a lot of pain in his right forearm, wrist and chest. He also had a laceration to his forehead. His daughter found him lying on the floor an hour later and immediately called an ambulance.

Mr Esposito was taken to the Emergency Department and, following X-rays, was diagnosed with a Colles' fracture, three fractured ribs and concussion. An ECG and blood tests revealed digitalis toxicity and hypokalaemia. The admitting medical officer attributed Mr Esposito's collapse to (a) postural hypotension caused by dehydration, and (b) the dizziness caused by the arrhythmia that resulted from digitalis toxicity.

Mr Esposito was discharged to his daughter's home seven days later, but it took many months for his fractures to heal and for him to regain his independence, confidence, strength and sense of wellbeing.

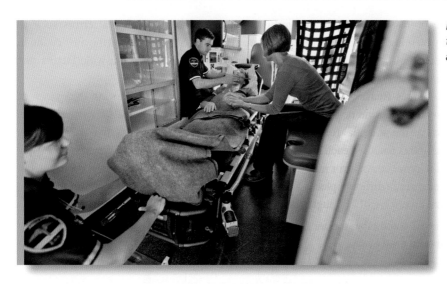

Mr Esposito returns to hospital via ambulance

Epidemiology of medication errors

Medication administration is a complex process involving counting, calculating, measuring, mixing and ensuring that the right person receives the right medicine in the right dose, at the right time, by the right route and for the right reason (Manias, 2014). The complexity of the medication administration process is compounded by polypharmacy, patient acuity, interruptions, use of electronic technologies, facility design and time constraints (Grigg, Garrett & Craig, 2011). The unpredictable and dynamic nature of the clinical environment further adds to this complexity.

Medication administration errors refer to giving the wrong drug or dose, by the wrong route, to the wrong patient or at the wrong time (Westbrook et al., 2010). Errors also include failure to adhere to established practices, standards or policies in any aspect of medication administration process, for example, failure to check a patient's identification, read the medication label/expiry date or accurately document medication administration (Westbrook et al., 2010).

Medication errors are the second most common type of incident reported in Australian hospitals (Johnson & Young, 2011), and the World Health Organization (2012) estimates that more than 50 per cent of all medications are prescribed, dispensed, administered or used inappropriately. However, it is likely that this is an underestimate as many errors are not reported (Johnson & Young, 2011). Medication errors cost the Australian healthcare system approximately $380 million per year in the public hospital system alone (Australian Institute of Health and Welfare, 2012).

> *Nurses are the last line of defence to protect against medication errors. It is vital that their practice is informed by evidence of effective interventions for reducing medication administration errors.*

REFLECTION

Q1   In this scenario, Madeline did every task she had been asked to do by the RN. Should anything else have been expected of her?

Q2   What interpersonal and situational factors influenced how this scenario unfolded?

Q3   How might the outcome for Mr Esposito have been different had Madeline had a requisite level of clinical reasoning skills?

Q4   What aspects of this adverse drug event were preventable?

Q5   Should this adverse drug event be documented and reported? If so … where, by whom, to whom and why?

Q6   The medical officer and nurse discussed whether Mr Esposito and his daughter should be told that he had experienced an adverse drug event. The nurse thought they should be told, but the doctor disagreed saying that telling Mr Esposito and his daughter would make them worry needlessly. What do you think and why?

> *The NSQHS Standards specify that each health service organisation must have processes for documenting adverse drug reactions in the healthcare record and in an organisation-wide incident reporting system (ACSQHC, 2016).*

> *Access this online module for insights into open disclosure following clinical errors: <www.ipeforqum.com.au/index.php/modules/young-min-lee>.*

Sometimes healthcare professionals adopt an overly simplistic approach to clinical errors such as adverse drug events by blaming the person who administered, prescribed or dispensed the medication in error. However, this does not take into account the multiple contextual and system-wide factors that create the conditions in which errors can occur.

It is helpful to use James Reason's 'Swiss Cheese Model' (2000) when reviewing the causes of adverse drug events such as the one described in Scenario 2.1. In Reason's model of system failure, every step in a process has the potential for failure, to varying degrees. The ideal system is like a stack of Swiss cheese slices. In this analogy, each hole is an opportunity for a process to fail, and each slice is a 'defensive layer' in the process. An error may allow a problem to pass through a hole in one layer, but in the next layer the holes are in different places and the problem should be caught. The fewer the holes, the more likely it is that an error will be caught or stopped.

Q7   Reflect on Scenario 2.1 and label Figure 2.1 with some of the errors that occurred and led to Mr Esposito's adverse drug event.

Figure 2.1
Adverse drug reaction—Reason's Swiss Cheese Model

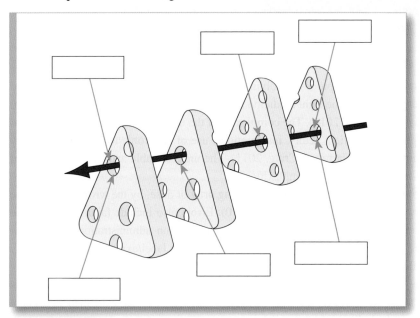

SCENARIO 2.2   What might have happened …

CHANGING THE SCENE

Let's imagine that we could rewind Scenario 2.1 and this time we'll see how Mr Esposito's outcomes are influenced by the use of clinical reasoning skills and person-centred care.

PERSON-CENTRED CARE

Why is person-centred care essential to safe medication practices? Review Chapter 9 of Critical Conversations for Patient Safety: An Essential Guide for Health Professionals (Levett-Jones et al., 2014) if unsure.

Person-centred health professionals are ethical, open-minded, empathetic, respectful and self-aware with a profound sense of moral agency (Levett-Jones et al., 2014). Person-centred care means seeing the *person,* not just the patient or their disease process. Integral to person-centred care is the nurse's understanding of the patient's beliefs and values, and respect for and appreciation of the patient's life history. Person-centred care is a holistic approach to healthcare that is grounded in a philosophy of personhood. Although there are varying definitions of person-centred care, each promotes self-determination, empowerment and a commitment to providing healthcare that is responsive to the needs and preferences of the individual (Rossiter, Scott & Walton, 2014). Attributes of person-centred care include the existence of a therapeutic relationship between the nurse and the person they are caring for, the provision of individualised care and evidence of patient participation. Person-centred care is central to safe medication practices (Bolster & Manias, 2010).

Something to think about …

Person-centred care and effective communication help nurses to develop an understanding of the patient as a person and to work collaboratively in a therapeutic relationship (Rossiter, Scott & Walton, 2014). Nurses who communicate effectively with their patients are better able to collect and validate assessment data, initiate appropriate nursing actions, evaluate the effectiveness of outcomes and prevent unsafe practice.

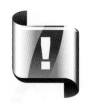

Mr Giuseppe Esposito, 81 years, was admitted to the medical ward of Griffith Community Hospital with dehydration as a result of suspected gastroenteritis. He had been vomiting and had diarrhoea for two days prior to admission. Intravenous fluids were commenced and his diarrhoea began to improve the following day, although some nausea persisted. Mr Esposito's IV was not resited when it 'tissued' later that evening.

Madeline Rose, a student nurse, was caring for Mr Esposito following his admission and spent time talking to him and his daughter, Bella. He asked Madeline to call him Giuseppe, and, as she got to know him, he began to tell her about his past.

Giuseppe had lived alone on his five-hectare farm in Yenda, approximately 10 kilometres from Griffith in New South Wales, since his wife Fiore's death a year ago. He arrived in Australia in 1944 from a village near the town of Verona. Like many of his fellow Italians, he came to Australia in search of *benessere* (prosperity). He worked as a labourer on road construction in order to buy and pay off his farm. It was a tough existence made worse by the racist taunts and other displays of vilification that he and the other Italian farmers endured. To this day, Giuseppe is embarrassed by his accent and he still feels very much like an 'outsider'.

Giuseppe and Fiore had three sons and one daughter, Bella. His sons now live in Sydney and Bella lives in Griffith. Giuseppe loves to spend time with his daughter and grandsons but they have busy lives and he sees them only once or twice a week. Bella worries about him and wishes he lived closer to town but he has refused to move. For most of Giuseppe's life his health has been reasonably good, although he has had some arrhythmias and hypertension over the past few years. Lately, Bella has been concerned that Giuseppe isn't taking care of himself properly and she thinks he is becoming a little forgetful. She believes that his gastroenteritis is a result of eating a chicken dish that had been in his refrigerator for more than a week.

At 0800, two days following Giuseppe's admission, Madeline was asked to administer his usual oral medications (frusemide 80 mg, digoxin 125 µg and enalapril 20 mg). It was a busy shift and the RN supervising Madeline was interrupted and asked to attend to another patient. She said, 'Keep going—I'll watch what you are doing from over here.'

Madeline, although new to the ward and feeling quite intimidated, was conscious that this contravened university and healthcare policies and was outside of her scope of practice. She replied, 'I'm sorry but I am not allowed to administer medications without direct supervision by a registered nurse.' The RN looked surprised but said, 'Oh … okay, I'll be there in a tick.'

While she waited, Madeline checked whether Giuseppe had any allergies and that there was a valid order for the medications. She also reviewed the *Australian Medicines Handbook* (Rossi, 2016) to find out more about the medications she was administering. Once the RN returned, Madeline administered the medications following the 'six rights' (right patient, right drug, right dose, right time, right route and right documentation). She asked Giuseppe to check his medications as she gave them to him, saying, 'I'm giving you your Lanoxin, Lasix and Renitec, is that right? Do you know what they're for, Giuseppe?' He nodded and replied, 'Yes, yes, they're for my ticker and my water.'

Q1 What other 'rights' are essential to medication safety?

Q2 What does a valid medication order require?

Q3 What three checks are required when administering medications?

Q4 Should Madeline have taken Giuseppe's vital signs prior to administering his medications? Why or why not?

> Words are, of course, the most powerful drug used by mankind (Rudyard Kipling).

> Cultural awareness: How might Giuseppe's personal history, culture and life experiences influence the way he interacts in healthcare environments?

> Research has identified that the occurrence and frequency of interruptions are significantly associated with the incidence of medication errors (Westbrook et al., 2010).

> The NMBA standards for practice (2016) specify that registered nurses must comply with legislation, regulations, policies, guidelines and other standards or requirements relevant to the context of practice.

> An individualised and person-centred approach to medication activities involves a dialogue between nurses and patients. This promotes patient safety by engaging the patient as a participative member of the medication team (Bolster & Manias, 2010).

Later that morning, the RN told Madeline that the bed was needed and asked her to quickly shower Mr Esposito, do his vital signs and get him ready for discharge.

1. CONSIDER THE PATIENT SITUATION

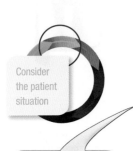

Consider the patient situation

In the first stage of the clinical reasoning cycle, the nurse begins to gain an initial impression. He or she takes notice of the patient's concerns and begins to think about the situation.

Madeline entered Giuseppe's room and explained that Bella would be in to pick him up soon but that she was going to take him to have a shower first. She also asked how he was feeling. He replied, 'I'm much better now that I don't have the "runs" ... I still feel sick in the stomach though, and I'm right off my food. I'll feel better when I get home, I should think. This gastro thing has really knocked me. My eyes are shot, too ... couldn't read the paper this morning.'

Madeline sat Giuseppe on the side of the bed as she collected his things for the shower. As he sat there, he said, 'Geez, I'm a bit dizzy, girly.' Madeline wasn't sure what to do but decided to leave Giuseppe sitting for a few minutes because she was concerned that if she took him to the shower he might fall.

> A simple question such as 'How are you feeling?' often elicits meaningful patient information. The problem is that in healthcare, as in everyday life, we don't always listen carefully to the person's response to this question.

2. COLLECT CUES/INFORMATION

(a) Review current information

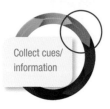

Collect cues/ information

During the second stage of the clinical reasoning cycle, the nurse begins to collect relevant information about the patient. He or she starts by reviewing the information that is currently available via the patient's clinical documentation, medical and nursing notes, handover report or other available information.

As Madeline began to think about why Giuseppe was feeling dizzy, she reviewed his charts. The fluid balance chart was incomplete, as it had not been maintained since the IV tissued the previous day. Madeline noticed that on the previous day Giuseppe was in a positive balance (2400 mL in—mostly IV fluids and small amounts of oral fluids; total output 700 mL—he had been voiding small amounts infrequently).

Giuseppe's observations had been relatively stable, but his pulse rate seemed to have decreased in the days since admission. Madeline was not sure what this meant. Giuseppe's blood pressure had been between 120/70 mmHg and 110/60 mmHg. His temperature had been 38°C on admission but 36.4–37°C over the last 24 hours. Giuseppe's respiratory rate had been 16–20 per minute. Madeline read Giuseppe's progress notes but there was no mention of him feeling dizzy before.

> It appears on face value that Giuseppe is in a positive balance. Do you think this is an accurate reflection of his fluid status? Why?

Madeline looked for Giuseppe's blood results, as she'd remembered hearing in handover that some tests had been done, but the results were not in his chart. She was curious but not that concerned, as she realised that she probably wouldn't be able to interpret the results anyway.

(b) Gather new information

The next stage of the clinical reasoning cycle is to collect relevant cues and information. This requires the nurse to determine which cues are relevant for a particular person at a particular point in time.

Madeline considered Giuseppe's dizziness and decided to take his blood pressure sitting and standing before getting him up for the shower. She used the manual sphygmomanometer attached to the wall beside his bed.

Q1   Why did Madeline take a sitting and a standing BP?

Q2   Why do you think Madeline chose to use the manual sphygmomanometer instead of the electronic one?

Q3   Giuseppe's blood pressure was 120/70 mmHg sitting and 110/60 mmHg standing. What might this reading indicate?

Madeline also checked Giuseppe's pulse rate; it was 64, weak and thready, and irregular. She confirmed this finding by checking Giuseppe's apical pulse for 60 seconds using a stethoscope. Taken apically, Madeline thought his pulse rate was 68 and very irregular.

Q4   Why did Madeline check Giuseppe's apical pulse?

Q5 From the list below, identify three other cues that you believe Madeline should have collected?

    a Appetite

    b Condition of oral mucosa

    c Oral intake

    d Pain

    e Cognitive state

    f Level of thirst

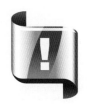

Something to think about …

When the correct cues are not collected, all of the actions that follow may be incorrect. Making decisions based on incomplete information is a leading cause of clinical errors. Early subtle cues, when missed, can lead to adverse patient outcomes (Levett-Jones et al., 2010).

Q6 Are there any questions you would have asked Giuseppe if you had been in this situation?

(c) Recall knowledge

While cue collection involves reviewing current information and gathering new information, it also requires you to recall related knowledge. This includes a broad and deep knowledge of physiology, pathophysiology, pharmacology, epidemiology, therapeutics, culture, context of care, ethics and law, and so on, as well as an understanding of evidence-based practice. For students this can be challenging, because it requires not only a strong foundation of knowledge but also the ability to synthesise and apply their knowledge to clinical situations that are often complex and fluid.

Madeline tried to recall what she had learnt about gastroenteritis, quality use of medicines and the medications Giuseppe was taking.

QUICK QUIZ!

To ensure that you have a good understanding of these important topics, test yourself with the following questions.

Q1 List the four key members of the medication safety team.

Q2 'Therapeutic index' refers to:

    a The way drugs are categorised into groups (e.g. analgesics)

    b The margin between effectiveness and toxicity of drugs

    c The register that is kept of drugs that are and are not therapeutic for particular patient groups

    d The relative potency of a medication

Q3 Vomiting and diarrhoea may cause a significant loss of which electrolyte from the gastrointestinal tract?

    a Calcium

    b Magnesium

    c Potassium

    d Sodium

Q4 Giuseppe takes the drug digoxin for his arrhythmia. If his serum digoxin levels are above the therapeutic range, he is at highest risk for developing digitalis toxicity if he also develops which of the following?

    a Hyponatraemia

    b Hypokalaemia

    c Vitamin B12 deficiency

    d Vitamin K deficiency

Q5 Digoxin is made from which flowering plant?

    a Rose

    b Sunflower

    c Foxglove

    d Opium

Q6 The organ responsible for the excretion of most drugs and their metabolites is the:

    a Liver

    b Gut

    c Kidney

    d Lungs

Q7 Dehydration results in:

    a An increased glomerular filtration rate

    b A decreased glomerular filtration rate

    c No change to the glomerular filtration rate

Q8 What is the action of the diuretic frusemide?

    a It blocks the absorption of sodium, chloride and water from the fluid in the Bowman's capsule, causing an increase in urine output (diuresis).

    b It blocks the absorption of sodium, chloride and water from the filtered fluid in the kidney tubules, causing an increase in urine output (diuresis).

    c It enhances the absorption of sodium, chloride and water from the filtered fluid in the kidney tubules, causing a decrease in urine output (oliguria).

    d It blocks the absorption of potassium, magnesium and water from the filtered fluid in the kidney tubules, causing an increase in urine output (diuresis).

Q9 Frusemide may cause serum potassium levels to:

    a Increase

    b Decrease

    c Stay the same

Q10 Enalapril should be used with caution in patients with:

    a Hypervolaemia (fluid overload)

    b Hypertension

    c Hypovolaemia and/or dehydration

    d Asthma

Prior to administering Giuseppe's medications, Madeline had reviewed the *Australian Medicines Handbook* (Rossi, 2016). She recalled reading that digoxin has a narrow therapeutic index and that adverse effects commonly include anorexia, nausea, vomiting, diarrhoea, blurred vision, visual disturbances, confusion, drowsiness, dizziness, nightmares, agitation, depression and ECG changes.

Q11 Which of these signs and symptoms did Giuseppe have?

3. PROCESS INFORMATION

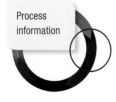

Process information

(a) Interpret

The next step of the clinical reasoning cycle is to interpret the data (cues) collected through careful analysis and to identify aberrations from normal. Always ask the question: 'Are these cues normal for this person, at this time and in this place?'

Q Which of the following would be considered to be within normal parameters for Giuseppe?

   a Temperature: 36.4–37°C

   b Apical pulse: 64 beats/min

   c Respiratory rate: 16–20 breaths/min

   d Blood pressure: 120/70 mmHg sitting and 110/65 mmHg standing

(b) Discriminate

At this stage, the nurse narrows down the information to what is most important.

Q From the list below, select five cues that you believe are *most relevant* to Giuseppe *at this time*.

   a Blood pressure

   b Respiratory rate

   c Blurred vision

   d Temperature

   e Dizziness

   f Pulse rate

   g Level of consciousness

   h Urine output

> *Research indicates that novice nurses tend to wait until they have identified a patient problem before they collect cues, whereas experts practise more proactively, collecting a wide range of relevant cues to prevent possible patient complications (Hoffman, Aitken & Duffield, 2009).*

(c) Relate

The next step for Madeline was to cluster together the cues that she had collected and try to make sense of them by looking for relationships or patterns. Some people call this stage 'connecting the dots' or 'putting two and two together'.

Q Label the following 'true' or 'false'.

   a Giuseppe may have been hypotensive due to insensible fluid loss (vomiting and diarrhoea).

   b Giuseppe's blurred vision was most likely an indication of deteriorating eyesight due to his age.

   c Giuseppe's dizziness and nausea could have been a side effect of one of his medications.

   d Giuseppe's irregular pulse may have been caused by his hypotension and negative fluid balance.

   e Giuseppe's tachycardia and hypotension may have been from anxiety and stress.

   f Giuseppe's negative fluid balance may have been caused by vomiting, diarrhoea and inadequate oral intake.

(d) Infer

In this stage of the clinical reasoning cycle, the nurse thinks about all the cues that have been collected and makes inferences based on the analysis and interpretation of those cues.

From what Madeline knew about Giuseppe's history, signs and symptoms, as well as the information she had recalled, she considered potential inferences.

Q Giuseppe could have been experiencing which of the following? (Select the two that you think are most correct.)

   a Signs and symptoms of dehydration

   b An exacerbation of his gastroenteritis

   c An allergic reaction to one of his medications

   d An adverse drug event

(e) Predict

Next the nurse must anticipate potential outcomes depending on a particular course of action (or inaction).

Madeline was worried and not sure what course of action to take. Because of her inexperience and uncertainty, she wanted to just 'wait and see'. However, she began to think about what might happen if she did nothing.

Q   If Madeline did nothing, what might happen to Giuseppe? Select the two correct answers.

    a   He could go into septic shock.

    b   His condition would probably improve over the next few days.

    c   He could experience serious complications once discharged.

    d   He could develop a life-threatening arrhythmia.

(f) Match

In this stage, the nurse matches the current situation to past situations or current patient to past patients using mental prompts such as: 'I remember when this happened before and …'; 'This is similar to …'; and 'Last time I saw this …'. However, keep in mind 'matching' is usually an expert thought process.

Over time, Madeline will develop a repertoire of experiences with which she can compare presenting clinical situations, but this will take repeated opportunities to engage in clinical reasoning (in real or simulated contexts).

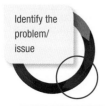

Identify the problem/issue

4. IDENTIFY THE PROBLEM/ISSUE

Diagnosing is the fourth stage of the clinical reasoning cycle when the nurse synthesises all of the information he or she has collected in order to identify critical patient problem(s). There are two types of nursing diagnoses: actual and risk. An actual diagnosis consists of the patient problem, the related aetiology (causal relationship between a problem and its related or risk factors) and supporting evidence (e.g. cues). A risk nursing diagnosis is a clinical judgment about a potential problem where the presence of risk factors indicates that a problem has the potential to develop unless nurses intervene appropriately (Levett-Jones & Fagen, 2015).

> *Diagnosing is a pivotal step in clinical reasoning as care planning and nursing interventions follow directly from this phase. Safe and effective healthcare depends upon an accurate communication and documentation of nursing diagnoses.*

Q   Develop one actual and one risk nursing diagnosis for Giuseppe?

5. ESTABLISH GOALS

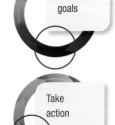

Establish goals

As a first-year student, Madeline was sure of only one thing at this stage—she needed help to work out what to do for Giuseppe and she needed it fast.

6. TAKE ACTION

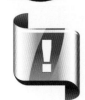

Take action

The next stage of the clinical reasoning cycle requires knowledge, clinical skills, effective communication skills and clinical reasoning ability. The nurse has to decide which actions take priority, and who should be notified and when (Levett-Jones et al., 2010).

Something to think about …

Too often nurses observe and document but fail to follow up on clinical abnormalities. For example, in a study by Thompson et al. (2008) it was reported that 50 per cent of cardiac arrests had clinical signs of deterioration recorded in the preceding 24 hours but were not acted upon. These types of situations can eventuate when nurses do not have adequate clinical reasoning skills.

Madeline realised that she had to notify the RN she was working with. She wasn't sure what was happening with Giuseppe but she was concerned enough to know that she had to tell someone. Because she felt uncomfortable telling the RN and worried that she might be seen to be 'making a mountain out of a molehill', she decided to use ISBAR (Identify, Situation, Background, Assessment, Request/ Recommendation) to structure her conversation.

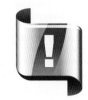

Something to think about …

At times the most appropriate nursing action is to relay your concerns about a deteriorating patient to senior staff. To do this, you need to be confident and skilled in communicating with members of the interprofessional healthcare team so that you can signal your need for immediate help when required. Use of acronyms such as ISBAR is effective in streamlining the way health professionals communicate and in increasing patient safety (Levett-Jones et al., 2010).

Q   Draw up a table like the one below and record the words Madeline could use to communicate her concerns about Giuseppe to the RN:

I	Identify	Self: name, position, location. Patient: name, age, gender.	
S	Situation	Briefly explain the reason for your concern.	
B	Background	Patient's medical diagnosis, relevant history, investigations, what has been done so far.	
A	Assessment	Summarise the patient's current condition or situation. Explain your assessment of the problem including your risk diagnoses for Giuseppe.	
R	Request/ recommendation	State your request.	

7. EVALUATE

In this stage of the clinical reasoning cycle, the effectiveness of one's actions is assessed.

Because of Madeline's clear, succinct and relevant communication, the RN felt compelled to review Giuseppe. She repeated the observations, including the apical pulse, and asked Giuseppe to describe how he was feeling again. She returned to the nurses' station and accessed Giuseppe's blood results on the intranet identifying that he was hypokalaemic and hypernatraemic.

The RN then conducted an ECG and identified a prolonged PR interval (this can be a sign of digitalis toxicity). The RN consulted the clinical pharmacist who was on the ward and phoned the medical officer.

Following a medical review, Giuseppe was transferred to the Coronary Care Unit. Oxygen, IV fluids with 20 mmol KCl (potassium chloride) and cardiac monitoring were initiated. A serum digoxin level was also ordered. It revealed digoxin levels of 3.8 nmol/L (or 3 µg/L)—the therapeutic range is 0.6–2.6 nmol/L (0.5–2 µg/L) (Rossi, 2016).

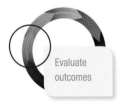

Evaluate outcomes

What is hypokalaemia and hypernatraemia? What may have caused this electrolyte imbalance?

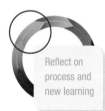

Communication errors are identified as the root cause of 70 per cent of sentinel events in healthcare settings (Joint Commission, 2004). Access this website to explore why interprofessional communication is essential to safe medication practices: <www.ipeforqum.com.au>.

When telling the afternoon staff what had happened to Giuseppe, the RN said to the nurses, 'I am so glad Madeline was on the ball. I dread to think what might have happened if we'd sent him home like that.'

Giuseppe's condition improved over the next three days and he was discharged under the care of his local GP. He agreed to stay with Bella for a few days before going back to his farm.

Giuseppe returns to his farm following discharge

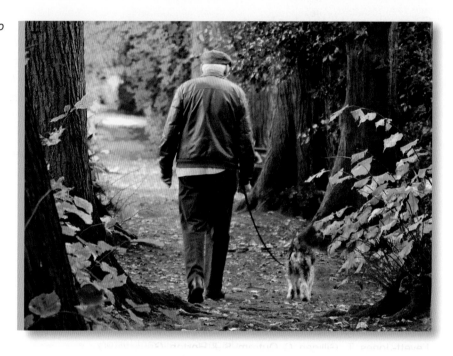

8. REFLECT

The final stage of the clinical reasoning cycle is 'reflection'. Reflection in this context refers to the process of 'looking back' and reviewing what you have learnt from the scenario. It also means 'looking forward' and deciding what you will do if presented with a similar situation in clinical practice.

Reflect on process and new learning

Consider the following questions:

Q1 What are three of the most important things that you have learnt from this scenario?

Q2 What actions will you take in clinical practice as a result of your learning from this scenario?

Q3 How will you demonstrate person-centred care when administering medications?

Q4 What have you learned from this scenario about communication, clinical leadership and teamwork that you can apply to your clinical practice?

FURTHER READING

Bolster, D. & Manias, E. (2010). Person-centred interactions between nurses and patients during medication activities in an acute hospital setting: Qualitative observation and interview study. *International Journal of Nursing Studies, 47*(2), 154–65.

Interprofessional Education for Quality Use of Medicine website: <www.ipeforqum@newcastle.edu.au>.

NPS Medicinewise Learning—Medication Safety Module. Accessed December 2016 at <www.nps. org.au/health-professionals/cpd/activities/online-courses/medication-safety-training>.

Reid-Searl, K., Moxham, L., Walker, S. & Happell, B. (2008). Shifting supervision: Implications for safe administration of medication by nursing students. *Journal of Clinical Nursing, 17*(20), 2750–57.

REFERENCES

Australian Commission on Safety and Quality in Health Care (ACSQHC). (2016). *National Safety and Quality Health Service Standards Version 2.* Draft, Sydney, Australia.

Australian Institute of Health and Welfare (AIHW). (2012). *Australian Hospital Statistics 2010-11.* Canberra: AIHW.

Bolster, D. & Manias E. (2010). Person-centred interactions between nurses and patients during medication activities in an acute hospital setting: Qualitative observation and interview study. *International Journal of Nursing Studies, 47*(2), 154–65.

Grigg, S. J., Garrett, S. K. & Craig, J. B. (2011). A process centered analysis of medication administration: Identifying current methods and potential for improvement. *International Journal of Industrial Ergonomics, 41*(4), 380–88.

Hoffman, K., Aitken, L. & Duffield, C. (2009). A comparison of novice and expert nurses' cue collection during clinical decision-making: Verbal protocol analysis. *International Journal of Nursing Studies, 46*(10), 1335–44.

Johnson, M. & Young, H. (2011). The application of Aronson's taxonomy to medication errors in nursing. *Journal of Nursing Care Quality, 26*(2), 128–35.

Levett-Jones, T. & Fagen, A. (2015). Diagnosing. In A. Berman, S. Synder, T. Levett-Jones et al. (Eds), *Kozier and Erb's Fundamentals of Nursing* (3rd edn). Sydney: Pearson.

Levett-Jones, T., Gilligan, C. Outram, S. & Horton, G. (2014). Key attributes of 'patient safe' communication. In T. Levett-Jones (Ed.), *Critical Conversations for Patient Safety: An Essential Guide for Health Professionals.* Sydney: Pearson.

Levett-Jones, T., Hoffman, K., Dempsey, Y., Jeong, S., Noble, D., Norton, C., ... Hickey, N. (2010). The 'five rights' of clinical reasoning: An educational model to enhance nursing students' ability to identify and manage clinically 'at risk' patients. *Nurse Education Today, 30*(6), 515–20.

Manias, E. (2014). Communicating to promote medication safety. In T. Levett-Jones (Ed.), *Critical Conversations for Patient Safety: An Essential Guide for Health Professionals.* Sydney: Pearson.

Nursing and Midwifery Board of Australia (NMBA). (2016). Registered nurse standards for practice. Retrieved from <www.nursingmidwiferyboard.gov.au/Codes-Guidelines-Statements/ Professional-standards.aspx>.

Reason, J. (2000). Human error: Models and management. *British Medical Journal, 320,* 768–70.

Reid-Searl, K., Moxham, L., Walker, S. & Happell, B. (2008). Shifting supervision: Implications for safe administration of medication by nursing students. *Journal of Clinical Nursing, 17*(20), 2750–57.

Rossi, S. (Ed.). (2016). *Australian Medicines Handbook* (3rd edn). Adelaide: Australian Medicines Handbook Pty Ltd.

Rossiter, R., Scott, R. & Walton, C. G. (2014). Key attributes of therapeutic communication. In T. Levett-Jones (Ed.), *Critical Conversations for Patient Safety: An Essential Guide for Health Professionals.* Sydney: Pearson.

Thompson, C., Dalgleish, L., Bucknall, T., Estabrooks, C., Hutchinson, A., Fraser, K., ... Saunders, J. (2008). The effects of time pressure and experience on nurses' risk assessment decisions: A signal detection analysis. *Nursing Research, 57*(5), 302–11.

Westbrook, J., Woods, A., Rob, M., Dunsmuir, W. & Day, R. (2010). Association of interruptions with an increased risk and severity of medication administration errors. *Archives of Internal Medicine, 170*(8), 683–90.

World Health Organization. (2012). *Reporting and Learning Systems for Medication Errors: Detecting, Analysing and Preventing Within Pharmacovigilance Centres.* Draft report of the FP7 funded project 'Monitoring Medicines'. Uppsala, Sweden: World Health Organization.

PHOTO CREDITS

CHAPTER 3

CARING FOR A PERSON WITH FLUID AND ELECTROLYTE IMBALANCE

TRACY LEVETT-JONES AND PETER SINCLAIR

LEARNING OUTCOMES

Completion of the activities in this chapter will enable you to:

○ explain why an understanding of fluid and electrolyte balance is essential to competent practice (**recall** and **application**)

○ identify the clinical manifestations of hypovolaemia, dehydration, hypervolaemia and electrolyte imbalance that guide the collection and interpretation of appropriate cues (**gather**, **review**, **interpret**, **discriminate**, **relate** and **infer**)

○ identify risk factors for fluid and electrolyte imbalance (**match** and **predict**)

○ review clinical information to identify the main nursing diagnoses for a patient with a fluid and electrolyte imbalance (**synthesise**)

○ describe the priorities of care for a patient with a fluid and electrolyte imbalance (**goal setting** and **taking action**)

○ identify clinical criteria for determining the effectiveness of nursing actions taken to manage fluid and electrolyte imbalance (**evaluate**)

○ apply what you have learnt about fluid and electrolyte imbalance to new situations (**reflection** and **translation**).

INTRODUCTION

The two linked scenarios introduced in this chapter focus on the care of an older person who experiences fluid and electrolyte imbalance. You will be introduced to Mr Arthur Barrett and follow his healthcare journey from admission, through the post-operative period, and to discharge. Alterations in fluid status are common in post-operative patients; they manifest rapidly and can have potentially fatal consequences, particularly in an older person with multiple co-morbidities. Maintaining the delicate fluid and electrolyte equilibrium of post-operative patients is essential to safe and effective nursing care. Excellent clinical reasoning skills will help you to recognise and manage people at risk of fluid and electrolyte imbalance early, with the aim of preventing deterioration and adverse patient outcomes.

KEY CONCEPTS

dehydration
hypovolaemia
hypervolaemia
electrolyte imbalance
kidney disease

SUGGESTED READINGS

P. LeMone, K. Burke, G. Bauldoff, P. Gubrud-Howe, T. Levett-Jones, T. Dwyer … D. Raymond (Eds). (2017). *Medical–Surgical Nursing: Critical Thinking in Person-Centred Care* (3rd edn). Melbourne: Pearson.

Chapter 3: Nursing care of people having surgery

Chapter 9: Nursing care of people with altered fluid, electrolyte and acid–base balance

Chapter 27: Nursing care of people with kidney disorders

SCENARIO 3.1 The fluid shift begins ...

SETTING THE SCENE

Mr Arthur Barrett is a 74-year-old man diagnosed with cancer of the colon. He had sought medical treatment after noticing rectal bleeding, and occasional constipation and diarrhoea. Noting that Mr Barrett was anaemic and that he had a family history of bowel cancer, his GP performed a digital rectal examination. Although unable to identify a palpable rectal mass, the GP referred Mr Barrett to a gastroenterologist and a colonoscopy was subsequently scheduled. The colonoscopy revealed left-sided colon cancer and a bowel resection was scheduled.

Access Australia's Health 2016 to find out more about the incidence, mortality, death rate and survival rate for colorectal cancer. Go to <www.aihw.gov.au/WorkArea/DownloadAsset.aspx?id=60129555788>.

The epidemiology of colorectal cancer

Epidemiology is the study of the distribution and determinants of disease, injury and other health-related outcomes in populations. In Australia, colorectal cancer is one of the cancers with the highest incidence in both men and women and this has remained largely unchanged over the past 20 years (*Australia's Health 2016*).

The aetiology and pathogenesis of colorectal cancer

Colorectal cancer is a malignant tumour that starts in the bowel wall. Usually, the tumour is confined locally for a relatively long period before spreading through the bowel wall and metastasising to lymph nodes and other parts of the body. The aetiology of colorectal cancer is complex and involves hereditary and environmental factors. Modifiable dietary and lifestyle factors have been estimated to account for 70 per cent of the risk for colorectal cancer in Western populations.

Person-centred care

If you do not know a person's past, then you cannot understand their present (Kerr & Wilkinson, 2005).

Mr Barrett was born in Geraldton, a country town in Western Australia. He was the oldest child of a large family, with four sisters and two brothers. Arthur left school at age 15 and worked on the land for a number of years before marrying Megan. They had two children, a son and a daughter. Arthur and Megan had a strong marriage and a happy life. Meg died three years ago from breast cancer and last year Arthur's son was killed in a farming accident. Once an active and jovial man, Arthur has been very lonely and sad since their deaths. This period of his life has been hard and he is struggling to come to terms with his recent diagnosis of bowel cancer.

Pre-operative care

Mr Barrett was admitted the day before his surgery as he was considered to be 'high risk'.

Admission observations

Temperature   36.7°C
Pulse rate   90
Respiratory rate   18
Blood pressure   150/90 mmHg

Co-morbidities

- COPD (chronic obstructive pulmonary disease) which Mr Barrett has had for 15 years. He uses a salbutamol inhaler and smokes occasionally.
- Osteoarthritis: Mr Barrett takes the over-the-counter (OTC), non-steroidal anti-inflammatory drugs (NSAIDs) ibuprofen and paracetamol PRN.
- Type 2 diabetes (diet-controlled).

Medical orders

Mr Barrett's doctor ordered the following:

- Two PicoPreps to be given the night before surgery
- Clear fluid diet until midnight and then nil orally
- Enoxaparin sodium 40 mg SCI
- Metronidazole 500 mg IV and cephalothin 2 g IV

Q1 Why was Mr Barrett considered to be 'high risk'?

Q2 What other information would you need if you were caring for Mr Barrett pre-operatively?

Q3 What risk assessments should be undertaken pre-operatively?

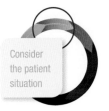

What are sodium phosphate bowel preparations such as Fleet Preps and PicoPreps, and why are they used with extreme caution in older people?

1. CONSIDER THE PATIENT SITUATION

Day 1 post-operatively

You are allocated to the care of Mr Barrett on the morning shift and receive the following handover:

We have Mr Arthur Barrett in room 22. He's 74 years old. He had a partial colectomy and formation of a colostomy secondary to bowel cancer. He's under Dr Ng. His surgery was uneventful and he was stable throughout. He has a morphine PCA and an IV of normal saline running at 84 mL/hr. His last reported pain score was 5/10. He didn't have a good night as his BP dropped and he needed two 300 mL fluid challenges. He's still dry though. He has an IDC on hourly measures and they have dropped progressively overnight. His urine output has been averaging about 25–30 mL/hr since midnight. He has a bellovac and it has drained 300 mL since yesterday. His wound has a dry dressing and it's intact. He has a drainage bag over the stoma—no drainage. His oxygen therapy is still at 6 L/min via a Hudson mask. His sats are OK. The obs are due again at 0800. He is on 4th hourly BGLs and they have been OK. His daughter should be in later today.

QUICK QUIZ!

This handover report uses a number of abbreviations and terminologies. Although this is useful for providing a lot of information concisely, it can cause problems if the terms are not clearly understood. Test your understanding of abbreviations and terminologies by selecting the correct response for each of the identified terms:

Q1 Partial colectomy:

    a Removal of the colon

    b Removal of a section of the large bowel

    c Removal of a section of the small bowel

Q2 PCA:

    a Patient care assistant

    b Pre-cancer anaesthetic

    c Patient-controlled analgesia

Q3 IVT:

    a Intra-operative therapy

    b Intravenous therapy

    c Intravascular therapy

Q4 Fluid challenge:

    a Administration of a large amount of IV fluids over a short period of time under close monitoring to evaluate the patient's response

    b Rapid ingestion of water under close monitoring to evaluate the patient's response

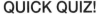

Consider
the patient
situation

Q5 Bellovac:

    a Urinary drainage system

    b Vacuum dressing

    c Vacuum drain

Q6 IDC:

    a Independent drainage catheter

    b Indwelling catheter

    c Intermittent drainage catheter

Q7 Stoma:

    a An opening into the body from the outside created by a surgeon

    b An opening out of the body from a fistula

Q8 BGL:

    a Blood glucose level

    b Basic saturation level

    c Blood gas levels

2. COLLECT CUES/INFORMATION

(a) Review current information

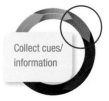

Now that you have considered Mr Barrett's situation, the next stage of the clinical reasoning cycle is to collect relevant cues and information. Start by reviewing Mr Barrett's current observations and comparing them to his pre-operative vital signs:

Temperature	37°C
Pulse rate	112 (weak and thready)
Respiratory rate	22
Blood pressure	90/50 mmHg
Oxygen saturation level	97%
Hourly urine output (average)	26 mL/hr
Specific gravity of urine	1.022
BGL	4 mmol/L

(b) Gather new information

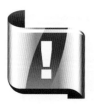

Something to think about …

Remember: When the correct cues are not collected, all of the actions that follow may be incorrect. Making decisions based on incomplete information is a leading cause of clinical errors. Early subtle cues, when missed, can lead to adverse patient outcomes (Levett-Jones et al., 2010).

Q   What other clinical information do you need? From the list below, identify four cues that you believe are *most* relevant to your assessment of Mr Barrett at this time.

    a Appetite (nil)

    b Condition of oral mucosa (dry and tongue furrowed)

    c Level of thirst (reports that he is very thirsty)

    d Pain 3 out of 10

    e Cognitive state (restless and anxious)

    f Colour (pale)

    g Skin condition (poor skin turgor)

(c) Recall knowledge

While cue collection involves reviewing current information and gathering new information about Mr Barrett, it also requires you to recall what you know about related physiology and pathophysiology.

QUICK QUIZ!

Test your knowledge of physiology and pathophysiology related to fluid balance.

To revise your knowledge of the renal system, access Meet the Kidneys! at the Khan Academy: <www.khanacademy. org/science/health-and-medicine/ human-anatomy-and-physiology>.

Q1   When a person's glomerular filtration rate drops:

   a   The anterior pituitary gland responds by secreting antidiuretic hormone

   b   The adrenal glands respond by secreting renin

   c   The adrenal glands respond by reducing the secretion of aldosterone

   d   The juxtaglomerular cells in the kidney respond by secreting renin

Q2   Antidiuretic hormone is secreted:

   a   By the anterior pituitary gland in response to increased serum albumin

   b   By the posterior pituitary gland in response to increased serum osmolality

   c   By the posterior pituitary gland in response to decreased serum sodium levels

   d   By the collecting ducts of the kidneys in response to dehydration

Q3   Oliguria:

   a   May be defined as an absence of urine production

   b   Is common after major surgery and, as such, is nothing for the nurse to be concerned about

   c   Is generally defined as more than 30 mL/hr of urine excretion and is uncommon in the immediate post-operative period

   d   Is generally defined as less than 30 mL/hr of urine excretion and, left untreated, may lead to acute kidney injury

Q4   When assessing a patient's fluid status, which of the following groups include the *most* important nursing observations?

   a   Weight, urine output, bowel sounds

   b   Chvostek's sign, fluid intake, blood pressure

   c   Serum potassium, bowel sounds, urine output

   d   Urine output, blood pressure, weight

Q5   Insensible fluid loss occurs through all of the following routes *except*:

   a   Skin

   b   Lungs

   c   Kidneys

   d   Gastrointestinal tract

Q6   Extracellular fluid loss refers to fluid loss from the interstitial fluid compartment and/or:

   a   Intravascular compartment

   b   Intracellular compartment

   c   Retention of fluid in the plasma

   d   Loss of magnesium and albumin from the kidneys

Q7   In assessing a patient with dehydration, you would expect the urine output to be:

   a   Increased with elevated specific gravity

   b   Increased with decreased specific gravity

   c   Decreased with elevated specific gravity

   d   Decreased with decreased specific gravity

Q8   A third-space fluid shift may occur as a result of all of the following *except*:

   a   Hypoalbuminaemia

   b   An allergic reaction

   c   Hypertension

   d   Hypovolaemia

3. PROCESS INFORMATION

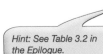

Process information

(a) Interpret

The next step of the clinical reasoning cycle is to interpret the data (cues) that you have collected by careful analysis and by applying your knowledge of fluid balance. By comparing normal versus abnormal, you will come to a more complete understanding of Mr Barrett's signs and symptoms.

Q1   Which of the following are considered to be within normal parameters for Mr Barrett?

   a   Temperature: 37°C

   b   Pulse rate: 112 beats/min

   c   Respiratory rate: 22 breaths/min

   d   Blood pressure: 90/50 mmHg

   e   Specific gravity of 1.022

In handover, a number of statements were made that need further clarification. Analyse each of the following statements and physiological parameters. Compare normal versus abnormal, and identify what you would consider 'normal' for Mr Barrett at this time.

Q2   'His sats (SaO_2) are OK.' A 'normal' oxygen saturation level for Mr Barrett would be:

   a   80–85%

   b   85–90%

   c   90–95%

   d   95–100%

Q3   'He has an IDC on hourly measures and these are still a bit low.' For Mr Barrett, a 'normal' urine output would be at least:

   a   41 mL/hr

   b   82 mL/hr

   c   60 mL/hr

   d   10 mL/hr

Hint: See Table 3.2 in the Epilogue.

Q4   'His BGLs are okay.' A 'normal' BGL for Mr Barrett would be:

   a   4–8 mmol/L

   b   2–4 mmol/L

   c   1–3 mmol/L

   d   8–10 mmol/L

(b) Discriminate

From the cues and information you now have, you need to narrow down the information to what is most important.

Q   From the list below, select four cues that you believe are *most relevant* to Mr Barrett's fluid status *at this time*.

   a   Blood pressure

   b   Respiratory rate

   c   Temperature

    d   Pulse

    e   Condition of wound

    f   Oxygen saturation level

    g   Condition of oral mucosa

    h   Level of consciousness

    i   Appetite

    j   Urine output

(c) Relate

It is important to cluster cues together and identify relationships between them (based on the information you have collected so far).

Q   Label the following 'true' or 'false':

    a   Mr Barrett is probably hypoxic as a result of the extended anaesthetic period and his COPD.

    b   Mr Barrett could be hypotensive and tachycardic from the pre-operative bowel prep.

    c   Mr Barrett could be tachycardic and hypotensive from a third-space fluid shift.

    d   Mr Barrett is febrile and tachycardic because of a post-operative wound infection.

    e   Mr Barrett could be oliguric from hypotension and the PCA.

> ### Something to think about …
> *A third-space fluid shift occurs when too much fluid moves from the intravascular space (blood vessels) into the interstitial space (the area between the cells), the bowel or the peritoneal cavity. Fluid sequestered in these spaces is physiologically useless and the loss of fluids from the intravascular compartment can lead to hypotension and reduced cardiac output (Strunden et al., 2011).*

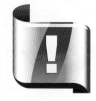

(d) Infer

It is time to think about all the cues that you have collected about Mr Barrett's condition, and to make inferences based on your analysis and interpretation of those cues.

Q   From what you know about Mr Barrett's history, surgery, signs and symptoms (as well as your knowledge about fluid balance), identify which of the following inferences are correct. (Select the two that apply.)

    a   Mr Barrett is normotensive and bradycardic.

    b   Mr Barrett is oliguric and tachycardic.

    c   Mr Barrett is hypertensive and afebrile.

    d   Mr Barrett is polyuric and hypotensive.

    e   Mr Barrett is hypotensive and afebrile.

(e) Predict

At this stage, you begin to consider the consequences of your actions or inaction by predicting potential outcomes for your patient.

Q   If you do not take the appropriate actions at this time, what could happen to Mr Barrett if his fluid imbalance is not corrected? (Select the three that apply.)

    a   Mr Barrett could go into shock.

    b   Mr Barrett's condition will gradually improve over the next few days.

    c   Mr Barrett could develop acute kidney injury.

    d   Mr Barrett could develop pulmonary oedema.

    e   Mr Barrett could die.

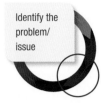

4. IDENTIFY THE PROBLEM/ISSUE

Now bring together (synthesise) all of the facts you've collected and inferences you've made to make a nursing diagnosis of Mr Barrett's main problems or issues.

Q1   Select from the following list the three correct nursing diagnoses for Mr Barrett.

a   Hypervolaemia related to fluid intake and surgical blood loss evidenced by tachycardia, hypertension and cognitive changes

b   Hypovolaemia related to third-space fluid shift evidenced by oliguria and elevated specific gravity of urine

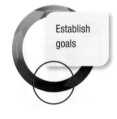

Do you know the difference between hypovolaemia and dehydration?

c   Dehydration related to GIT fluid losses (PicoPrep) and limited oral fluid intake evidenced by decreased skin turgor, dry mucous membranes and thirst

d   Hypovolaemic shock related to excess fluid output and inadequate fluid intake

e   Acute kidney injury related to third-space fluid shift evidenced by oliguria and elevated specific gravity of urine

f   Hypovolaemia related to inadequate fluid intake and surgical blood loss evidenced by tachycardia, hypotension and cognitive changes

Hint: Think about the causes and consequences of third-space fluid shifts.

Q2   Identify four factors that led to Mr Barrett's deterioration.

5. ESTABLISH GOALS

Establish goals

The therapeutic goal for the management of hypovolaemia and dehydration is to return the intravascular fluid compartment to normal in order to prevent the potentially life-threatening complication of hypovolaemic shock.

Q   Before implementing any actions to improve Mr Barrett's condition, it is important to clearly specify what you want to happen and when. From the list below, choose the most important and realistic short-term goals for Mr Barrett's management at this time.

a   For Mr Barrett to be normotensive with urine output at least 30–40 mL/hr within the next 24 hours

b   For Mr Barrett to be normotensive with urine output greater than 80–100 mL/hr within the next 2 hours

c   For Mr Barrett to be normotensive with urine output at least 40–45 mL/hr within the next 2–4 hours

d   For Mr Barrett to be normotensive with urine output greater than 80–100 mL/hr within the next 24 hours

6. TAKE ACTION

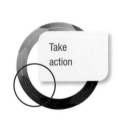

Take action

Nursing 'action' is the behaviour following on from a judgment or decision. This stage of the cycle requires knowledge, clinical skills, effective communication skills and sophisticated clinical reasoning ability. The nurse has to decide which actions take priority, who should be notified and who is best placed to undertake the nursing action(s). At all times, the nurse's practice must be informed by a sound evidence base and relevant policies and guidelines (Levett-Jones et al., 2010).

Note: All of these actions are important, but you need to select those that are most important to the management of Mr Barrett's deteriorating condition at this time!

Q1   The treatment of hypovolaemia and dehydration consists of restoring fluid volume, correcting any electrolyte imbalances and monitoring for improvement or deterioration in the person's condition. From the list below, choose the five *most immediate actions* you should take at this stage.

a   Notify Mr Barrett's doctor of his condition.

b   Monitor Mr Barrett's level of consciousness.

c   Monitor Mr Barrett's pain score.

d   Monitor the condition of Mr Barrett's drain, stoma and wound.

e   Check that the IV cannula is not kinked or blocked.

f   Administer a fluid challenge and increase Mr Barrett's IV fluid rate *as ordered*.

g   Monitor Mr Barrett's vital signs and oxygen saturation level.

h   Strictly monitor Mr Barrett's hourly urine output.

Q2   In the table below, match the rationales for care to the corresponding nursing action.

Nursing action	Rationale
Document all nursing observations and actions accurately and contemporaneously	Anxiety and restlessness may indicate worsening fluid status
Daily weight (same scales, same clothes)	To increase fluid intake
Check cognitive status regularly	To maintain psychosocial wellbeing
Monitor haemodynamic status closely	Values including sodium, potassium, urea, creatinine and haematocrit are important indicators of fluid status and renal function
Regular position change	To manage dry mouth and tongue and to promote patient comfort
Maintain patent IV access and monitor IV site regularly	This is the best indication of fluid status
Encourage oral fluids as ordered/tolerated by patient	To monitor changes in fluid status
Maintain oxygen therapy via nasal prongs or Hudson mask and hourly oxygen sats	To ensure adequate oxygen delivery
Review biochemistry and haematology as ordered	To identify improvement or deterioration in Mr Barrett's condition
Reassure patient	To ensure clear, accurate and timely communication between all health professionals caring for Mr Barrett
Provide regular oral care	To prevent pressure areas due to dry skin
Check specific gravity of urine	To ensure fluids are administered as ordered

7. EVALUATE

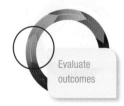

Evaluate outcomes

It is now 1100, two hours since Mr Barrett was given a 300 mL fluid challenge and had his IV rate increased to 125 mL/hr. Each of Mr Barrett's signs and symptoms provide you with cues to make a determination of whether or not your nursing actions have been effective and whether his condition is improving.

Q1   Rate each of the following signs and symptoms as either:

•   Unchanged

•   Improving

•   Deteriorating

Cognitive status: patient restless and anxious

Level of thirst: patient reports some thirst

Pulse rate: 90 beats/min

Urine output: 36 mL/hr

Oral mucosa: mouth is dry and tongue furrowed

Oral intake: tolerating sips of water

Blood pressure: 110/70 mmHg

Colour: pale

Skin condition: skin turgor poor

Q2 You now need to synthesise these parameters to decide whether Mr Barrett's fluid status has improved overall. Which of the following statements are most correct?

    a Mr Barrett's fluid status has improved significantly.

    b Mr Barrett's fluid status has improved significantly but still requires careful monitoring.

    c Mr Barrett's fluid status has improved slightly but still requires careful monitoring. You will need to contact the doctor again if further improvement is not seen in the next four hours.

    d Mr Barrett's fluid status has not improved but you will monitor his condition carefully for the next four hours.

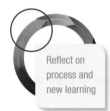

8. REFLECT

The final stage of the clinical reasoning cycle is 'reflection'. Reflect on your learning from this scenario and consider the following questions:

Q1 Could Mr Barrett's deterioration have been prevented? If so, how?

Q2 What are three of the most important things that you have learnt from this scenario?

Q3 What actions will you take in clinical practice as a result of your learning from this scenario?

SCENARIO 3.2   The pendulum swings in the other direction

CHANGING THE SCENE

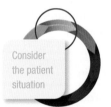

1. CONSIDER THE PATIENT SITUATION

Day 2 post-operatively

It is now 1430 hours and Mt Barrett is day 2 post-op. You are the registered nurse responsible for his care.

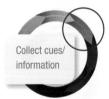

2. COLLECT CUES/INFORMATION

(a) Review current information

You review Mr Barrett's charts and identify the following:

Temperature	37°C
Pulse rate	121 beats/min (full, bounding and irregular)
Respiratory rate	32 breaths/min
Blood pressure	184/95 mmHg
Oxygen saturation level	90%
Hourly urine output (average)	15–30 mL/hr
BGL	6.9 mmol/L

(b) Gather new information

When you enter Mr Barrett's room at 1500 hours to take his observations, you note that he has a dry irritating cough, and is talking to himself, plucking at the bed sheets and attempting to get out of bed. When you ask, 'Are you alright, Mr Barrett?', he does not look at you but holds his head and mumbles, 'My head hurts.' Then he vomits a small amount of clear fluid.

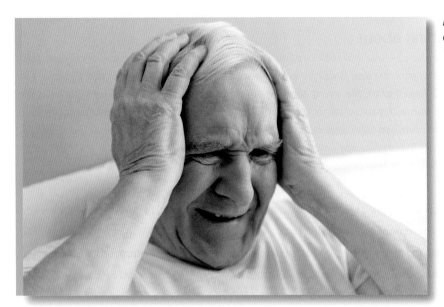

Mr Barrett complaining that his 'head hurts'

The nurse caring for the patient in the next bed shakes her head and says to you, 'Just what we need today, another one with dementia.'

Q1 This nurse's comment is an example of (select two correct answers):

    a Ascertainment bias

    b Diagnostic momentum

    c Pattern matching

    d Intuition

Q2 From the following list, select the seven clinical assessments that are *most relevant* at this stage.

    a Glasgow Coma Scale: 14

    b Pain score: 6

    c Temperature: 37.2°C

    d Level of consciousness: responsive but slightly confused

    e Mini-mental assessment: N/A

    f Oxygen saturation level: 90%

    g Condition of wound: dressing dry and intact, no ooze, no redness around the area

    h Respiratory rate: 32 breaths/min

    i IV rate: 125 mL/hr

    j Urine specific gravity: 1.001

(c) Recall knowledge

QUICK QUIZ!

Q1 When the inflammatory stage of wound healing resolves (24–72 hours post-operatively), what is likely to happen to your patient?

    a Plasma from the interstitial compartment typically returns to the circulating blood volume.

    b Plasma from the intravascular compartment typically returns to the intracellular compartment.

    c Plasma from the intracellular compartment typically returns to the intravascular compartment.

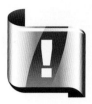

Something to think about …

Third-spacing has two phases—loss and reabsorption. In the loss phase, increased capillary permeability leads to the movement of proteins and fluids from the intravascular space to the interstitial space. This phase lasts 24 to 72 hours after the event that precipitated the increased capillary permeability (e.g. surgery, trauma, burns, sepsis or ascites). During the reabsorption phase, tissues begin to heal, fluid shifts back into the intravascular space and hypovolaemia resolves. Patients should be monitored carefully at this stage as hypervolaemia can occur as many litres of interstitial fluid move back to the intravascular space (Simmons Holcombe, 2009, p. 10).

Q2 Type 2 diabetes can influence fluid balance. Label the following 'true' or 'false'.

    a   Diabetes can cause impaired renal function.

    b   Hypoglycaemia results in increased serum osmolarity, resulting in nocturnal diuresis.

    c   Hyperglycaemia results in increased serum osmolarity, resulting in excessive diuresis.

    d   Diabetes can cause impaired liver function.

Q3 Confusion in the older post-operative person can result from which of the following? (Select the six correct responses.)

    a   Melaena

    b   Constipation

    c   Urinary tract infection

    d   Pain

    e   Atrial fibrillation

    f   Leukopaenia

    g   Fluid and electrolyte imbalance

    h   Infection

    i   Hypoxia

    j   Haemoptysis

Q4 Fluid shifts can contribute to tachypnoea because:

    a   Hypovolaemia causes anxiety.

    b   Dehydration causes carbon dioxide retention.

    c   Insensible fluid losses cause hypoxia.

    d   Fluids shifts into the alveolar spaces causing pulmonary oedema and impacting on oxygenation levels.

Q5 Which of the following is *true* of altered sodium (Na^+) levels?

    a   Decreased sodium concentration can be a consequence of over-hydration.

    b   Decreased sodium levels are a consequence of dehydration and excessive dietary intake.

    c   Decreased sodium concentration can be a consequence of dehydration and excessive exercise.

    d   Increased sodium levels are a consequence of excessive vomiting and diarrhoea.

Q6 Older people are at risk of fluid imbalance because they have an increased likelihood of all of the following *except*:

    a   Impaired renal function

    b   Chronic dehydration

    c   Morbid obesity

    d   Malnutrition

3. PROCESS INFORMATION

Process information

(a) Interpret

Q1   Based on Mr Barrett's current signs and symptoms, do you think he is in a positive or a negative fluid balance?

Pathology results—Arthur Barrett

	Pre-op	Day 1	Day 2	Normal values
Sodium	140 mmol/L	138 mmol/L	128 mmol/L	136–144 mmol/L
Potassium	3.9 mmol/L	3.6 mmol/L	3.3 mmol/L	3.6–5.0 mmol/L
Urea	3.0 mmol/L	4.1 mmol/L	2.9 mmol/L	3.6–8.4 mmol/L (55+ years)
Creatinine	130 µmol/L	130 µmol/L	400 µmol/L	110 µmol/L (males)

Interpret the information on the above pathology chart and answer the following questions.

Q2   Today (day 2), is Mr Barrett hypernatraemic or hyponatraemic?

Q3   Today (day 2), is Mr Barrett hyperkalaemic or hypokalaemic?

Q4   What do Mr Barrett's urea and creatinine levels indicate?

Q5   Hyponatraemia can cause which of the following signs and symptoms? (Select the four correct answers.)

> Can you define the terms 'hyponatraemia' and 'hypokalaemia'?

    a   Constipation

    b   Confusion

    c   Headaches

    d   Polyuria

    e   Nausea and vomiting

    f   Abdominal cramps

    g   Thirst

    h   Muscle weakness

    i   Low-grade fever

Q6   Which of the signs and symptoms of hyponatraemia is Mr Barrett exhibiting? (Select the three correct answers.)

    a   Confusion

    b   Abdominal cramps

    c   Headache

    d   Nausea and vomiting

    e   Muscle weakness

Q7   Hypokalaemia can cause which of the following signs and symptoms? (Select six correct answers.)

> Mr Barrett's hyponatraemia and hypokalaemia have probably resulted from the increased fluid volume rather than an actual loss of electrolytes.

    a   Nausea

    b   Irregular pulse

    c   Arrhythmias

    d   Diarrhoea

    e   Cardiac arrest

    f   Decreased bowel sounds

g   Irritability

h   Cramps

i   Hypotension

j   Polyuria

Q8   Which of the signs and symptoms of hypokalaemia is Mr Barrett exhibiting? (Select one correct answer.)

a   Irregular pulse

b   Decreased bowel sounds

c   Cramps

d   Polyuria

(b) Discriminate, (c) Relate and (d) Infer

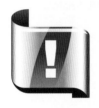

Something to think about …

Nurses have a unique advantage in the identification of deteriorating patients. Rather than 'treat' and 'retreat', nurses are a constant presence when caring for patients. They detect trends, can compare normal vs abnormal, and recognise gaps in the information at hand. Their ability to recognise clinically 'at risk' patients is crucial. By recognising early warning signs you will be able to identify patients at risk of serious adverse events.

Q   With reference to the table below, identify the four clinical indicators that are early warnings of serious adverse outcomes for Mr Barrett.

The NSQHS Standards highlight the importance of early recognition of patient deterioration. However, serious adverse events, such as unexpected death, or cardiac or respiratory arrests, are often preceded by observable physiological abnormalities which aren't always recognised or managed appropriately (ACSQHC, 2016).

Early warning signs
SpO$_2$: 90–95%
Urine output: <200 mL over 8 hours
Glasgow Coma Scale (GCS): <9–11 or a fall in GCS by >2
Changes in cognition
Respiratory rate: 5–9 or 31–40 breaths/min
Systolic blood pressure: 80–100 mmHg or 181–240 mmHg
Pulse rate: 40–49 or 121–140 beats/min
Chest pain
Newly reported pain or uncontrolled pain
Blood glucose level: 1–2.9 mmol/L

Source: Adapted from T. Jacques, G. Harrison, M. McLaws & G. Kilborne (2006). Signs of critical conditions and emergency responses (SOCCER): A model for predicting adverse events in the inpatient setting. *Resuscitation, 69*(2), 175–83.

(e) Predict

Positive patient outcomes depend on close surveillance and timely identification of deterioration, followed by prompt and effective nursing actions.

Q   If you do not take the appropriate actions at this time, what could happen to Mr Barrett if his fluid imbalance is not corrected? (Select the four that apply.)

a   Mr Barrett could die.

b   Mr Barrett could go into shock.

c   Mr Barrett could become hypoxic.

d   Mr Barrett's condition will gradually improve over the next few days.

e   Mr Barrett could develop pulmonary oedema.

(f) Match

Q   Have you ever seen someone with the same signs and symptoms as Mr Barrett? If so, what was done to manage the situation?

4. IDENTIFY THE PROBLEM/ISSUE

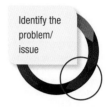
Identify the problem/ issue

Q1   Based on all of the information that you have about Mr Barrett, complete these nursing diagnoses:

a   Hypervolaemia related to excess IV fluids evidenced by _____ and _____.

b   Hypervolaemia related to the reabsorption phase of the third-space fluid shift and return of fluids from the interstitial space to the intravascular component, evidenced by hypertension and _____.

c   Early-stage pulmonary oedema related to _____ evidenced by _____, _____ and _____.

d   Electrolyte imbalance related to hypervolaemia evidenced by _____, _____ and irregular pulse.

Q2   What factors contributed to Mr Barrett's deterioration?

5. ESTABLISH GOALS

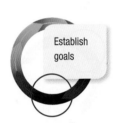
Establish goals

Before implementing any actions to improve Mr Barrett's condition, it is important to clearly specify what you want to happen and when.

Q   From the list below, choose the four most important goals for Mr Barrett's management at this time.

a   Mr Barrett to be self-caring and ambulant

b   Vital signs to be within normal parameters

c   Oral food and fluid intake established

d   Oxygen saturation level >94%

e   Cognitive status improving

f   Stoma functioning

g   Urine output satisfactory

h   Lung sounds normal

I   Electrolytes returning to normal levels

6. TAKE ACTION

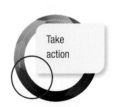
Take action

Q1   From the list below, choose the five most *immediate* actions you would take at this stage. *Note*: Many of these actions are correct but you need to focus on immediate priorities.

a   Contact attending doctor immediately to request medical review.

b   Administer an antiemetic.

c   Administer oxygen 6–8 L/min.

d   Document vital signs QID.

e   Sit Mr Barrett in a semi-Fowler's position.

f   Check weight each day.

g   Decrease IV rate TKVO pending medical orders.

h   Monitor cognitive status.

Hint: Think ABC!

Timing is critical in clinical reasoning. Critical incidents occur not only when early signs and symptoms fail to be recognised or acted upon but also when nursing/ medical interventions are commenced too late.

i   Monitor for improvement in serum electrolytes.

j   Regular position change to prevent pressure areas.

k   Take an ECG.

Q2   Using ISBAR (Identity, Situation, Background, Assessment, Request/Recommendation), document how you would communicate with Mr Barrett's doctor or the Rapid Response Team Leader if you were to phone them.

Q3   From the list below, choose the three nursing actions that you anticipate taking following a clinical review.

a   Increase IV rate following doctor's orders.

b   Administer a diuretic (probably frusemide IV) following doctor's orders.

c   Give anginine tablets following doctor's orders.

d   Reduce IV rate as ordered by medical officer.

e   Take blood for biochemistry and haematological profile.

f   Prepare to give a fluid challenge.

> *Another useful acronym, particularly when you have concerns about a particular course of action, is CUS:*
> - *I am Concerned about my patient's condition.*
> - *I am Uncomfortable with your plan of action.*
> - *I am worried this will impact on my patient's Safety.*

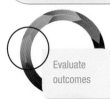

Evaluate outcomes

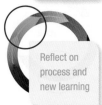

Reflect on process and new learning

> *The NMBA's Registered Nurse Standards for Practice (2016) state that registered nurses must evaluate and monitor progress towards expected goals, revise the care plan based on the evaluation, and discuss further priorities with the relevant person(s).*

7. EVALUATE

Q   List eight signs and symptoms that will indicate to you that Mr Barrett's condition has improved following clinical review and initiation of appropriate nursing actions.

8. REFLECT

Reflective practice is a crucial professional activity and one that is intrinsic to learning. Reflection is a deliberate, orderly and structured intellectual activity. It allows you to process and critically review your learning experience with a view to refinement, improvement or change.

Contemplate what you have learnt from this scenario and how this learning will inform your practice. Respond to the following three questions with reference to Mr Barrett:

Q1   How could Mr Barrett's deterioration have been prevented?

Q2   What have you learnt from the scenario that you can apply to your future practice?

Q3   Why are older post-operative patients at risk of fluid and electrolyte imbalance?

Now read the epilogue and consider the following questions:

Q4   What actions should nurses take to promote kidney health in the community and in healthcare contexts?

Q5   What actions will you take in clinical practice to identify people at risk of kidney disease?

EPILOGUE

The two scenarios presented in this chapter illustrate situations that are all too common in clinical practice. Mr Barrett's deterioration resulted from several factors, including a failure to recognise the seriousness of his condition and to establish his baseline kidney function pre-admission. Identification of pre-existing kidney disease is critical as it enables the treating team to reduce the risk of further kidney damage (e.g. by minimising exposure to nephrotoxic medications) and prevent additional post-operative complications.

Consider what might have happened had Mr Barrett been reviewed by a Practice Nurse in the GP clinic five years prior to his diagnosis of colorectal cancer. Would he have been considered to be at risk of chronic kidney disease (CKD) based on the modifiable and non-modifiable CKD risk factors outlined in Table 3.1.

Table 3.1 *Risk factors for CKD*

What are the risk factors for CKD?	
Not a risk factor	NSAID usage, COPD, alcohol consumption, sedentary lifestyle
CKD risk factors	• Diabetes • High blood pressure • Age over 60 years • Smoking • Obesity • Family history of kidney disease • Aboriginal or Torres Strait Islander origin • Established cardiovascular disease • History of acute kidney injury

Mr Barrett had five risk factors for CKD: four modifiable (diet-controlled diabetes, history of hypertension, smoking and BMI 31.4) and one non-modifiable (age). Once a person at risk of CKD has been identified, further screening should be conducted using the Kidney Health Check (Johnson & Mathew, 2010). This simple three-step process includes (1) a blood test to measure eGFR; (2) a urine albumin:creatine ratio (ACR) to check for the presence of albuminuria; and (3) blood pressure measurement.

Glomerular filtration rate (GFR) is determined through a formula that takes into consideration the person's serum creatinine level, age and gender. In Australia, whenever a biochemistry screen is ordered, the estimated glomerular filtration rate (eGFR) is tested to screen for and detect early kidney damage. The eGFR is also used to categorise the stages of chronic kidney disease (see Figure 3.1).

A person is diagnosed as having CKD if their eGFR is <60 mL/min/1.73 m^2 for a period of three months or longer, with or without evidence of kidney damage; or if they have evidence of kidney damage (with or without decreased GFR) for longer than three months (i.e. microalbuminuria, proteinuria, haematuria, or pathological or anatomical abnormalities). Timely identification of CKD can prevent

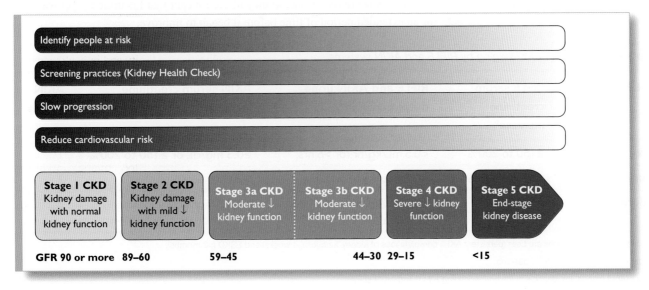

Figure 3.1
The chronic kidney disease trajectory

Source: Used with permission of University of Newcastle.

complications, slow disease progression and reduce cardiovascular risk, as well as reducing mortality and morbidity (Johnson & Mathew, 2010).

Do you want to learn more about identifying, screening and managing CKD in the primary care setting? Check out <http://kidney.org. au/cms_uploads/docs/ ckd-management-in-gp- handbook-3rd-edition. pdf>.

Let's imagine Mr Barrett had a Kidney Health Check five years ago and his blood pressure was 130/82 mmHg and ACR 7.8 mg/mmol (indicating microalbuminuria). A creatinine level of 110 µmol/L at the age of 69 would have given Mr Barrett an eGFR of 58 mL/min/1.73 m^2. With a repeat eGFR confirming this level three months later, Mr Barrett would have been diagnosed with stage 3a CKD and he would have been closely monitored for further decline in kidney function, particularly acute increases in serum creatinine and/or decreases in urine output. Importantly, knowledge of Mr Barrett's pre-existing kidney disease would have enabled the treating team to reduce the risk of acute kidney injury (AKI) when he was admitted to hospital for surgery.

AKI can be precipitated by numerous factors, including nephrotoxic medications, sepsis and hypovolaemia (Stewart et al., 2009). The presence of CKD during any acute insult to the kidneys results in further decreased renal function; this is called 'acute on chronic kidney disease', sometimes referred to as 'acute on chronic'. It is important to remember that eGFR is not valid in AKI as its measurement is reliant on a steady-state creatinine (Bennett, Sinclair & Schoch, 2017). Consequently, classification systems that consider levels of severity based on serum creatinine increases and urine output are used (see Table 3.2).

Using the criteria shown in Table 3.2 in Scenario 3.1, Mr Barrett's urine output dropped to between 25 and 30 mL/hr for at least eight hours. According to the **R**isk, **I**njury, **F**ailure, **L**oss, **E**nd-Stage Kidney Disease (RIFLE) and Acute Kidney Injury Network (AKIN) staging criteria, this put him *at risk of* AKI due to hypoperfusion to his kidneys. Continued hypoperfusion and associated renal tissue hypoxia resulted in damage to his renal parenchyma and the development of acute tubular necrosis.

In Scenario 3.2, when Mr Barrett was day 2 post-operatively, his condition changed from hypovolaemia to hypervolaemia as a result of the over-correction of his fluid status, resolution of his third-space fluid shift and his kidneys being unable to maintain homeostasis. For over 12 hours, Mr Barrett's urine output remained at less than 0.5 mL/kg/hr but the severity of his condition was not recognised. His specific gravity was 1.001, demonstrating that his renal tubules were no longer able to concentrate the glomerular filtrate, damage to his renal parenchyma had occurred and Mr Barrett was experiencing pre-renal AKI (see Table 3.2).

With the development of pulmonary oedema, he was placed on fluid restriction and IV frusemide was administered. Consequently, his urine output began to improve. However, delays in identification and management of Mr Barrett's acute on chronic kidney disease meant that his urine output was less than 30 mL per hour for an extended period of time before it began to improve.

Table 3.2 *Comparison of AKI staging by RIFLE and AKIN systems*

RIFLE stages[a]	RIFLE serum creatinine increase[b]	RIFLE and AKIN urine output criteria[c]	AKIN serum creatinine increase[d]	AKIN stages
Risk	≥150 to 200%	<0.5 mL/kg/hr for >6 hrs	≥0.3 mg/dL or ≥150 to 200%	1
Injury	>200 to 300%	<0.5 mL/kg/hr >12 hrs	>200 to 300%	2
Failure	>300%	<0.3 mL/kg/hr for ≥24 hrs or anuria ≥12 hrs	>300%[D] or acute RRT	3

a The remaining RIFLE stages are Loss (persistent AKI = complete loss of kidney function >4 weeks) and ESKD (>3 months).

b Serum creatinine increase from baseline.

c Urine output criteria are identical in the corresponding RIFLE and AKIN stages.

d Increase in Cr> 4 mg/dL and acute rise ≥0.5 mg/dL

One of the major post-operative priorities for any individual, regardless of whether they have pre-existing kidney disease, is to ensure the continued perfusion of the kidneys. This is achieved through avoiding insults to the kidney, vigilant monitoring and the careful management of fluid status throughout a person's hospital stay, and particularly in the first 72 hours post-operatively.

By day 3 post-operatively, Mr Barrett's urine output had improved and he was discharged from hospital seven days later. However, his pre-operative baseline creatinine increased from 130 μmol/L to 210 μmol/L. He was referred to a nephrologist for follow-up and three months later blood tests confirmed the deterioration in his kidney function, with his eGFR declining to 27 mL/min/1.73 m^2. This indicated that Mr Barrett had progressed to stage 4 CKD and renal replacement therapy options (i.e. dialysis) had to be considered.

Mr Barrett's clinical deterioration was preventable. Had the healthcare professionals caring for him identified his underlying CKD earlier, recognised that he was predisposed to AKI and managed his post-operative complications in a timely manner, acute on chronic kidney disease would not have resulted. Mr Barrett's story should be used as a precedent to highlight how clinical reasoning errors and failure to escalate in a timely manner can lead to serious and preventable adverse patient outcomes.

FURTHER READING

Johnson, D. W. & Mathew, T. (2010). How to treat chronic kidney disease. *Australian Doctor*, March, 27–34.

Strunden, M. S., Heckel, K., Goetz, A. E. & Reuter, D. A. (2011). Perioperative fluid and volume management: Physiological basis, tools and strategies. *Annals of Intensive Care*, *1*(2), 1–8.

REFERENCES

Australian Commission on Safety and Quality in Health Care (ACSQHC). (2016). *National Safety and Quality Health Service Standards Version 2.* Draft, Sydney, Australia.

Australian Institute of Health and Welfare (AIHW). (2016). *Australia's Health 2016.* Australia's Health Series No. 15. Cat. No. AUS 199. Canberra: AIHW.

Bennett, P., Sinclair, P. & Schoch, M. (2017). Chapter 27: Caring for people with kidney disorders. In P. LeMone, K. Burke, T. Dwyer, T. Levett-Jones, L. Moxam, K. Reid-Searl, … D. Raymond (Eds), *Medical–Surgical Nursing: Critical Thinking in Client Care* (3rd edn). Sydney: Pearson.

Jacques, T., Harrison, G., McLaws, M. & Kilborne, G. (2006). Signs of critical conditions and emergency responses (SOCCER): A model for predicting adverse events in the inpatient setting. *Resuscitation, 69*(2), 175–83.

Johnson, D.W. & Mathew, T. (2010). How to treat chronic kidney disease. *Australian Doctor*, March, 27–34.

Kerr, D. & Wilkinson, H. (2005). *In the Know: Implementing Good Practice–Information and Tools for Anyone Supporting People with a Learning Disability and Dementia.* Brighton: Pavilion Publishing.

Levett-Jones, T., Hoffman, K., Dempsey, Y., Jeong, S., Noble, D., Norton, C., … Hickey, N. (2010). The 'five rights' of clinical reasoning: An educational model to enhance nursing students' ability to identify and manage clinically 'at risk' patients. *Nurse Education Today, 30*(6), 515–20.

Nursing and Midwifery Board of Australia (NMBA). (2016). *Registered Nurse Standards for Practice.* Retrieved from <www.nursingmidwiferyboard.gov.au/Codes-Guidelines-Statements/Professional-standards.aspx>.

Simmons Holcombe, S. (2009). Third-spacing: When body fluids shift. *Nursing 2009, 4*(2), 9–12.

Stewart, J., Findlay, G., Smith, N., Kelly, K. & Mason, M. (2009). *Adding Insult to Injury: A Review of the Care of Patients Who Died in Hospital with a Primary Diagnosis of Acute Kidney Injury (Acute Renal Failure): A Report by the National Confidential Enquiry into Patient Outcome and Death.* London: National Confidential Enquiry into Patient Outcome and Death.

Strunden, M., Heckel, K., Goetz, A. & Reuter, D. (2011). Perioperative fluid and volume management: physiological basis, tools and strategies. *Annals of Intensive Care, 1*(2), 1–8.

PHOTO CREDIT

CHAPTER 4

CARING FOR A PERSON EXPERIENCING PAIN

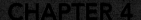

TRACY LEVETT-JONES AND CAROLINE PHELAN

LEARNING OUTCOMES

Completion of the activities in this chapter will enable you to:

○ explain why an understanding of pain is essential to competent practice (**recall** and **application**)

○ identify the clinical manifestations of acute and persistent pain that are used to guide the collection and interpretation of cues (**gather**, **review**, **interpret**, **discriminate**, **relate** and **infer**)

○ examine myths related to pain management (**recall**)

○ explain the benefits of pre-emptive and multimodal analgesia (**recall**)

○ identify complications from poorly managed pain (**match** and **predict**)

○ review clinical information to identify the main nursing diagnoses for someone experiencing acute or persistent pain (**synthesise**)

○ describe the priorities of care for a patient with acute or persistent pain (**goal setting** and **taking action**)

○ identify clinical criteria for determining the effectiveness of nursing actions taken to prevent and manage pain (**evaluate**)

○ adopt a holistic approach to pain management (**taking action**)

○ apply what you have learnt about pain management to clinical practice (**reflection** and **translation**).

INTRODUCTION

In this chapter, you will be introduced to Mrs Grace Simpson, a 74-year-old woman admitted to hospital with a hip fracture following a fall at home. It is the therapeutic management of Mrs Simpson's pain, both in the acute care setting and following discharge, that is the focus of the two scenarios.

For many years, pain was accepted as inevitable, and indifference to its seriousness was common. Contemporary approaches to pain now recognise that effective pain management is a fundamental human right and integral to ethical, professional and cost-effective clinical practice (Macintyre et al., 2010). Pain management requires sophisticated clinical reasoning skills, a sound knowledge base, highly developed clinical skills and a commitment to person-centred care.

Pain is a complex, individual, multifactorial experience influenced by a person's culture, previous pain experiences, beliefs, mood and coping ability. Although pain may be an indicator of injury and tissue damage, it may also be experienced in the absence of an identifiable cause. Response to pain and the degree of disability it causes varies between people. Similarly, individuals respond differently to the management strategies used to alleviate pain. Complications resulting from poorly managed pain are significant, widespread and at times life-threatening. Research has identified a link between acute pain, especially when not managed appropriately, and persistent pain that lasts for months or years (National Pain Strategy, 2010). Sound clinical reasoning skills will help you to recognise and appropriately manage your patients' pain, thus preventing short- and long-term complications from poorly managed pain.

KEY CONCEPTS

acute pain
persistent (chronic) pain
pre-emptive pain management
multimodal pain management
pain myths
pain management plan

SUGGESTED READINGS

P. LeMone, K. Burke, G. Bauldoff, P. Gubrud-Howe, T. Levett-Jones, T. Dwyer ... D. Raymond (Eds). (2017). *Medical–Surgical Nursing: Critical Thinking in Person-Centred Care* (3rd edn). Melbourne: Pearson. Chapter 8: Nursing care of people in pain

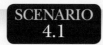

SCENARIO 4.1   Caring for a person experiencing acute pain

SETTING THE SCENE

Mrs Grace Simpson was admitted to hospital following a fall in which she fractured her right neck of femur. She fell at home and was not discovered until her son returned from work six hours later. Mrs Simpson's surgeon told her family that the fracture was related to her history of osteoporosis. Mrs Simpson had a knee replacement 12 months ago and has a history of angina.

Falls and injury—a National Health Priority Area

Injury prevention and control is a National Health Priority Area, with trauma-related injuries a leading cause of mortality and morbidity, resulting in significant healthcare costs (Australian Institute of Health and Welfare, 2011). However, the social cost of injuries is also significant due to the resultant levels of permanent disability.

Fall-related hospitalisation is common in older people. In 2011–12, 96 385 people aged 65 and over were hospitalised for a fall-related injury; of these, 68 per cent were women. There are also higher numbers of hip fractures in women and the average length of hospital stay following a hip fracture is longer for women (Australian Institute of Health and Welfare, 2016).

Osteoporosis

Osteoporosis means 'porous bones'; it is a musculoskeletal disorder in which the bone density thins and weakens, resulting in an increased risk of fracture. The most common sites of fracture are the bones of the spine, hip and wrist. The prevalence of osteoporosis among those aged 50 and over is 23 per cent of women and 6 per cent of men (Australian Institute of Health and Welfare, 2014). This is because there is a sharp decline in the female hormone oestrogen after menopause. This hormone plays a vital role in maintaining bone mass density and the decreased production accelerates calcium loss in bones.

Fracture of the hip is one of the most serious outcomes of osteoporosis. In 2011–12, 19 000 people aged 50 and over were hospitalised due to a hip fracture, of whom 71 per cent were aged 80 and over and 72 per cent were women (Australian Institute of Health and Welfare, 2014). Such fractures can cause significant pain, disability and reduced quality of life. They are also associated with an increased risk of premature death (Bliuc et al., 2013). The direct and indirect costs of osteoporosis in Australia are estimated to be $2754 million per annum (Watts, Abimanyi-Ochom & Sanders, 2013).

Acute pain

> Adjuvant medications are those used in pain management whose initial purpose was for another condition. Examples include antidepressants and anticonvulsants, which can be used for the treatment of neuropathic pain.

Acute pain occurs across the life span, and the majority of patients within the acute hospital setting will experience pain. It is estimated that 90 per cent of patients could obtain effective, safe relief of acute pain with currently available treatments; however, 50 per cent of hospitalised patients have unacceptable levels of pain due to poor assessment and/or under-treatment (National Pain Strategy, 2010).

Acute pain is defined as pain that has a recent onset and limited duration. This is in contrast to persistent or chronic pain, which persists beyond the time of healing of the original injury (Macintyre et al., 2010). Pain generated from damage of the tissues, skin, ligaments and visceral organs is referred to as 'nociceptive' pain. This type of pain generally responds well to simple analgesics and opioids. Pain generated from damage to the nervous system itself is referred to as 'neuropathic' pain. This type of pain is much more difficult to treat and often requires adjuvant medications.

Person-centred care

Mrs Simpson grew up in the Blue Mountains in New South Wales and was a primary school headmistress for many years. She is a widow and lives with her eldest son, Alan. Mrs Simpson is the matriarch of her family, loved and respected by her children and grandchildren. Although fiercely independent and stoic in many ways, Mrs Simpson is acutely aware that her body is 'letting her down' even though mentally she remains 'sharp as a tack'.

1. CONSIDER THE PATIENT SITUATION

It is now 0800 hours and Mrs Simpson is day 1 post-operatively. You are given the following handover report:

0700 hours: Mrs Simpson, day 1, has a morphine PCA. She was given a single-shot nerve block in theatre but this wore off in recovery. She was quite unsettled and complained of pain on and off during the night. She vomited twice and ondansetron was given at 0300. She seems a bit more settled now and has drifted off to sleep. Obs stable, but BP a bit elevated. Urine output OK. Wound dressing dry and intact. IV 8-hourly.

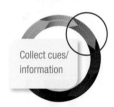

Consider the patient situation

Handover practices are often highly variable and unreliable. Breakdown in the transfer of information or in communication at handover has been identified as a preventable cause of patient harm (Iedema, 2014).

2. COLLECT CUES/INFORMATION

(a) Review current information

You review Mrs Simpson's charts and note that her blood pressure is 145/90 mmHg, pulse rate 98 and urine output 35–40 mL/hr. On the PCA chart, a lockout period of 10 minutes and a dose of 1 mg/mL are documented. You identify that Mrs Simpson made multiple and repeated PCA attempts during the night (not all of them successful). She was using about 4 mg of morphine per hour until 0400 and from then on used less than 1 mg/hr. When assessed during the night, Mrs Simpson reported pain scores of between 5 and 8 using a numerical rating scale.

Collect cues/ information

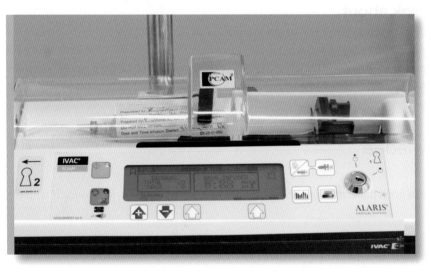

PCA showing 20 attempts but only 8 mg infused

Q The information you have to date leads you to think that overnight Mrs Simpson:

a Has pushed her PCA button too many times

b Has not pushed her PCA button enough

c Has needed a dose of morphine more frequently than the lockout period would allow

d Has needed a smaller dose of morphine than was prescribed

(b) Gather new information

You decide to assess Mrs Simpson's pain.

Q1 What are the two most accurate methods of assessing a person's pain?

a Asking the patient to describe and locate their pain

b Careful observation of physiological signs

c Asking the patient to rate their pain using a visual or numerical rating scale

d Reviewing the patient's chart

PCA pumps have been shown to be more effective in treating pain than intermittent IM or IV injections, providing increased patient control over pain relief and lower levels of pre-operative anxiety (Patak et al., 2013).

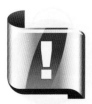

Something to think about ...

Margo McCaffery's well-accepted and much used definition of pain states that pain is whatever the patient says it is, existing whenever the patient says it does (McCaffery, Rolling Ferrell & Paseo, 2000). This definition implies that the patient is in the best position to describe and inform the nurse about his or her pain. Nurses must therefore elicit the patient's assessment of their pain, accept and believe that assessment, and take appropriate actions to manage the pain.

It is essential to reflect on and question one's assumptions and preconceptions about people who are experiencing pain, as failure to do so may negatively impact on your clinical reasoning ability and consequently your patient's clinical outcomes.

Q2 Why is pain often referred to as the fifth vital sign?

   a To ensure that nurses remember to assess their patient's pain when they undertake routine observations

   b To emphasise the importance of regular assessment and ongoing management of pain

   c So that pain assessment is always accurate and complete

   d To allow pain scores to be communicated from one nurse to another

You observe that Mrs Simpson is pale and drawn in appearance. When you ask her about her pain, she reveals that she is reluctant to use the PCA as one of the night nurses told her that she should be feeling better by now, that she could become addicted or even stop breathing, and that the morphine was causing her nausea.

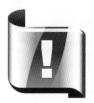

Something to think about ...

Nurses' beliefs cause them to process clinical situations and act in particular ways. Their overarching philosophies serve as perspectives that condition the ways in which they judge and ultimately deal with patients experiencing pain. In a study by McCaffery, Rolling Ferrell and Paseo (2000), nurses' opinions of their patients and their personal beliefs about pain significantly influenced the quality of their pain assessment and management.

(c) Recall knowledge

QUICK QUIZ!

To ensure that you have a good understanding of the key concepts related to pain, test yourself with the following questions.

Q1 Morphine is:

   a A non-steroidal anti-inflammatory (NSAID)

   b An antiemetic

   c An opioid analgesic

   d An antipyretic

Q2 Pain can result in stimulation of the stress response. For each of the following, indicate the response you would expect from acute pain by marking ↑ or ↓.

   a Heart rate

   b Serum cortisol level

   c Blood pressure

   d Gastric motility

   e Risk of deep vein thrombosis

Q3 Which of the following instructions should nurses give their patients regarding use of a PCA?

   a Use the PCA every hour on the hour.

   b Use the PCA only when the pain is severe.

   c Avoid overuse of the PCA because of the risk of addiction.

   d Use the PCA regularly to prevent and manage pain.

Q4 If a patient with a PCA was drowsy and unable to keep their eyes open, what would you do?

   a Administer oxygen and notify the nurse in charge.

   b Administer oxygen and initiate a rapid response call.

   c Administer oxygen and check the vital signs.

   d Immediately discontinue the PCA and select an alternative analgesic.

Q5 Examples of opioids are:

   a Codeine

   b Paracetamol

   c Ketoprofen

   d Oxycodone

   e Tramadol

   f Morphine

   g Digesic

   h Ibuprofen

3. PROCESS INFORMATION

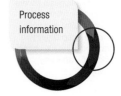

(a) Interpret

The next step of the clinical reasoning cycle is to interpret the data (cues) that you have collected by careful analysis, all the while applying your knowledge about pain.

Q Select 'true', 'false' or 'infrequently' for the following dose-related side effects of morphine.

   a Over-sedation

   b Nausea and vomiting

   c Drug dependency/addiction

   d Drug tolerance

   e Pruritus

   f Respiratory depression

   g Hypotension (due to vasodilation)

   h Decreased urine output

   i Full and bounding pulse, tachycardia

   j Pupillary dilation

   k Narcosis

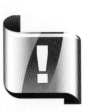

Something to think about …

It is not unusual for nurses to be overly concerned about the risks of respiratory depression and opioid addiction when caring for people who have a PCA. In reality, these side effects are uncommon. Patients in severe pain can tolerate very high doses of opioids without becoming excessively sedated or experiencing respiratory depression. Although you would check Mrs Simpson's respiratory rate and oxygen saturation level on room air regularly, you can be confident that if she is awake and conversing she is not likely to be experiencing respiratory depression.

Similarly, while tolerance may occur with long-term use of opioids, addiction is rare in the normal course of events for post-operative patients. Research shows that addiction occurs in less than 1 per cent of hospitalised patients treated with opioids (Patak et al., 2013). It is important to be clear about making the distinction between tolerance and addiction. Tolerance occurs when the body no longer responds as well to the opioid's pain-relieving properties at the current dose. For example, some cancer patients with severe pain may need increasing amounts of morphine to maintain an adequate level of pain relief. Addiction, on the other hand, is an overwhelming compulsion to continue use of the drug even when pain relief is no longer needed.

(b) Discriminate and (c) Relate

Q There are many myths about pain and pain management. From the following, identify those that are 'true' and those that are 'false'.

a Young children can usually be relied on to report on their own pain levels.

b 'Clock watching', 'knowing too much' and asking for more medication often indicate narcotic addiction.

c Severe pain always presents with physiological signs.

d Women typically have a lower pain threshold than men.

e Pre-emptive analgesia is more effective than PRN analgesia.

f Pain is an inevitable consequence of injury and cannot be completely relieved.

g 'No pain, no gain' is a correct assumption.

h People with dementia are unable to rate their pain levels.

i Older men are stoic about pain.

j It is important to use pre-emptive analgesia to prevent rather than treat pain.

> *Nurses should pre-empt their patient's pain and provide analgesia before rather than after pain develops, for example, prior to deep breathing and coughing exercises or painful dressing changes.*

(d) Infer

Q A continuing pain score of 5–8 is:

a Indicative of a low pain threshold and of significant concern

b Not unusual for a person who has had major surgery

c Indicative of severe pain that is poorly managed

d Typical for a person who is day 1 post-operatively and nothing to be concerned about

> *The NMBA's Code of Ethics (2008) states that 'nurses value respect and kindness for self and others'. People experiencing pain often feel vulnerable, powerless and fearful. Nurses must therefore prevent rather than just treat pain, and ensure that their patients are informed, educated and supported.*

(e) Match

Nurses have a professional, ethical and legal responsibility to manage pain effectively. Have you ever been in a clinical situation where you felt concerned about how a patient's pain was managed? If so, what actions did you take or should you have taken?

(f) Predict

Q Complications of poorly managed acute pain may include which of the following? (Select the six correct answers.)

a Hypercoagulopathy

b Delayed wound healing

c Pneumonia

d Bleeding tendencies

e Impaired immune response

f   Paralytic ileus

g   Improved wound healing

h   Increased gastric motility

i   Persistent pain

4. IDENTIFY THE PROBLEM/ISSUE

Q   Mrs Simpson is currently experiencing a number of problems. From the following list, select three *incorrect* nursing diagnoses.

a   Poor pain tolerance associated with inaccurate use of PCA, evidenced by pallor, tachycardia, hypertension and pain score of 5–8

b   Exacerbation of acute pain related to provision of misinformation about PCA use, evidenced by pain scores of 5–8, pallor, intermittent sleeping overnight, nausea, tachycardia and hypertension

c   Acute post-operative pain related to a low pain threshold evidenced by pain scores of 5–8

d   Post-operative pain related to inappropriate PCA use, evidenced by reluctance to use PCA and incorrect understanding of potential PCA side effects

e   Acute pain related to tissue injury secondary to surgery, evidenced by restlessness, pallor, tachycardia, hypertension and pain score of 5–8

f   Post-operative pain related to inaccurate PCA prescription, evidenced by PCA observations, pain scores of 5–8, intermittent sleeping pattern overnight, nausea, tachycardia and hypertension

g   Risk of addiction related to excessive PCA use

h   Risk of delayed wound healing associated with poor acute pain management

Why is pre-operative patient education about pain management strategies essential?

5. ESTABLISH GOALS

Q1   In regard to Mrs Simpson's pain, your goals should include which of the following? (Select all that apply.)

a   That she reports her pain severity as 0 on a 0 to 10 scale

b   That she reports her pain severity as less than 4 on a 0 to10 scale

c   That her level of pain allows her to take deep breaths and participate in activities of daily living (ADLs) without any discomfort

d   That her level of pain allows her to participate in activities of daily living (ADLs) without too much discomfort

Q2   You are concerned that, by encouraging Mrs Simpson to use her PCA more often, her nausea and vomiting will recur. Which of the following will achieve the goal of managing Mrs Simpson's pain while reducing her nausea and vomiting? (Select the three correct answers.)

a   Anti-emetics should be administered prophylactically.

b   Opioids should be titrated slowly and steadily.

c   The morphine PCA should be discontinued.

d   Anti-emetics should be administered PRN.

e   Simple medications should be administered to reduce the need for opioids and because they have a synergistic effect.

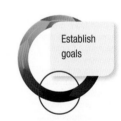

Simple analgesics include paracetamol and NSAIDS. On occasion, adjuvant medications are also prescribed.

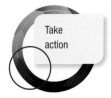

Take action

6. TAKE ACTION

Currently Mrs Simpson's pain is not at a satisfactory level. You decide to undertake a more comprehensive physical assessment and a detailed pain assessment because you want to be sure that her pain is related to the site of surgery only. You are aware that Mrs Simpson's pain could be caused by a number of other problems (e.g. full bladder, internal bleeding).

Q1 Using the PQRST method of pain assessment, categorise each of the questions below with a P, a Q, an R, an S or a T.

P = Provokes

Q = Quality

R = Radiates

S = Severity

T = Time

a   Did it start elsewhere and is now localised to one spot?

b   How severe is the pain on a scale of 1 to 10?

c   Is it sharp, dull, aching, stabbing, burning, crushing?

d   What time did the pain start? How long has it lasted? What is causing the pain?

e   Does anything make it worse?

f   Where is the pain?

g   What does it feel like? Ask your patient to describe the pain.

h   Does the pain radiate or is it just in one place?

i   How does it affect ADLs, sleep, concentration, relationships, mood?

Q2 Put the following list of nursing actions in the order in which you would carry them out.

a   Provide education about the use of the PCA.

b   Make Mrs Simpson more comfortable in the bed.

c   Obtain an order for simple medications such as IV paracetamol.

d   Adjust PCA lockout to five minutes (following medical orders).

e   Check if Mrs Simpson has been ordered any other medications for pain.

f   Obtain an order for oxycontin 10 mg orally BD for when Mrs Simpson is able to tolerate oral fluids.

g   Contact pain team (if available) or medical officer.

> A pain team provides a multi-disciplinary approach to pain management. It consists of health professionals who are specifically trained in the assessment and management of pain. The team is also responsible for staff training, quality control and auditing.

    As a result of your assessment, you determine that Mrs Simpson's pain is most likely related to her surgery. Because there are no contraindications, you reassure Mrs Simpson that it is quite safe for her to use her PCA regularly. The pain team orders paracetamol and changes the PCA lockout to five minutes. Oral oxycodone immediate release is prescribed for when the PCA is removed.

Q3 You are aware that multimodal analgesia has which of the following effects? (Select the three correct responses.)

a   Increases the need for opioids by 20–30%

b   Reduces the risk of over-sedation and respiratory depression from excessive narcotics

c   Increases pain relief, while minimising the potential for side effects due to reduced reliance on a single drug

d   Increases the risk of complications such as constipation, pruritus and post-operative nausea and vomiting

e   Reduces the need for opioids by 20–30%

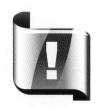

Something to think about ...

The concept of multimodal analgesia involves the use of different classes of analgesics and different sites of analgesic administration to provide better pain relief with reduced analgesic-related side effects. This method of pain management interrupts the pain transmission pathway at numerous points, from the peripheral to the central nervous system. Multimodal analgesia often employs combinations of COX-2 specific inhibitors, local anaesthetics, opioids, non-steroidal anti-inflammatory drugs and paracetamol. Both NSAIDs and paracetamol reduce the total daily requirements of opioids, although paracetamol may be better tolerated in the older post-operative patient (Macintyre et al., 2010).

7. EVALUATE

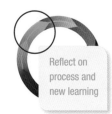

Evaluate outcomes

Q   Once you have given the prescribed IV paracetamol and changed the PCA lockout to five minutes, it is essential to reassess Mrs Simpson's pain to determine the effect of the analgesics. Which of the following are true statements?

   a   Mrs Simpson's report of pain and response to interventions are the best indicators of treatment effectiveness.

   b   Mrs Simpson's behaviour and physiological status are the best indicator of analgesia effectiveness.

   c   Mrs Simpson should be advised to wait until her pain reaches a score of 4 before using the PCA.

   d   Mrs Simpson's pain should be reassessed 30 to 60 minutes later.

   e   Pain assessment using the 0 to 10 scale is the preferred way of determining the effectiveness of analgesics.

   f   Mrs Simpson's pain should be reassessed four hours later.

8. REFLECT

Reflect on process and new learning

In the last stage of the clinical reasoning cycle, it is important to consider what you have learnt and how your learning will inform your future practice. Reflect on your learning from this scenario and consider the following questions:

Q1   What are three of the most important things that you have learnt about acute pain management from this scenario?

Q2   In what way is patient education important to effective pain management?

Q3   Why is a contemporaneous and evidenced-based approach to pain management essential for effective pain management?

Q4   Why is pain management legally and ethically imperative?

Q5   Has this scenario changed your attitude towards pain management? If so, how?

Q6   What actions will you take in your clinical practice as a result of your learning from this scenario?

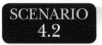

SCENARIO 4.2   Caring for a person experiencing persistent pain

CHANGING THE SCENE

Scenario 4.1 was situated in an acute orthopaedic ward and the focus was on the management of acute pain. Once Mrs Simpson's pain had been effectively addressed, her post-operative recovery progressed without further complications. Seven days following her surgery, Mrs Simpson was transferred to a rehabilitation unit. During the two weeks of rehabilitation and with daily physiotherapy and hydrotherapy, she gradually became more ambulant and independent. Mrs Simpson's home was assessed by an occupational therapist to ensure that it was safe for her to return home. Rails and a shower chair were installed in the bathroom and a rail was installed to help her negotiate the stairs to her back door.

It is now four months since Mrs Simpson returned home. Her family has noticed that she 'just isn't herself'; she is often 'teary' and tells them that she is frightened she might fall again, especially when Alan (her son) is at work. Mrs Simpson confides in her son that, although her hip is getting better, it is the unremitting pain in her lower back that is making her miserable. Alan phones the GP, as he is becoming increasingly concerned about his mother's pain and the impact it is having on her quality of life. The GP informs him that his mother has severe osteoarthritis, a degenerative condition that is common in older people. However, the GP believes that Mrs Simpson is 'not as stoic as some older people' and that she has 'quite a low pain threshold'. He feels that the analgesics he prescribed should be adequate and he suggests to Alan that because his mother is not keeping busy she is spending too much time thinking about her pain. Alan accepts this advice but wants someone to see his mother at home. The GP, somewhat reluctantly, agrees to organise a community nurse to visit.

> The GP's attitude is an example of **fundamental attribution error**, that is, the tendency to be judgmental and to blame patients for their illnesses rather than examine the situational factors that may be responsible (Croskerry, 2003).

Osteoarthritis

Osteoarthritis is one of the most common forms of arthritis. It is a degenerative condition that is caused mainly by accumulated wear of the cartilage. Cartilage cushions the ends of bones where they meet to form a joint. As the cartilage degenerates, the normal function of the joint is disrupted, causing pain. The disease affects mainly the hands, spine and weight-bearing joints such as the hips, knees and ankles. In Australia, osteoarthritis affects more than 1.6 million Australians and is a major cause of disability, psychological distress and poor quality of life. Osteoarthritis most commonly develops between the ages of 45 and 90, and women are more commonly affected than men (Australian Institute of Health and Welfare, 2010a, pp. 186–90). In 2010, osteoarthritis accounted for over $1.2 billion of health expenditure in Australia (Australian Institute of Health and Welfare, 2010b).

> 'Pain is often under-reported by older people, under-recognised by health care professionals and undertreated. Inadequately treated painful conditions in older people may present as mood and behavioural changes, reduced socialisation, impaired mobility, reduced function, and loss of independence' (National Pain Strategy, 2010, p. 16).

Persistent (chronic) pain

One in five Australians has persistent pain, and one in three people over the age of 65 experiences pain every day (National Pain Strategy, 2010). The annual cost of persistent pain in Australia is $34.3 billion. However, application of evidence-based treatments could halve the cost of persistent pain to the Australian economy, a saving of $17 billion per annum (National Pain Strategy, 2010).

1. CONSIDER THE PATIENT SITUATION

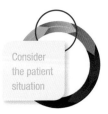

Consider the patient situation

You are the community nurse asked to visit Mrs Simpson to discuss her pain and possible management options. When you arrive, Mrs Simpson offers to make you a cup of tea. You accept, seeing this as an opportunity to begin to assess her functional capacity.

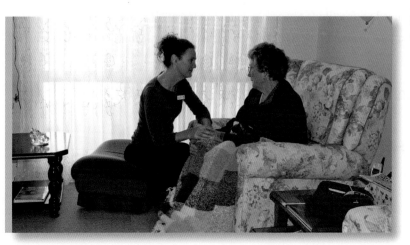

Community nurse visiting Mrs Simpson

2. COLLECT CUES/INFORMATION

(a) Review current information

As you drink your tea, Mrs Simpson begins to share her story with you …

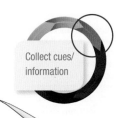

Her mother died at the age of 75 following a fall and a fractured femur; this plays on Mrs Simpson's mind a lot as she is nearly the same age. When Mrs Simpson was first discharged from hospital, she attended hydrotherapy sessions three or four times a week, but it was very expensive and getting in and out of the community transport vehicle was difficult and painful. Her grandchildren used to call in quite often on their way home from work, but lately she has told them not to bother as she is 'fine' and really 'too tired' for visitors in the afternoon. Mrs Simpson sits on her own most of the day with a hot-water bottle on her back. She doesn't sleep well and her pain has made her feel as if life is just too difficult. She wonders how much more she can take. Mrs Simpson's GP prescribed panadeine forte—one to be taken at night—and he advised her to take paracetamol during the day if she 'really needs it'.

The NSQHS Standards emphasise that safe care must be delivered based on a comprehensive care plan and in partnership with patients, carers and families (ACSQHC, 2016).

You observe that Mrs Simpson is pale and drawn in appearance and that she briefly grimaces when she moves in her chair. Her responses to your questions are given quietly and with little facial expression.

(b) Gather new information

You decide to assess Mrs Simpson's pain.

Q1 What are the four most accurate methods of assessing Mrs Simpson's pain in this situation?

a Asking Mrs Simpson to describe and locate her pain

b Observing Mrs Simpson's behaviours and facial expressions

c Asking Mrs Simpson to tell you what provokes her pain and makes it feel better

d Asking Mrs Simpson to score her pain using a numerical rating scale

e Using a validated assessment tool such as the Brief Pain Inventory (see p. 63)

f Taking Mrs Simpson's vital signs

g Reviewing reports from the physiotherapist and occupational therapist about Mrs Simpson's functional capacity

Intensity rating scales alone are not as useful in the person with persistent pain as scales which measure both intensity and the amount of interference to everyday activities that the pain causes.

Q2 Persistent pain often results in which five of the following?

a Grimacing on movement

b Fatigue

c Laughing

d Sleep deprivation

e Listlessness

f Restlessness

g Depression

h Irritability

i Pain score of 7 to 8 out of 10

(c) Recall knowledge

QUICK QUIZ!

To ensure that you have a good understanding of the key concepts related to persistent pain, test yourself with the following questions.

Q1 Persistent pain is pain that lasts longer than:

a 12 months

b 2 years

c 1 month

d 3 months

Q2   Label the following 'true' or 'false':

a   Persistent pain always has an identifiable cause.

b   Persistent pain often occurs in the absence of identifiable tissue injury.

c   Persistent pain is more prevalent in men than women.

d   Persistent pain rarely occurs in young people.

e   The majority of people with persistent pain remain in full-time employment.

Q3   Of the people who experience persistent pain:

a   33% cannot identify an event that caused their pain

b   Most will be able to recall the event that led to their pain

c   10% cannot identify an event that caused their pain

d   All will be able to recall the event that led to their pain

Q4   Identify the seven main causes of persistent pain from the list below.

a   Lower back pain

b   Neurological conditions

c   Headache and migraines

d   Arthritis

e   Mental illness

f   Cancer

g   Gastrointestinal conditions

h   Post-surgical pain

j   Work-related accidents

Q5   Physical activity:

a   Is harmful for people with pain

b   Should be avoided if someone has persistent pain

c   Must be undertaken only if weight loss is required

d   Should be encouraged but be undertaken within a person's physical limits

Q6   Complete the following table.

	Acute pain	Persistent pain
Diagnosis	Usually clear	
Duration		
Pain descriptors	Sharp, stabbing	

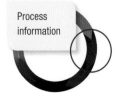

3. PROCESS INFORMATION

(a) Interpret

The next step of the clinical reasoning cycle is to interpret the data (cues) that you have collected by careful analysis, while at the same time applying your knowledge about persistent pain.

Review Mrs Simpson's Brief Pain Inventory:

Completed form of the Brief Pain Inventory

STUDY ID #:_ _ _ _ _ _ _ _ _   HOSPITAL #: _ _ _ _ _ _ _ _ _

DO NOT WRITE ABOVE THIS LINE

The Modified Brief Pain Inventory

Date:_ _ _ _ / _ _ _ _ / _ _ _ _   Time:_ _ _ _ _ _ _

Name: _ _ _ _ _ _ _ _ _ _ _ _ _ _ _ _ _   _ _ _ _ _ _ _ _ _ _ _ _ _ _   _ _ _ _ _ _ _ _ _ _ _ _ _ _
　　　　　　　　　Simpson　　　　　　　　　　　　　*Grace*
　　　　　　　　　　Last　　　　　　　　　　　　　　First　　　　　　　　　　Middle Initial

1. Throughout our lives, most of us have had minor aches and pains from time to time. Have you had pain, other than these everyday kinds of pain, today?

    　　　　　　　1. (Yes)　　　　　　2.　No

2. Please rate your pain by circling the one number that best describes your pain *at its worst* in the past 24 hours:

    0　　1　　2　　3　　4　　5　　6　　7　　(8)　　9　　10
    　　No　　　　　　　　　　　　　　　　　　　　　Worst pain
    　　pain　　　　　　　　　　　　　　　　　　　　possible

3. Please rate your pain by circling the one number that best describes your pain *at its least* in the past 24 hours:

    0　　1　　2　　3　　(4)　　5　　6　　7　　8　　9　　10
    　　No　　　　　　　　　　　　　　　　　　　　　Worst pain
    　　pain　　　　　　　　　　　　　　　　　　　　possible

4. Please rate your pain by circling the one number that best describes your pain *on average*:

    0　　1　　2　　3　　4　　5　　(6)　　7　　8　　9　　10
    　　No　　　　　　　　　　　　　　　　　　　　　Worst pain
    　　pain　　　　　　　　　　　　　　　　　　　　possible

5. Please rate your pain by circling the one number that best describes your pain *right now*:

    0　　1　　2　　3　　4　　5　　(6)　　7　　8　　9　　10
    　　No　　　　　　　　　　　　　　　　　　　　　Worst pain
    　　pain　　　　　　　　　　　　　　　　　　　　possible

6. What treatments or medications are you receiving for your pain?

    Panadeine forte and panadol

7. In the past 24 hours, how much relief have pain treatments or medications provided?

    0%　　(10)　　20　　30　　40　　50　　60　　70　　80　　90　　100%
    No　　　　　　　　　　　　　　　　　　　　　　　　　　　Complete
    relief　　　　　　　　　　　　　　　　　　　　　　　　　relief

8. On the diagram, shade the area where you feel pain. Put an X on the area that hurts the most.

Page 1 of 2

STUDY ID #:_ _ _ _ _ _ _ _ _ _   HOSPITAL #: _ _ _ _ _ _ _ _ _ _

DO NOT WRITE ABOVE THIS LINE

Date:_ _ _ _ / _ _ _ _ / _ _ _ _   Time:_ _ _ _ _ _

Name: _ _ _ _ _ _ _ _ _ _ *Simpson* _ _ _ _ _ _   _ _ _ _ _ _ _ _ *Grace* _ _ _ _ _ _ _ _   _ _ _ _ _ _ _ _ _ _ _ _ _ _
                               Last   First   Middle Initial

9.   Circle the one number that describes how, during the past 24 hours, pain has interfered with your:

A.   *General activity*

0   1   2   3   4   5   6   ⑦   8   9   10
Does not   Completely
interfere   interferes

B.   *Mood*

0   1   2   3   4   ⑤   6   7   8   9   10
Does not   Completely
interfere   interferes

C.   *Walking ability*

0   1   2   3   4   5   6   7   ⑧   9   10
Does not   Completely
interfere   interferes

D.   *Relations with other people*

0   1   2   3   ④   5   6   7   8   9   10
Does not   Completely
interfere   interferes

E.   *Sleep*

0   1   2   3   4   ⑤   6   7   8   9   10
Does not   Completely
interfere   interferes

F.   *Enjoyment of life*

0   1   2   3   4   5   6   ⑦   8   9   10
Does not   Completely
interfere   interferes

Measures:

Pain severity (BPI): 6/10 (add first four numbers and divide by 4)
Pain interference (BPI): 6/10 (add last six numbers together and divide by six)

Page 2 of 2

The Brief Pain Inventory (BPI) was developed to assess pain in people with cancer but it is now widely used for people with all types of persistent pain, including osteoarthritis (Williams, Smith & Fehnel, 2006). It is a self-administered test which looks at the severity of a person's pain (averaging the worst and least pain with the current pain) and the extent to which the pain interferes with a person's life (examining how pain influences walking, mood, sleep, the ability to concentrate and the person's relationship with others).

It is important to remember that pain assessment tools do not always capture fluctuations in pain, like those that can occur in osteoarthritis. A comprehensive pain history should be taken as well.

Q1 With reference to Mrs Simpson's Brief Pain Inventory, label the following 'true' or 'false'.

a Mrs Simpson's pain severity score is 3.

b Mrs Simpson's pain interference score is 6.

c Mrs Simpson's analgesics have little impact on her level of pain.

d Mrs Simpson's pain ranges from 2 to 9.

Q2 On the body map on the Brief Pain Inventory, Mrs Simpson indicated the location of her pain. How would you report this pain?

a As localised

b As radiating

c As referred

(b) Discriminate and (c) Relate

Q With reference to Mrs Simpson's Brief Pain Inventory results, generally Mrs Simpson's pain interferes most with which of the following?

a Walking

b Housework

c Relationships

d Enjoyment of life

e Sleep

f Mood

g General activity

> It is generally accepted that people in persistent pain will have higher mood interference scores than the general population; however, older people do not always report their mood accurately.

(d) Infer

Q With reference to Mrs Simpson's Brief Pain Inventory results, what is your interpretation of the impact of Mrs Simpson's pain on her quality of life (QOL)?

a Pain is having a slight impact on Mrs Simpson's QOL.

b Pain is having a moderate impact on Mrs Simpson's QOL.

c Pain is having a severe impact on Mrs Simpson's QOL.

(e) Match

Have you ever experienced persistent pain or do you know someone who has? Reflect on the physical and psychosocial impact of that pain and how it influenced the person's (or your) quality of life.

(f) Predict

What are the potential consequences for Mrs Simpson if her pain were to be dismissed, ignored or inadequately managed.

Something to think about …

Ongoing pain can be difficult to live with and older people suffer more complications associated with under-managed pain. Sadly, health professionals too often accept pain in the older person as an inevitable consequence of ageing, and fail to take into account the impact of pain on the person's physical and emotional wellbeing.

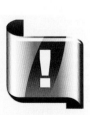

Q   From the list below, identify seven issues associated with poorly managed persistent pain.

a   Social isolation

b   Depression

c   Pneumonia

d   Weight loss

e   Dementia

f   Loss of muscle strength

g   Increased sensitivity to light

h   Suicidal thoughts

i   Improved physical fitness

4. IDENTIFY THE PROBLEM/ISSUE

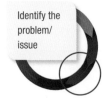

Identify the problem/issue

Q   From the information you have gathered and interpreted about Mrs Simpson's pain, complete the nursing diagnoses below.

a   Persistent pain related to osteoarthritis of _____, as evidenced by Mrs Simpson's pain severity report of _____.

b   Disruption of social and family relationships related to persistent pain, evidenced by Mrs Simpson's pain interference score of _____.

c   Persistent pain related to osteoarthritis, evidenced by consistent pain for _____ months, grimacing, _____, _____ and _____.

5. ESTABLISH GOALS

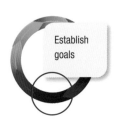

Establish goals

Even though there may not be a 'cure' for persistent pain, there are many ways to help manage the pain and improve Mrs Simpson's quality of life. The primary goal of persistent pain management is to reduce any disability caused by the pain; to achieve or maintain fitness, movement and function; and for Mrs Simpson to be able to continue with normal everyday activities.

In regards to Mrs Simpson's pain, the management goals should be SMART:

Specific

Measureable

Achievable

Realistic

Timely

It is important to ask Mrs Simpson to begin by identifying three goals, one short-term (achievable within two weeks), one medium-term (achievable within two months) and one long-term (achievable within six months). The goals need to be specific and realistic, and most importantly they must be goals of Mrs Simpson's, something she herself wants to achieve. It is best to link goals, so that those that are completed in the short term can contribute to the realisation of the longer-term goals. The goals may not initially have a pain focus; for example, Mrs Simpson enjoys learning about her genealogy, but she has not been able to document her family tree as she finds sitting and concentrating difficult because of her pain. Therefore, the plan of care should provide strategies that will help Mrs Simpson achieve this goal.

People with persistent pain require a structured approach and a pain management plan that takes into account the areas mentioned above. Mrs Simpson's plan is best developed by her with your assistance; that way it will be more personally meaningful. The plan should identify the actions to be taken by Mrs Simpson to achieve her goals and the actions required of healthcare professionals to support her to do so.

Q   The following plan provides examples of possible goals for Mrs Simpson. Complete the table by adding one more short-, medium- and long-term goal for Mrs Simpson. (*Note*: The 'actions' columns will be completed later in the scenario.)

Pain Management Plan for Mrs Grace Simpson

Goal	Review date	Mrs Simpson's actions	HCP actions
Short term 1. Sitting for up to five minutes without flaring pain 2. Hanging out the washing without flaring pain	2 weeks		
Medium term 1. Sitting for up to 20 minutes without flaring pain 2. Joining local seniors Tai Chi club and attending once a week 3.	2 months		
Long term 1. Sitting for up to 40 minutes without flaring pain 2. Attending the local library's genealogy classes 3.	6 months		

6. TAKE ACTION

Approaches to persistent (chronic) pain management

Our knowledge of the mechanism of pain, how it affects the body and how to prevent and manage it, has developed greatly in the past 30 years. We now understand that pain, no matter what type, is produced in the brain. Acute pain lasting for less than three months is generally considered to be associated with acute tissue damage or injury. After three months, tissue injury has usually healed and therefore pain that persists beyond this point is less about tissue or structural damage and more about sensitivity in the nervous system. Persistent or chronic pain is therefore more complex to treat and requires a different management approach from that of acute pain.

Persistent pain is best addressed by taking a broad approach and reviewing all the things that can affect the nervous system and may be contributing to a person's pain. Passive approaches to treatment are less effective than active approaches for people in persistent pain.

Medical management

Medication is very useful in the management of acute pain but may have a limited role in the ongoing management of persistent pain. Medications that allow the person to become active and maintain function are initially useful but should be tapered and ceased. Other medical interventions, such as

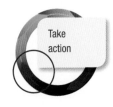

Take action

Watch this TED talk on 'The mystery of chronic pain': <www.ted.com/talks/elliot_krane_the_mystery_of_chronic_pain?utm_source=tedcomshare&utm_medium=referral&utm_campaign=tedspread>.

> The understanding of the processes behind the development of persistent pain has evolved over the past 30 years and there is now a greater emphasis on the use and benefits of pre-emptive pain management.

surgery, may not be useful in the treatment of persistent pain, and surgeons will take into consideration the underlying biological issues as well as broader approaches to persistent pain.

Thoughts and emotions

Ongoing pain can cause stress, anxiety and depression. It is important to remember that these emotions will, in turn, affect the person's pain and can in some circumstances make the pain worse. Both pain and these thoughts and emotions are produced in the brain, so looking at ways to reduce stress and manage anxiety and depression can wind down the nervous system and reduce pain.

Diet and lifestyle

Lifestyle can have a positive or negative effect on the nervous system. Diet and lifestyle may contribute to nervous system wind-up and contribute to pain. Smoking, alcohol, fatty foods and low levels of activity create physical ill-health and affect the nervous system.

The person's story

There is often a deeper meaning to a person's ongoing pain and it is worthwhile allowing them to explore this if they wish. By looking at all the things that were happening in their lives when the pain started, such as their relationships, life circumstances and emotional wellbeing, a person may be able to identify a deeper meaning to their pain, and this awareness may be included in their treatment approach. It is important to remember that a person should be *invited* to examine their personal story and not be forced to do so.

Activity

For many people in pain, physical activity is reduced or decreased and function can be lost. Activity is physically, mentally and emotionally therapeutic. It is important for people with persistent pain to undertake activity at a sensible pace and within their comfort levels without fear and without their brain using pain to stop them. Over time, people with persistent pain will gradually improve function and fitness and be able to achieve much more with their bodies.

Interprofessional collaboration

The management of persistent pain is a complex process and often includes a layered approach, involving a number of healthcare professionals. Most pain centres have pain specialists, psychologists, nurses and physiotherapists, while some also include dieticians, occupational therapists, social workers, and complementary and alternative therapy practitioners. All of these healthcare professionals work together to assess the person's needs and help them develop a realistic management plan. It is also important to consider both pharmacological and non-pharmacological approaches.

Pharmacological management of persistent pain

Mrs Simpson is currently taking panadeine forte 1 nocte and paracetamol PRN during the day. After consultation with Mrs Simpson's GP and the pain service, this is changed to paracetamol six-hourly and oxycodone in small doses for breakthrough pain. The aim of these medications is to enable Mrs Simpson to undertake activities of daily living and to improve her ability to undertake physical activity.

The pain service advises that the oxycodone should be trialled for a week to determine its effectiveness and potential side effects. They recommend that this medication should not be used as a long-term management strategy. Mrs Simpson is asked to maintain a pain diary (see p. 70). This will enable the community nurse, the pain service and Mrs Simpson's GP to track her progress and the effectiveness of the medications prescribed.

The pain service also advises Mrs Simpson to take glucosamine, as research shows that it stops the progression of osteoarthritis, decreases pain and improves function (Towheed et al., 2005).

However, they advise that it takes time to take effect and must be taken daily over a two-week period at least.

It is also recommended that Mrs Simpson take omega 3, as it has anti-inflammatory properties and may improve mood and general wellbeing (Goldberg & Katz, 2007). Again this must be taken daily and for a period of at least two weeks before any benefits become obvious. The best source of omega 3 is a diet high in large oily fish, such as salmon, but dietary supplements may also be used.

Non-pharmacological management of persistent pain

During her admission in the rehabilitation unit, Mrs Simpson was reviewed by a physiotherapist who identified that she had poor posture and poor abdominal tone; her sitting tolerance was less than three minutes and her walking tolerance was less than 10 metres.

You refer Mrs Simpson to the physiotherapist from the pain service and he teaches Mrs Simpson stretching and strengthening exercises for her lower limbs, abdomen and back. Mrs Simpson is given a daily program and her progress will be reviewed each week. The physiotherapist suggests that Mrs Simpson consider Tai Chi classes, as they improve strength and flexibility and also allow older people to remain socially connected. Tai Chi has been shown to have a positive effect on a person's muscle strength and may improve balance, which has been a major concern for Mrs Simpson (Logghe et al., 2010). Improving her balance will also decrease Mrs Simpson's fear of falling.

Mrs Simpson is also referred to the psychologist who works with the pain service so that she has the opportunity to explore some of the issues surrounding her pain. It is important to reinforce that her pain is not 'in her head' but 'real' and causing her distress. This distress in turn can exacerbate her pain. Providing Mrs Simpson with an opportunity to learn techniques to manage stress, anxiety and low mood may be beneficial for her pain management.

Q   Now go back to the pain management plan and complete the two 'actions' columns (that of Mrs Simpson and that of the healthcare professionals).

7. EVALUATE

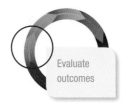

Evaluate outcomes

Evaluation of the effectiveness of the pain management plan may take up to six weeks. The plan will need regular review and may need revision. Remember that, just as the plan was developed in collaboration with Mrs Simpson, its effectiveness will also be determined by her.

Maintaining a pain diary will allow Mrs Simpson to take control of her management plan and allow health professionals to review the impact of the strategies that are implemented.

Evaluation of the effectiveness of the medication regime includes assessing the benefits and side effects, including the impact on general wellbeing. The role of the community nurse is to review the pain diary and to begin to taper and cease opioids when Mrs Simpson's pain score reaches less than 4 out of 10. The Brief Pain Inventory should be used to evaluate changes in pain severity and pain interference. Seeking input from other members of the pain service will also be important in the evaluation of the pain management plan.

It is now four weeks since your initial visit to Mrs Simpson. Review Mrs Simpson's pain diary and evaluate the effectiveness of her current pain management plan and related strategies.

Grace Simpson

Five-Day Medication and Pain Diary—Grace Simpson

Please fill this diary in over five consecutive days. Include a pain score, aids used, prescribed and over-the-counter drugs, and other substances taken (e.g. alcohol and caffeinated drinks). Note any side effects.

Rate your pain on a score of 0 to 10

0   1   2   3   4   5   6   7   8   9   10
No pain   Worst pain imaginable

Date	Time	Pain score before	Substance/ aid	Notes/observations
13/9	10 am	6	oxycodone	I began to feel better by 1 pm
13/9	3 pm	5	paracetamol	Pain score 3 by 4.30 pm
13/9	9 pm	6	oxycodone	Couldn't sleep. Still awake at 11.30 pm
14/9	7 am	6	oxycodone	Very stiff and sore
14/9	10 am	5	stretches	Less stiff but still sore
	1 pm	3		
	5 pm	6	paracetamol	Keep forgetting to take
	8 pm	7	oxycodone	Overdid it today; very sore
15/9	7 am	5	paracetamol	
	10 am	5	stretches	Less stiff but still in a little pain
	12 pm	4	paracetamol	Pain score 3 by 2 pm
	6 pm	6	paracetamol and oxycodone	Sat in chair all afternoon and now more pain
	8 pm	3		Feeling better
	9 pm	2	paracetamol and oxycodone	

Q1 Mrs Simpson's pain diary indicates that:

  a Mrs Simpson is not taking her medications as instructed

  b Mrs Simpson has increased her physical activity

  c Mrs Simpson completed her stretches on 13/9 and 14/9

  d Mrs Simpson has reached all her short-term goals

Q2 Mrs Simpson's pain diary indicates that:

  a Paracetamol is ineffective

  b Caffeine exacerbates Mrs Simpson's pain

  c Oxycodone has a negative impact on Mrs Simpson's pain score

  d Stretching reduces Mrs Simpson's pain score

8. REFLECT

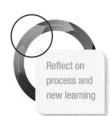

Reflect on process and new learning

In the last stage of the clinical reasoning cycle, it is important to consider what you have learnt and how your learning will inform your future practice. Reflect on your learning from this scenario and consider the following questions:

Q1 What are three of the most important things that you have learnt about persistent pain management from this scenario?

Q2 In what way is therapeutic communication and person-centred care important for effective assessment of persistent pain?

Q3 In what way is interprofessional communication and teamwork important for effective management of persistent pain?

Q4 What actions will you take in your clinical practice as a result of your learning from this scenario?

EPILOGUE

The comprehensive and interprofessional approach taken to address Mrs Simpson's persistent pain resulted in a gradual but consistent improvement. Within two months, she had resumed her genealogy classes and was once again enjoying spending time with her grandchildren. Although Mrs Simpson still had some pain on and off during the day, her sleep pattern improved considerably. Sadly, a year later when Alan took his mother her morning cup of tea, he was shocked to discover that she had died in her sleep. The autopsy revealed a massive stroke. When going through her papers, Alan discovered this poem written by his mother in the last weeks of her life. He read it at her funeral:

A new day wakening; the glow of sunrise

Sparking on cobwebs strung with dewdrops

Faint, wafting perfumes as multi-hued flowers unfurl

Songbirds display their talents

For those who would listen

Trees with branches entwined

Swaying to the caress of a gentle breeze

The hours march on gathering along their way

The laughter of children

Friendly words, helping hands, passing smiles

Minutes filled with useful, caring endeavours

Memories of loves ones, happy times, proud moments

A diversity of music, books, art

Wonderment at the beauty of nature

So that at days end we may

Pull up the coverlet of sleep

And rest finally and peacefully in God's arms.

FURTHER READING

International Association for the Study of Pain: <www.iasp-pain.org>.

REFERENCES

Australian Commission on Safety and Quality in Health Care (ACSQHC). (2016). *National Safety and Quality Health Service Standards Version 2.* Draft, Sydney, Australia.

Australian Institute of Health and Welfare (AIHW). (2016). *Falls in Older People.* Accessed December 2016 at <www.aihw.gov.au/injury/falls/>.

Australian Institute of Health and Welfare (AIHW). (2014). *Estimating the Prevalence of Osteoporosis.* Cat. No. PHE 178. Canberra: AIHW. Accessed December 2016 at <www.aihw.gov.au/WorkArea/DownloadAsset.aspx?id=60129548481>.

Australian Institute of Health and Welfare (AIHW). (2011). *Injury Prevention and Control.* Accessed December 2016 at <www.aihw.gov.au/injury-prevention-and-control-health-priority-area/>.

Australian Institute of Health and Welfare (AIHW). (2010a). *Australia's Health 2010: In Brief.* Cat. No. AUS 126. Canberra: AIHW. Accessed December 2016 at <www.aihw.gov.au/publication-detail/?id=6442468375>.

Australian Institute of Health and Welfare (AIHW). (2010b). *A Snapshot of Arthritis in Australia 2010.* Arthritis Series No. 13. Cat. No. PHE 126. Canberra: AIHW. Accessed December 2016 at <www.aihw.gov.au/publication-detail/?id=6442468397&libID=6442468395>.

Bliuc, D., Nguyen, N., Nguyen, T., Eisman, J. & Center, J. (2013). Compound risk of high mortality following osteoporotic fracture and refracture in elderly women and men. *Journal of Bone and Mineral Research, 28*(11), 2317–24.

Croskerry, P. (2003). The importance of cognitive errors in diagnosis and strategies to minimize them. *Academic Medicine, 78*(8), 1–6.

Goldberg, R. J. & Katz, J. (2007). A meta-analysis of the analgesic effects of omega 3 polyunsaturated fatty acid supplementation for inflammatory joint pain. *Pain, 129*(1–2), 210–23.

Iedema, R. (2014). Clinical handover. In T. Levett-Jones (Ed.), *Critical Conversations for Patient Safety: An Essential Guide for Health Professionals.* Sydney: Pearson.

Logghe, I., Verhagen, A., Rademaker, A., Bierma-Zeinstra, S., van Rossum, E., Faber, M. & Koes, B. (2010). The effects of Tai Chi on fall prevention, fear of falling and balance in older people: A meta-analysis. *Preventative Medicine, 51*(3–4), 222–27.

Macintyre, P., Schug, S., Scott, D., Visser, E. & Walker, S. (APM:SE Working Group of the Australian and New Zealand College of Anaesthetists and Faculty of Pain Medicine). (2010). *Acute Pain Management: Scientific Evidence* (3rd edn). Melbourne: ANZCA & FPM. Accessed December 2016 at <www.anzca.edu.au/resources/college-publications/Acute%20Pain%20Management/books-and-publications/Acute%20pain%20management%20-%20scientific%20evidence%20-%20third%20edition.pdf>.

McCaffery, M., Rolling Ferrell, B. & Paseo, C. (2000). Nurses' personal opinions about patients' pain and their effect on recorded assessments and titration of opioid doses. *Pain Management Nursing, 1*(3), 79–87.

National Pain Strategy. (2010). Australian and New Zealand College of Anaesthetists. Accessed March 2017 at <www.painaustralia.org.au/images/pain_australia/NPS/National%20Pain%20Strategy%202011.pdf>.

Nursing and Midwifery Board of Australia (NMBA). (2016). *Registered Nurse Standards for Practice.* Retrieved from <www.nursingmidwiferyboard.gov.au/Codes-Guidelines-Statements/Professional-standards.aspx>.

Nursing and Midwifery Board of Australia (NMBA). (2008). *Code of Ethics.* Accessed December 2016 at <www.nursingmidwiferyboard.gov.au/Codes-Guidelines-Statements/Professional-standards.aspx>.

Patak, L., Tait, A., Mirafzali, L., Morris, M., Dasgupta, S. & Brummett, C. (2013). Patient perspectives of patient-controlled analgesia (PCA) and methods for improving pain control and patient satisfaction. *American Society of Regional Anesthesia and Pain Medicine, 38*(4), 326–33. doi: 10.1097/AAP.0b013e318295fd50

Towheed, T., Maxwell, L., Anastassiades, T., Shea, B., Houpt, J., Welch, V., ... Wells, G. (2005). Glucosamine therapy for treating osteoarthritis. *Cochrane Database of Systematic Reviews,* (2), CD002946. Accessed December 2016 at <www.thecochranelibrary.org>.

Watts, J., Abimanyi-Ochom, J. & Sanders, K. (2013). *Osteoporosis Costing All Australians: A New Burden of Disease Analysis 2012 to 2022.* Sydney: Osteoporosis Australia.

Williams, V., Smith, M. & Fehnel, S. (2006). The validity and utility of the BPI interference measures for evaluating the impact of osteoarthritic pain. *Journal of Pain Symptom Management, 31,* 48–57.

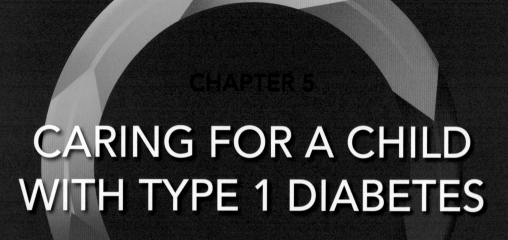

CHAPTER 5

CARING FOR A CHILD WITH TYPE 1 DIABETES

LORETTO QUINNEY, KERRY REID-SEARL, VERONICA MILLS AND BREE WALKER

LEARNING OUTCOMES

Completion of the activities in this chapter will enable you to:

- explain why an understanding of diabetes mellitus is essential to competent practice (**recall** and **application**)
- outline the clinical manifestations of hypoglycaemia and diabetic ketoacidosis (DKA) that guide the collection and interpretation of appropriate cues (**gather**, **review**, **interpret**, **discriminate**, **relate** and **infer**)
- identify risk factors for a child with type 1 diabetes (**match** and **predict**)
- review the clinical information to identify the main nursing diagnoses for a child with type 1 diabetes who experiences hypoglycaemia and DKA (**synthesise**)
- describe the priorities of care for a child experiencing hypoglycaemia and DKA (**goal setting** and **taking action**)
- identify clinical indicators for determining the effectiveness of nursing actions taken to manage hypoglycaemia or DKA (**evaluate**)
- apply what you have learnt to new situations (**reflection** and **translation**).

INTRODUCTION

This chapter focuses on the care of a child who has type 1 diabetes mellitus. You will follow the journey of Haley Milangu, a 9-year-old girl, from her initial diagnosis to discharge, and then readmission with a serious and life-threatening metabolic complication of diabetes.

Children are not 'little adults'; they have unique needs and respond in individual ways to the care provided. Thus, the care of the acutely ill child requires vigilance, commitment and well-developed clinical reasoning skills in order to identify and manage clinical deterioration.

When caring for a child, nurses must consider the societal factors that impact on the child and their family, as well as the related psychosocial factors. This is referred to as 'family-centred care'; it is an approach that acknowledges that the family is the constant in the child's life and the expert on his or her needs.

This chapter also emphasises the importance of cultural safety to the provision of quality care and addresses some of the misconceptions about Aboriginal peoples. Culturally safe nursing care means making decisions based on principles of social justice and includes an acceptance of human diversity (Douglas et al., 2014).

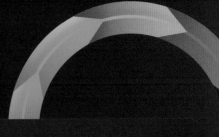

KEY CONCEPTS

diabetes
hypoglycaemia
hyperglycaemia
diabetic ketoacidosis
cultural safety
family-centred care

SUGGESTED READINGS

P. LeMone, K. Burke, G. Bauldoff, P. Gubrud-Howe, T. Levett-Jones, T. Dwyer . . . D. Raymond (Eds). (2017). *Medical–Surgical Nursing: Critical Thinking in Person-Centred Care* (3rd edn). Melbourne: Pearson. Chapter 19: Nursing care of people with diabetes mellitus

J. Mould, C. Rudd, & A. Wilkinson. (2014). Communicating with children and families. In T. Levett-Jones (Ed.), *Critical Conversations for Patient Safety: An Essential Guide for Health Professionals*. Sydney: Pearson.

A. Siafarikas & S. O'Connell. (2010). Type 1 diabetes in children: Emergency management. *Australian Family Physician, 39*(5), 290–93. Accessed December 2016 at <http://search.proquest.com/docview/216293325?accountid=8194>.

Caring for a child diagnosed with type 1 diabetes

SETTING THE SCENE

Haley Milangu is a 9-year-old girl who lives with her parents, Jenny and Bob, her two brothers, Jim and Charlie, and her grandmother, Doris. They live on a cattle property 60 kilometres from Mepunda in central Queensland, which is a five-hour drive from the nearest regional hospital. Healthcare is provided by a nurse practitioner (NP) and remote area nurses (RANs) at the community health centre, with fortnightly visits from a GP.

Over the last month, Jenny has noticed that Haley has become increasingly unwell, and is constantly thirsty and often hungry. She has been passing urine frequently and getting up to the toilet two or three times a night. More recently, Haley has had episodes of abdominal pain and her mother has noticed she has lost weight. Haley has a close network of friends at school and the highlight of her week was playing soccer in her little league team, although lately she has lost interest in physical activities and seems to be tired much of the time.

With her level of concern increasing, Jenny takes Haley to the community health centre. After obtaining the history from Jenny, the NP performs a blood glucose level (BGL) test and a urinalysis. Haley's BGL is 20 mmol/L and her urinalysis shows large amounts of glucose and a trace of ketones. The NP contacts the paediatrician at the regional hospital and arranges for Haley to be transported by air and admitted to the hospital, accompanied by her mother.

The epidemiology of type 1 diabetes mellitus

> Access the Diabetes Australia website to learn more about the incidence of diabetes in Australia: <www.diabetesaustralia.com.au/en/Understanding-Diabetes/Diabetes-in-Australia/>.

Diabetes is the world's fastest growing chronic disease, with 246 million people currently affected (Diabetes Australia, 2017). Of these, 10 to 15 per cent of people have type 1 diabetes, with the majority having type 2. Although type 1 diabetes can occur at any age, it is more common in children and young people. Australia has one of the highest incidences of type 1 diabetes with approximately 1000 children 14 years and under diagnosed every year (Australian Institute of Health and Welfare, 2014). In the past, type 2 diabetes was unusual in children, but it is becoming more common in this age group as a result of increased obesity and lack of exercise (Australian Bureau of Statistics, 2011). Despite ongoing awareness, the incidence of both type 1 and type 2 diabetes continues to rise and nearly a million Australians have been diagnosed with diabetes since 2011 (Parrish, 2017).

The aetiology and pathogenesis of type 1 diabetes

> For more information about the aetiology, pathogenesis and management of diabetes, access <http://diabetesnsw.com.au/diabetes-nsw-launches-online-resource-for-schools/>.

There have been no modifiable risk factors for type 1 diabetes identified as yet; however, it is thought that a combination of environmental and genetic factors are responsible (Diabetes Australia, 2017). At this stage, there is no cure or way of preventing type 1 diabetes.

The disease processes of type 1 and type 2 diabetes have some similarities but also important differences. Refer to the table below which compares the key factors that differentiate these diseases.

	Type 1 diabetes	Type 2 diabetes
Origin of diagnosis	Autoimmune disease related to insulin deficiency; inconclusive direct causes but related to genetic, environmental and idiopathic factors	Metabolic disease related to insulin resistance, heredity factors, obesity (central adipose), physical inactivity and metabolic syndrome
Early signs	Blood sugar level (finger prick) usually >12 mmol/L, weight loss, polydipsia, polyuria, polyphagia, glycosuria, blurred vision and tiredness	Blood sugar level (finger prick) usually >12 mmol/L, tiredness, malaise, polyuria (especially at night), polydipsia, weight loss/gain, blurred vision and frequent slow-healing infections; sometimes asymptomatic

	Type 1 diabetes	Type 2 diabetes
Body weight	Mostly normal or thin	Mostly overweight or obese
Usual age at onset	Usually children/teens/young adults: 5–25 years (majority 5–14 years)	Usually adults >40 years (Although uncommon in children, those diagnosed with type 2 diabetes—usually around puberty—generally have a family history of diabetes, are overweight and are physically inactive.)
Onset	Rapid (days to weeks); often acute presentation with weight loss and ketoacidosis	Slow (1–5 years); many people are not diagnosed for up to 20 years or more
Ketones	High at diagnosis, then absent after insulin therapy starts	Usually negative but can be positive in pregnancy or if insulin is deficient
Treatment	Always requires insulin to sustain life (subcutaneous injection usually via insulin pens or insulin pumps); requires dietary management, regular BGL monitoring and daily exercise	Usually requires oral hypoglycaemic medications, dietary management, regular BGL monitoring, daily exercise and weight loss; SCI insulin may be required some time after onset
Glucose channel/ receptors	Insulin opens glucose receptors and helps absorb glucose into cells to be utilised by the body for energy production. (This is impeded when the endogenous production of insulin ceases.)	People with T2D are unable to open glucose receptors and absorb glucose; therefore, glucose cannot be utilised for energy production. Consequently, high levels of glucose stay in the blood stream.
Cure	None (Pancreatic transplant and closed loop pump therapy will potentially decrease the mundane daily management demands.)	There is no cure for type 2 diabetes, although extreme weight loss (usually via gastric surgery) can result in 'remission'. Physical exercise, maintaining a healthy weight and dietary management are always required.

Sources: Adapted from <www.diabetesaustralia.com.au/Understanding-Diabetes/What-is-Diabetes/Type-1-Diabetes/> and <www.diabetesaustralia.com.au/Understanding-Diabetes/What-is-Diabetes/Type-2-Diabetes/>.

Type 1 diabetes is an autoimmune disease that occurs when there is a gradual destruction of the insulin-producing beta cells in the islets of Langerhans in the pancreas. This results in a gradual and progressive decline in the production of insulin needed to assist the transport of glucose from the blood into the cells where it is utilised as energy. Blood glucose levels then rise and, because there is a lack of glucose available for cellular metabolism, the body uses fat stores as an alternative. A by-product of fat oxidation by the liver is the formation of ketone bodies, resulting in ketonaemia and ketonuria (Craig et al., 2014). The presence of ketones alters the acid–base balance and the person develops metabolic acidosis. Additionally, the presence of high levels of glucose shifts the osmolarity of the blood, and the kidneys increase urine output as a consequence. Thus, the person with type 1 diabetes usually presents with a combination of the following signs and symptoms: polydipsia (excessive thirst), polyuria (excessive urination), polyphagia (excessive hunger), dehydration, lethargy, tiredness, unexplained weight loss, delayed wound healing, pruritus, skin infections, blurred vision, mood swings, headaches, dizziness and leg cramps. Treatment consists of replacing the body's insulin with a regime of injected insulin (Diabetes Australia, 2017).

Admission to the Emergency Department

At 1200 hours, Haley arrives at the hospital's Emergency Department (ED) where she is assessed by nursing staff and the paediatrician. Her initial assessment includes vital signs, blood glucose and ketone levels, capillary refill, skin turgor, weight, height, level of consciousness and pain score. Dr James, the paediatrician, assesses Haley and organises for her transfer to the Paediatric Unit at 1500 hours. You are the paediatric nurse who will be responsible for Haley's care. You receive the following handover from the ED nurse.

Handover report

I	Identify	*My name is Tyler Jones and I am the RN from ED. This is Haley Milangu and her mother, Jenny. Haley is 9 years old.*
S	Situation	*Haley was flown in from Mepunda at 1200 hrs and has been diagnosed with type 1 diabetes.*
B	Background	*Haley presented with a history of polyuria and polydipsia, as well as abdo pain and weight loss. She has had increasing tiredness.* *Haley's mother, Jenny, took her to the community health centre this morning; her BGL was 20 mmol/L and urinalysis showed large glucose and a trace of ketones. The NP contacted Josh James, the paediatrician, and Haley was brought to the ED.*
A	Assessment	*On arrival at the ED, Haley's BGL was 17.0 mmol/L and ketones 1.5 mmol/L. Urinalysis showed large glucose and ketones.* **Admission observations:** Temperature — 37.1°C (tympanic) Pulse rate — 96 Blood pressure — 100/60 mmHg Respiratory rate — 30 Capillary refill — <2 secs Skin turgor — skin fold evident for 1 sec *Haley weighs 22 kg, which is slightly below average weight range for her age; and her height is 132 cm, which is slightly above average.* *Haley had a stat dose of 3 u/s NovoRapid at 1240 hrs. Bloods for serology have been taken.*
R	Request/ recommendation	*Haley has an IV cannula in her left cubital fossa. It was inserted at 1230.* **Medical orders:** 4-hourly obs Full diet, with carb counting IVT normal saline 30 mL/hr BGLs prior to meals, including morning and afternoon tea, at 2100 and 0200 hrs; and a urinalysis each shift. Check ketones using finger prick test with every BGL until negative or trace levels reached. If BGL >15 mmol/L, contact MO for further orders. SCI NovoRapid, a short-acting insulin, and 'Lantus' (glargine insulin), a long-acting insulin, but report all BGLs to the doctor prior to the dose being decided. *Can you arrange for the diabetic educator to see Haley and her mother today?* *Notify Dr James if you have any concerns.*

Having received the handover from the ED nurse, you introduce yourself to Haley and Jenny and begin a 'rapid assessment'. You visually inspect Haley and take her vital signs and a BGL:

For a more detailed understanding of insulin and delivery devices, refer to this website: <www.diabetesaustralia.com.au/insulin>.

Temperature	37°C (tympanic)
Pulse rate	90
Blood pressure	102/58 mmHg
Respiratory rate	25
BGL	12 mmol/L
SpO$_2$	98% on room air

You then begin the formal admission process, which includes a physical assessment, risk assessment and history taking.

Communicating with children

Hospitals are alien places to most children and the way in which Haley is greeted and settled into the Paediatric Unit can have a significant impact on Haley and her family. Haley may react strongly and unpredictably to smells, sounds, people and procedures. She may have concerns about separation from her family and isolation from activities she enjoys. She may also be worried about unfamiliar people touching and examining her. Hence, therapeutic communication skills are central to establishing an effective rapport with Haley and her family, and in developing a trusting partnership.

Family-centred care

Until now, the primary concern has been to monitor and stabilise Haley. However, when caring for a child it is important to remember that the child and his or her family (in all the many ways 'family' can be defined) should be considered as a single unit. This is defined as 'family-centred care'.

It is imperative to understand the societal factors that impact on families and the psychosocial and physical health and wellbeing of their members. Family-centred care takes into account that the family is the anchor point in the child's life. From this vantage point, nurses adopt strategies that promote collaboration between the family and healthcare professionals and recognise that the entire family are care recipients (Walton, 2014).

While there are immediate practicalities to contend with, there will also be ongoing challenges for all members of the Milangu family. Additionally, each member of the family will respond in an individual way to the circumstances of Haley's diagnosis.

Q1 Using the family background information provided below, consider the potential impact of Haley's diagnosis on the members of her family and how they can be supported to adjust and manage this situation.

> *Bob manages the cattle property the family lives on. He is an Aboriginal man with a strong spiritual connection to the land and his heritage. He and his wife have been concentrating on reducing overhead debt and the only road vehicle they own is an old four-wheel drive that requires frequent maintenance.*
>
> *Jenny is a qualified accountant. She runs a business from home doing the tax returns and business statements for several local property owners.*
>
> *Haley has been a fit and active girl until recently. She is captain of the school soccer team and plays in the regional representative side. Haley works hard to achieve above-average grades for her schoolwork. She is popular and has a strong network of friends at school.*
>
> *Doris is Bob's mother and she lives with the family on the property. Doris has type 2 diabetes mellitus, poor vision and stage 2 chronic kidney disease. She had a mild stroke last year. Every alternate Friday, Jenny drives Doris and several of the senior members of the outlying communities to the Aboriginal Medical Service in Mepunda for their checkups.*
>
> *Jim is Haley's older brother. He is 13 years old and works at a neighbouring station after school for two afternoons a week doing odd jobs. His dad picks him up from the station at around 6 pm. Jim has been selected for the under-16 football team.*
>
> *Charlie is Haley's 4-year-old younger brother. He attends play group at the local community centre four mornings a week and will begin school next year.*

Patient education

Haley's management plan includes regular monitoring of BGLs to achieve glycaemia control, and education for Haley and her parents on:

- how to measure BGL's correctly
- the role of HbA1c (glycosylated haemoglobin) in metabolic control of diabetes
- insulin administration (including monitoring injection sites)

> The NMBA's Registered Nurse Standards for Practice (2016) state that registered nurses must communicate effectively and be respectful of each person's dignity, culture, values, beliefs and rights.

> What are some important communication strategies that the nurse could implement to allay potential anxiety when Haley first presents to the Unit? Watch <www.youtube.com/watch?v=39bZYNnpH9k&sns=em> for more insight into communicating with children.

> Family-centred care enhances the family's confidence and capacity to care for their child's future health needs and a wide body of evidence details the benefits of this approach (Mould, Rudd & Wilkinson, 2014).

> The NSQHS Standards emphasise the importance of consumer-centred healthcare and the inclusion of patients and families as partners in shared decision making (ACSQHC, 2016).

> What is the relationship between Doris's chronic conditions and her type 2 diabetes? It is important to understand the aetiology and pathogenesis of this disease, as 1 in 10 of your patients is likely to have type 2 diabetes.

> HbA1c is an index of the diabetic client's blood glucose estimation over the previous 2- to 3-month period and is considered the most widely accepted measure for evaluation of glycaemic control (Rewers et al., 2014).

- nutrition and carbohydrate counting
- meal planning
- recognising and managing hyper- and hypoglycaemia
- sick-day management
- the importance of exercise

Q2   Why is it necessary for Haley to monitor her carbohydrate intake?

> *Smart et al. (2010) advocate that carbohydrate counting is a skill that children with type 1 diabetes can learn. Educating children about their diabetes is vital for successful management. Refer to the following link for some useful resources for children in understanding their condition: <www.health. qld.gov.au/publications/ best_practice/16855. pdf>.*

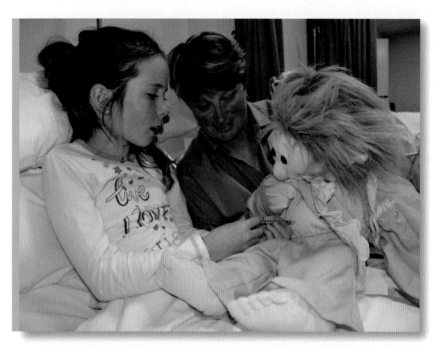

The nurse uses a puppet to actively engage Haley and teach her about insulin injections

Refer to the clinical pathway in the table below for an overview of the education required for a child newly diagnosed with type 1 diabetes.

Stages of care	Expected condition of child	Care and education required	Clinician responsible
On admission (day 1)	**Subjective** Child will be drowsy, lethargic, anxious and usually hungry as fatigue reduces. **Objective** Treatment depends on acuity. Insulin infusion with hourly BGLs and twice daily blood tests. Expected BGL: 13–20 mmol/L Expected ketones: positive >1.5 mmol/L	Initial assessment: vital signs including capillary refill, BGL and ketones. Orientate child and family to the ward; outline what to expect and the initial plan. Provide a brief overview of diabetes and demonstrate the BGL monitor. Provide child with the Juvenile Diabetes Research (JDRF) backpack which has a BGL monitor and information book. *Note:* If child is too unwell, education will be postponed.	Ward RN Refer to diabetes educator and social worker. *For more information about this backpack and booklet, access <www.jdrf.org.au/type-1-diabetes/community-resources-program>.*
Day following admission (day 2)	**Subjective** Child will be less tired but remain hungry, irritable and sometimes teary.	If potassium levels are >5.0 mmol/L and ketones <1.4 mmol/L, the insulin infusion will cease and subcutaneous insulin will commence.	Ward RN Paediatric consultant Paediatric registrar

Stages of care	Expected condition of child	Care and education required	Clinician responsible
	Objective Expected BGLs: 9–20 mmol/L Ketones: negative	Usual regime is a long-acting insulin at night and a short-acting insulin for each meal. BGL testing will continue before and after each meal. Education about how to take BGLs and self-administer insulin will start as soon as child and family feel ready.	Diabetes educator, dietitian and social worker will visit the child and family to establish a collaborative education plan.
Day before discharge (day 3)	Patient and family should be more relaxed and confident. Child will be looking forward to going home and becoming increasingly independent in managing diabetes. Expected BGLs: 3–16 mmol/L Ketones: negative	BGL monitoring continues seven times per day. The child (and family) should be able to do this independently. The child learns self-injection (with assistance from the ward RN or educator). The child is likely to experience a hypoglycemic episode during their first admission and an important part of preparing for discharge is ensuring the family can deal with potential emergencies. Day leave is encouraged for the child and family to have a trial with independently managing insulin and BGL monitoring.	Ward RN Diabetes educator will explain blood tests (e.g. HBA1c), sick-day management, hypoglycaemia education plan and register the child with the National Diabetes Services Scheme (NDSS). The diabetes educator will provide a carbohydrate-to-insulin ratio and the dietitian will provide education on carbohydrate counting. The medical team will review insulin requirements.
Day of discharge (day 4)	The child and family are usually looking forward to discharge. Expected BGLs: 3–12 mmol/L Ketones: negative	The medical team check that the child and family are independent with the following: • Self-injection of insulin • Operation of BGL monitor and checking ketones • Recognising signs of hypoglycaemia and management of a hypoglycaemic episode • Recognising hyperglycaemia and taking appropriate actions • Sick-day management • Suitable food choices, serving sizes and carbohydrate counting	Diabetes educator will assist with reviewing all skills and provide contact information. Dietitian will provide final review of carbohydrate counting. Medical team will review insulin requirements, provide prescriptions and make a daily plan for contact until outpatient appointment.

It is now two days since Haley's admission and she is progressing well. Her BGLs are becoming more stable and the nurses and diabetic educator are teaching her to monitor her own BGLs and administer her own insulin. However, Haley becomes distressed during one of the teaching sessions and says, 'I don't want any more needles. Why can't I just have tablets like Nanna does for her diabetes?'

Q1 How would you explain to Haley why she needs injections when her grandmother doesn't?

Q2 How could you help Haley openly discuss her fears and frustrations?

> *Children are sometimes told that needles just feel like a mosquito sting or that a cannula is a tiny straw going in their hand—analogies that are not helpful. How could you explain concepts such as subcutaneous injections, venepuncture or cannulation? (Mould, Rudd & Wilkinson, 2014).*

Research by Hanas et al. (2011) reveals that inconvenience, inaccuracy, pain, anxiety and social unacceptability all present barriers for children when learning to administer insulin.

Initially, Haley's insulin was administered by the nurses. She took particular notice of how two nurses always checked the dose of her insulin together. Haley asks you why she has two different types of insulin in the morning and evening but only one injection prior to meals.

Q3 What explanation will you give Haley for this?

Haley remembered the diabetes educator telling her mum about a pump that replaces the need for regular insulin injections and, distressed about all her needles, she asks you why she can't 'just have the pump now'.

Q4 How would you respond to Haley?

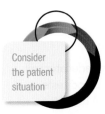

1. CONSIDER THE PATIENT SITUATION

On the afternoon of day 3, Haley is allowed to leave the Paediatric Unit for a few hours to attend her cousin's birthday party. Haley and her dad know that they need to be back by 1800 in time for her dinner and insulin.

2. COLLECT CUES/INFORMATION

(a) Review current information

Haley returns to the ward at 1800 hours and her vital signs are checked:

Temperature	37.1°C (tympanic)
Pulse rate	84
Blood pressure	100/76 mmHg
Respiratory rate	20
SpO$_2$	100% on room air

For more information about insulin delivery in children and adolescents, refer to Hanas et al. (2011).

Refer to the following resource for information about the advantages, disadvantages and management of insulin pumps: Caring for Diabetes in Children and Adolescents: <http://video.rch.org.au/diabetes/Diabetes_Book_Third_Edition.pdf>.

Haley tells you all about the party and says she 'feels fine'. Bob tells you that Haley did not eat much apart from some popcorn and a drink of soda water. She is still excited about playing with her cousins and doesn't eat much of her dinner.

When it is time for Haley to check her BGL, she organises the equipment under your supervision. As she is about to undertake the measurement, another child calls out from the bathroom for help and you respond to the needs of the other child. When you return, Haley has completed the BGL and the monitor reads 16 mmol/L.

You check the insulin with another RN and, following the six rights of safe medication administration, you administer three units of NovoRapid, a short-acting insulin, as prescribed. Half an hour later, Bob comes and tells you that Haley is not feeling well.

How could this situation have been managed differently?

(b) Gather new information

Q1 Short-acting insulin is clear in appearance and begins to work:

   a Immediately

   b Within 20 minutes

   c Within 30 minutes

   d Within 1 hour

Q2 You return to Haley's room. What cues would you collect at this time?

(c) Recall knowledge

QUICK QUIZ!

To ensure that you have a good understanding of the key concepts related to the care of diabetes, test yourself with the following questions.

Q1 A normal BGL is:

   a 2.5 to 3.5 mmol/L

   b 4.0 to 8.0 mmol/L

   c 5.0 to 10.0 mmol/L

Q2 Symptoms of hyperglycaemia *do not* include which of the following?

   a Higher levels of concentration

   b Moodiness

   c Muscle cramps

   d Tiredness

Q3 Symptoms of hypoglycaemia may include which of the following?

   a Kussmaul breathing and acetone-smelling breath

   b Polyuria and glycosuria

   c Pallor, sweating and irritability

   d Oliguria and ketonuria

Q4 Contamination of the skin from glucose can give a false BGL reading when using a finger prick technique.

   a Never

   b Often

   c Sometimes

Q5 Insufficient blood obtained on a glucometer test strip may result in:

   a A false low reading

   b A false high reading

   c Will make no difference at all

Q6 Label the following as 'true' or 'false'.

   a Hypoglycaemia is a high-priority situation.

   b Hyperglycaemia can happen within minutes.

   c A hypoglycaemic child may have a seizure.

   d Hypoglycaemia can happen within minutes.

   e Hypoglycaemia evolves over hours and sometimes days.

3. PROCESS INFORMATION

(a) Interpret

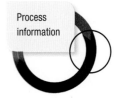

Process information

Q From the following list, identify which of Haley's cues are normal and which are abnormal. This will require careful analysis and application of your knowledge of type 1 diabetes.

   a Cold and clammy skin

   b Pallor

   c Irritability

   d Hunger

   e Nausea

   f Temperature: 36.9°C (tympanic)

    g   Pulse rate: 114

    h   Blood pressure: 96/54 mmHg

    i   Respiratory rate: 22

    j   BGL: 2.2 mmol/L

    k SpO_2: 98% on room air

(b) Discriminate

Q   Which of the above cues are of greatest concern at this time?

(c) Relate and (d) Infer

It is now time to cluster the cues together, identify relationships between them and make inferences based on those relationships.

Q   Consider the following statements in relation to your assessment of Haley. Label the following as 'true' or 'false'.

    a   Haley could have a low BGL and tachycardia because she ate cakes and sweets at the party.

    b   Haley could be pale and sweaty because she caught a virus from one of her cousins.

    c   Haley could be irritable and tachycardic because she is overtired.

    d   Haley could be irritable and tired because of her low BGL.

    e   Haley could be nauseated because she ate cakes and sweets at the party.

    f   Haley could have a low BGL because she was not given enough insulin when she returned from the party.

    g   When Haley came back from the party, her BGL measurement may have been inaccurate, leading to the administration of an inaccurate insulin dose.

    h   Haley could be pale and sweaty because of her low BGL.

(e) Predict

Q   Select three outcomes that could occur if you do not take immediate action in relation to Haley's signs and symptoms.

    a   Haley's condition will gradually improve.

    b   Haley could become unconscious.

    c   Haley will develop an infection.

    d   Haley could have a seizure.

    e   Haley could become cognitively impaired.

    f   Haley's blood glucose could continue to rise, causing her to go into a hyperglycaemic coma.

(f) Match

Q   Have you ever seen someone with the same signs and symptoms as Haley? If so, what was the problem and what was done to manage the situation?

4. IDENTIFY THE PROBLEM/ISSUE

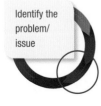

Identify the problem/issue

Q   Re-examine the information you have about Haley and then identify the three correct nursing diagnoses for Haley:

    a   Hypoglycaemia related to inadequate carbohydrate intake, as evidenced by BGL of 2.2 mmol/L, pallor and irritability

    b   Hyperglycaemia related to inadequate carbohydrate intake, as evidenced by BGL of 2.2 mmol/L, pallor and irritability c   Hyperglycaemia related to an underlying infection, as evidenced by temperature and tachycardia

d   Hypoglycaemia related to inadequate insulin administration, as evidenced by high BGL

e   Hypoglycaemia related to excessive insulin administration, as evidenced by BGL of 2.2 mmol/L, pallor and irritability

f   Risk of hypoglycaemic shock related to BGL of 2.2 mmol/L

g   Risk of DKA related to BGL of 2.2 mmol/L

h   Risk of seizure related to BGL of 2.2 mmol/L

5. ESTABLISH GOALS

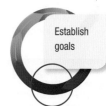

Q   Before initiating any actions, it is important to be clear about your goals for Haley. Select the correct nursing goal from the following.

a   For Haley's BGL to be between 4 and 8 mmol/L within the next 24 hours

b   For Haley's BGL to be between 8 and 12 mmol/L within the next 12 hours

c   For Haley's BGL to be between 2 and 4 mmol/L within the next 2 hours

d   For Haley's BGL to be between 4 and 8 mmol/L within the next 30 minutes

6. TAKE ACTION

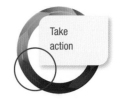

You realise that you need to deal with the immediate issue of Haley's hypoglycaemia; later you will need to determine the cause of this situation.

Q   Select two *immediate* priorities for Haley's care from the list below.

a   Leave Haley in the care of her father while you go to phone the paediatrician.

b   Administer glucagon subcutaneously.

c   Give a repeat dose of insulin.

d   Ask one of the other nurses to find a sandwich or some biscuits for Haley.

e   Give Haley some oral glucose (e.g. glucose lollies, lemonade or orange juice) and repeat 15 minutes later if needed.

f   Contact the medical officer using ISBAR and ask him or her to insert an IV so that you can administer IV glucose 5% to Haley.

g   Monitor Haley's condition closely and carefully.

7. EVALUATE

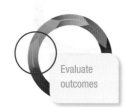

Q1   Which *two* statements provide evidence that your nursing actions have been effective in managing Haley's situation appropriately.

a   Following administration of insulin, Haley's BGL is 12 mmol/L.

b   Fifteen minutes after consuming the glucose drink, Haley's BGL is 4.4 mmol/L.

c   Forty-five minutes after consuming the glucose drink, Haley's BGL is 3.0 mmol/L.

d   Two hours after consuming the glucose drink, Haley's BGL is 3.0 mmol/L.

e   Haley's observations return to normal within 1 hour.

Once Haley's condition is stable, you consider what may have precipitated her hypoglycaemic episode when she had been so stable over the last few days. Although you are aware that Haley's carbohydrate intake was not high prior to this event, the insulin dose you administered was titrated to her BGL of 16 mmol/L. You begin to wonder whether the BGL could have been inaccurate.

Q2   What factors can contribute to an inaccurate BGL result?

At handover, when you are reporting on how Haley had a hypoglycaemic event when she returned from the party, one of the nurses makes the comment, 'Typical. Those people don't know how to look after their kids.'

Q3   This is an example of which clinical reasoning error?

Q4   How would you respond to this comment?

8. REFLECT

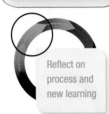

Reflect on process and new learning

After talking to Haley and her dad later in the evening, you discover that at the party one of her cousins tripped and spilt a jug of cordial over the table and Haley had helped to clean it up. Haley does not recall washing her hands after this happened and prior to checking her BGL. Bob tells you that he is really anxious about Haley having another 'hypo'.

Q1   What have you learnt from this scenario that will help you to support and educate Haley and Bob about how to prevent and manage hypoglycaemic events in the future?

Q2   What actions will you take in your future practice as a result of what you have learnt from this scenario?

SCENARIO 5.2   Caring for a child with diabetic ketoacidosis (DKA)

CHANGING THE SCENE

With her family's support, Haley progresses well in managing her diabetes and she is discharged on day 4. Part of Haley's discharge plan requires Jenny to be in regular contact with the paediatrician and diabetic educator. However, despite close attention and careful monitoring, Haley's condition deteriorates six weeks later.

At 0700, Jenny tries to wake Haley for school but finds her difficult to rouse. There is a large amount of vomit in the bed. Haley's younger brother has also woken with vomiting and diarrhoea. Bob immediately drives Haley to the community health centre. The remote area nurse organises for Haley's emergency transfer to the regional hospital by air.

1. CONSIDER THE PATIENT SITUATION

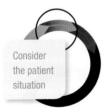

Consider the patient situation

You are the RN on the morning shift in the ED and receive the following handover from the retrieval nurse:

Handover report

This is 9-year-old Haley Milangu who was diagnosed six weeks ago with type 1 diabetes. She was very difficult to wake this morning—probably DKA. Other siblings have symptoms of GI upset.

Initial observations:

Temperature	38.4°C (tympanic)
Pulse rate	123
Blood pressure	95/72 mmHg
Respiratory rate	32 (regular and deep)
BGL	28 mmol/L
SpO$_2$	100%

Haley's skin is hot and flushed and she is complaining of a dry mouth. Her breath has an acetone smell. She is aware of where she is but slips into a deep sleep easily and needs to be roused. This seems to be getting worse. An IV of normal saline has been started and we gave Haley a stat dose of 6 units of NovoRapid an hour ago.

Diabetic ketoacidosis (DKA)

Diabetic ketoacidosis (DKA) is a potentially life-threatening complication of diabetes mellitus where a cascade of pathophysiology is generated from the absence of insulin. It is the result of inadequate insulin and usually (but not always) associated with an extremely elevated serum glucose level. DKA can occur as the first manifestation of diabetes in previously undiagnosed patients, or as an acute exacerbation of the disease initiated by stress, insufficient insulin intake, illness or infection (McFarlane, 2011) .

In undiagnosed diabetics, a lack of insulin results in the inability to transfer glucose across the cell membrane, so there is a high concentration of glucose in the blood. The elevated serum glucose results in the kidney increasing the volume of urine excreted to maintain osmolarity and a serious fluid imbalance can result (Siafarikas & O'Connell, 2010). In patients with known diagnosis, DKA can manifest secondary to an infection, stress or change in metabolism such as occurs in puberty. In these circumstances, the body releases counter-regulatory hormones such as glucagon, catecholamines, growth hormone and serum cortisol, which significantly impede the effectiveness of insulin (London et al., 2016).

Absence of glucose as a cellular energy source causes the body to 'implement a safety strategy' to maintain cellular function, so protein and fat are used as energy sources (Parrish, 2017). The utilisation of fat as an energy source results in the build-up of the liver metabolite, ketones. The accumulation of ketones results in metabolic acidosis, and the life-threatening condition known as DKA can develop. An acidotic state will cause a change in the respiratory pattern as the body compensates and tries to correct the shift in pH. Electrolyte levels are often affected and, in particular, hypokalaemia can occur (Craig et al., 2014). This is caused by a movement of potassium out of the intracellular space into the extracellular space to correct the acidosis. The potassium is then excreted by the kidneys, resulting in an overall body deficit of potassium. Although serum potassium levels may initially be normal or high, levels will drop as the insulin treatment causes the potassium to shift back into the cells and the patient will be at risk of life-threatening hypokalaemia (McFarlane, 2011). Haley's condition may be further complicated by the potassium loss that occurs with gastrointestinal upsets.

For further information about DKA, review pp. 581–85 of LeMone et al. (2017).

2. COLLECT CUES/INFORMATION

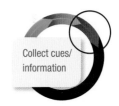

Collect cues/ information

(a) Review current information

You review the information provided by the retrieval nurse to gain a deeper understanding of Haley's condition. You also leave a phone message for the paediatrician.

(b) Gather new information

You then conduct a set of admission observations.

Admission observations:

Temperature	38.4°C (tympanic)
Pulse rate	140
Blood pressure	80/50 mmHg
Respiratory rate	32 (regular and deep)
Capillary BGL	30 mmol/L
Capillary ketones	1.2 mmol/L
SpO_2	100% on room air

Q   What other information do you need to collect at this time? From the list below, select the four cues that are of *least* importance at this time:

a   Appetite

b   BMI

c   Condition of oral mucosa

d   Cognitive state

    e   Urine output

    f   Serum urea and electrolytes

    g   Level of thirst

    h   Serum glucose

    i   Serum ketones

    j   Respiratory pattern

    k   FBC

(c) Recall knowledge

Test your knowledge of Haley's current condition and related terminology.

QUICK QUIZ!

Q1 GI refers to:

    a   Glucose intolerance

    b   Gastrointestinal

    c   Gut intestinal

Q2 U/E refers to:

    a   Usual enquiry

    b   Urea and electrolytes

    c   Urine and electrodes

Q3 Haley's pattern of breathing is called 'Kussmaul breathing'. It is a physiological response to:

    a   High levels of glucose

    b   Metabolic acidosis

    c   Deteriorating cerebral perfusion

    d   Altered electrolyte levels

Q4 An elevated WBC may indicate which of the following? (Select the two most correct answers.)

    a   A sign of ketosis

    b   Underlying infection

    c   An elevated metabolic rate

    d   A stress response to DKA

Q5 Which of the following pathways *do not* occur in diabetic ketoacidosis (DKA)?

    a   Hyperglycaemia → glycosuria → polyuria → dehydration → marked electrolyte loss

    b   Hyperglycaemia → cellular dehydration → diminished level of consciousness

    c   Fat breakdown → ketone accumulation → pH shift to acidosis

    d   Hyperglycaemia → increased viscosity of the blood → decreased urine output

Q6 The three main causes of DKA are:

    a   Too much insulin, infection, lack of fluid intake

    b   Noncompliance, ignorance, early discharge

    c   Lack of exercise, unstable home environment, lack of education

    d   Inadequate or missed insulin dose, illness or infection, and undiagnosed or untreated diabetes

Q7 Normal arterial pH is:

   a 7.25–7.33

   b 7.35–7.43

   c 7.45–7.53

   d 7.55–7.63

These questions require a solid knowledge base. If unsure of any of the answers, refer to your textbook or <www.health.qld. gov.au/improvement/ networks/docs/diabetic-ketoacidosis.pdf>.

3. PROCESS INFORMATION

Process information

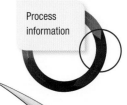

(a) Interpret

The next step in the clinical reasoning cycle is to interpret the data that you have collected about Haley.

Q1 Which of the following are within normal parameters for Haley?

   a Temperature: 38.4°C (tympanic)

   b Pulse rate: 140

   c Blood pressure: 80/50 mmHg

   d Respiratory rate: 32 (regular and deep)

   e BGL: 30 mmol/L

   f SpO_2: 100% on room air

   g U/A: large glucose and large ketones

   h Sleepy and difficult to rouse

   i Sweet-smelling breath

   j Poor capillary refill

This part of the clinical reasoning cycle aligns with the NSQHS Standards which emphasise the need for systems and processes to effectively recognise when a patient's condition is deteriorating, and respond appropriately (ACSQHC, 2016).

Q2 The pathology report reveals the following. Which of these are not within normal limits for Haley?

   a WBC: 18.9×10^9/L

   b Haemoglobin (Hb): 125 g/L

   c Urea: 6.3 mmol/L

   d Blood ketones: 4.2.2 mmol/L

   e Serum potassium (K^+): 3.8 mmol/L

   f Serum sodium (Na^+): 140 mmol/L

   g pH: 7.18

   h CO_2: 44 mmHg

   i HCO_3: 16

   j pO_2: 92 mmHg

(b) Discriminate

Q From the list below, identify the clinical indicators that are of greatest importance.

   a Temperature

   b Pulse rate

   c BP

   d Respiratory rate and depth

   e Smell of sweet breath

   f Capillary refill

   g pH

h CO_2

i BGL

j Ketones

k K^+

l Urea

m Condition of oral mucosa

n WBC

o Sleepy, requiring loud stimuli to wake her

(c) Relate and (d) Infer

It is now time to cluster the cues together, identify relationships between them and begin to make inferences about Haley's current condition.

Q Which of the following statements are true?

a Haley's sweet-smelling breath could be related to something she has eaten.

b Haley's sweet-smelling breath is related to ketone production in the liver.

c Haley's temperature and tachycardia may mean she has an infection.

d Haley's pH and CO_2 could indicate respiratory acidosis.

e The condition of Haley's oral mucosa is related to her fluid status.

f Haley's pH and CO_2 indicate metabolic alkalosis.

g Haley's respiratory rate and depth is how the body maintains a normal pH in metabolic acidosis.

h Haley's rapid respirations have no association with DKA.

i Haley's elevated WBC could be linked to an infection which is altering her blood glucose levels.

j Haley's pH and CO_2 indicate metabolic acidosis.

k Because Haley has an elevated BGL, her pancreas must be working effectively.

(e) Predict

Q If you do not take the appropriate actions at this time, what could happen to Haley? (Select three correct answers.)

a Haley could go into a diabetic coma and die.

b Haley's condition will continue to deteriorate.

c Haley's condition will gradually improve over the next few days.

d Haley could experience cerebral oedema.

e Haley could experience a hypoglycaemic episode.

f Haley could experience a cerebral vascular accident.

(f) Match

Q Have you ever seen someone with the same signs and symptoms as Haley? If so, what was done to manage the situation?

4. IDENTIFY THE PROBLEM/ISSUE

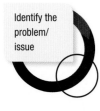

Identify the problem/issue

Q1 Complete the following nursing diagnoses for Haley.

a Dehydration related to _____ and vomiting, evidenced by glycosuria, _____, _____ and hypotension.

   b Ineffective breathing pattern related to metabolic acidosis, as evidenced by
       _____, _____, CO_2 and HCO_3.

   c Risk of electrolyte imbalance caused by _____.

   d Risk of coma related to _____ and cellular dehydration.

Q2 Identify four factors that could have led to Haley's deterioration.

5. ESTABLISH GOALS

Q Identify four immediate goals for Haley's management at this time. Identify what you want to happen and when.

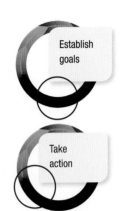

Establish goals

Take action

6. TAKE ACTION

This stage of the clinical reasoning cycle includes all that you do as a nurse in delivering care: practical skills, intellectual activities and effective communication skills. However, you are aware that you cannot do everything at once and that Haley's condition is serious. As Haley's paediatrician has not replied to your phone message, you decide to notify the paediatric medical team and using ISBAR request an immediate review of Haley.

Q1 What are the six priority issues for Haley at this time.

   a Diuretic therapy

   b Resolving acidosis

   c Antihypertensive therapy

   d Fluid replacement

   e Electrolyte replacement

   f Anticoagulation therapy

   g Management of hyperglycaemia

   h Maintenance of airway

   i Monitoring for cerebral oedema

Q2 Haley is reviewed and the subsequent medical orders are listed in the table on the next page, along with related nursing actions. Match the actions to the appropriate rationales.

The NSQHS Standards highlight the importance of effective and timely communication between patients, carers and families, and multi-disciplinary teams to promote patient safety (ACSQHC, 2016).

For further information about the management of DKA, refer to <www.health.qld.gov.au/improvement/networks/docs/diabetic-ketoacidosis.pdf>.

7. EVALUATE

Q1 List six signs and symptoms that would indicate that Haley's condition has improved.

Q2 List five potential complications of DKA that you will closely monitor her for.

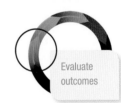

Evaluate outcomes

8. REFLECT

Q1 What actions will you take in clinical practice as a result of your learning from this scenario?

Q2 How do you think that your own beliefs, values and assumptions influence your ability to provide culturally safe care for Aboriginal people?

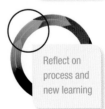

Reflect on process and new learning

EPILOGUE

Haley was transferred to ICU and her condition remained serious for some time. An arterial line was inserted to enable painless blood sampling and regular analysis of electrolyte and acid–base status. Two large-bore IV lines were inserted to enable delivery of fluids, electrolytes and IV insulin. Haley remained on neurological observations until her condition had stabilised, but she did not develop cerebral oedema. She was transferred to the paediatric ward two days later.

Medical order/nursing action	Rationale
Document all nursing observations and actions accurately and contemporaneously	To ensure appropriate expertise and resources are allocated to Haley
Check neurological status hourly	To identify electrolyte imbalances so that an ongoing titration of treatment to Haley's condition can occur
Monitor fluid status closely	To ensure adequate oxygen delivery
ECG and cardiac monitoring	To ensure adequate oxygen delivery
Maintain patent IV access and monitor IV site regularly	To enable the titration of intravenous dextrose so that BGL is maintained between 5 and 10 mmol/L (within acceptable parameters)
Maintain oxygen therapy via Hudson mask and hourly oxygen saturations	To promote a therapeutic relationship and maintain psychosocial wellbeing
Reassure Haley and her family	To correct fluid and electrolyte imbalances
Set up an insulin infusion to be commenced once K^+ improves, then titrate with S.Glucose and S.Ketone levels *according to doctor's orders*	To determine hydration status and enable administration of appropriate IV fluids
Hourly capillary BGL and ketones	To determine the average plasma glucose concentration over a period of time and so gain insight into how well controlled the disease is
Commence IV with N/Saline 0.9% with 20 mmol KCl as per medical orders	To provide adequate insulin to clear ketones and correct acidosis
Repeat ABGs in 2 hours	To identify improvement or deterioration in Haley's condition
Check glycosylated haemoglobin (HbA1c)	To identify improvement or deterioration in Haley's cognition
Prepare IV of 5% dextrose but do not commence unless ordered	To monitor response to insulin treatment and to identify appropriate management strategies
Ensure patent airway at all times	To ensure cannula remains patent
Transfer Haley to ICU	Hyperkalaemia may cause cardiac dysrhythmias
Hourly vital signs	To monitor respiratory and acid–base status and adjust management appropriately
Repeat U&Es in 2 hours	To provide effective communication between the health team and facilitate the delivery of appropriate individualised care; to provide an accurate and timely written evaluation of Haley's progress and health outcomes and progress

Haley and her family had continuing education about the management of her diabetes and, in particular, about the appropriate action to take if she became ill. A plan of 'sick-day rules' was developed which included an alternative regime of how much extra insulin to take when blood glucose levels were uncontrolled, advice on appropriate foods and fluids, methods of managing fever or infection and emergency contact numbers.

Haley recently celebrated her 10th birthday and has been able to manage her condition with no further episodes of hyperglycaemia. She is attending school and has returned to playing soccer. Haley continues to travel to the regional hospital for consultation with her paediatrician bi-monthly and has a teleconference on alternate months. The family has made contact with a local diabetes educator via a GP care plan. Together with Haley and her family, the GP and diabetes educator have developed a plan to give Haley necessary background education so that she can start using an insulin pump within the next three months.

FURTHER READING

Ambler, G. & Cameron, F. (2010). *Caring for Diabetes in Children and Adolescents* (3rd edn). Australia: Blue Star Print Group. Accessed at <http://video.rch.org.au/diabetes/Diabetes_Book_Third_Edition.pdf>.

REFERENCES

Australian Bureau of Statistics. (2011). *Diabetes in Australia: A Snapshot of 2007–2008*. Accessed October 2011 at <www.abs.gov.au/ausstats/abs@.nsf/mf/4820.0.55.001>.

Australian Commission on Safety and Quality in Health Care (ACSQHC). (2016). *National Safety and Quality Health Service Standards Version 2*. Draft, Sydney, Australia.

Australian Institute of Health and Welfare (AIHW). (2014). *Type 2 Diabetes in Australia's Children and Young People: A Working Paper*. Diabetes Series No. 21. Cat. No. CVD 64. Canberra: AIHW.

Australian Institute of Health and Welfare (AIHW). (2011). *The Health and Welfare of Australia's Aboriginal and Torres Strait Islander People: An Overview 2011*. Canberra: AIHW.

Craig, M. E., Jefferies, C., Dabelea, D., Balde, N., Seth, A. & Donaghue, K. C. (2014). Definition, epidemiology, and classification of diabetes in children and adolescents. *Pediatric Diabetes*, *15*(Suppl 20), 4–17.

Diabetes Australia. (2017). *Diabetes in Australia*. Accessed January 2017 at <www.diabetessa.com.au/type-1/newly-diagnosed.html>.

Douglas, M. K., Rosenkoetter, M., Pacquiao, D. F., Callister, L. C., Hattar-Pollara, M., Lauderdale, J., … Purnell, L. (2014). Guidelines for implementing culturally competent nursing care. *Journal of Transcultural Nursing*, doi: 10.1177/1043659614520998.

Hanas, R., de Beaufort, C., Hoey, H. & Anderson, B. (2011). Insulin delivery by injection in children and adolescents with diabetes. *Pediatric Diabetes*, *12*(5), 518–26.

London, M., Ladewig, P., Ball, J., Bindler. C. & Cowen, K. J. (2016). *Maternal and Child Nursing Care* (5th edn, Chapter 55, pp. 1621–39). New Jersey: Pearson.

McFarlane, K. (2011). An overview of diabetic ketoacidosis in children. *Paediatric Nursing*, *23*(1), 14–9.

Mould, J., Rudd, C. & Wilkinson, A. (2014). Communicating with children and families. In T. Levett-Jones (Ed.), *Critical Conversations for Patient Safety: An Essential Guide for Health Professionals*. Sydney: Pearson.

Nursing and Midwifery Board of Australia (NMBA). (2016). *Registered Nurse Standards for Practice*. Accessed at <www.nursingmidwiferyboard.gov.au/Codes-Guidelines-Statements/Professional-standards.aspx>.

Parrish, T. (2017). Nursing care of people with diabetes mellitus. In P. LeMone, K. Burke, G. Bauldoff, P. Gubrud-Howe, T. Levett-Jones, M. Hales, … K. Reid-Searl (Eds), (2017). *Medical–Surgical Nursing: Critical Thinking for Person-Centred Care* (Australian edn). Sydney, NSW: Pearson.

Rewers, M., Pillay, K., De Beaufort, C., Craig, M., Hanas, R., Acerini, C. & Maahs, D. (2014). Assessment and monitoring of glycemic control in children and adolescents with diabetes. *Pediatric Diabetes*, *15*, 102–14.

Siafarikas, A. & O'Connell, S. (2010). Type 1 diabetes in children: Emergency management. *Australian Family Physician*, *39*(5), 290–93.

Smart, C., Ross, K., Edge, J., King, B., McElduff, P. & Collins, C. (2010). Can children with type 1 diabetes and their caregivers estimate the carbohydrate content of meals and snacks? *Diabetic Medicine*, *27*, 348–53.

Walton, M. K. (2014). Person and family-centred care. *British Journal of Nursing*, *23*(17), 949. doi:10.12968/bjon.2014.23.17.949

CHAPTER 6

CARING FOR A PERSON EXPERIENCING RESPIRATORY DISTRESS AND HYPOXIA

KERRY HOFFMAN, AMANDA WILSON AND VANESSA McDONALD

LEARNING OUTCOMES

Completion of the activities in this chapter will enable you to:

○ explain why an understanding of ventilation, respiration, hypoxia and oxygenation is essential to competent practice (**recall** and **application**)

○ identify the clinical signs of respiratory distress and hypoxia that guide the collection and interpretation of cues (**gather, review, interpret, discriminate, relate** and **infer**)

○ identify risk factors for respiratory distress (**match** and **predict**)

○ use clinical information to identify the main nursing diagnoses for a person with respiratory distress and hypoxia (**synthesise**)

○ describe the priorities of care for a person with respiratory distress and hypoxia (**goal setting** and **taking action**)

○ identify clinical criteria for determining the effectiveness of nursing actions taken to manage respiratory distress and hypoxia (**evaluate**)

○ apply what you have learnt about respiratory distress and hypoxia to clinical situations (**reflection** and **translation**).

INTRODUCTION

This chapter focuses on the care of Mr Trent Fulton, a 35-year-old man with a history of asthma who is diagnosed with community-acquired pneumonia. Respiratory diseases are the most common conditions treated by Australian General Practitioners (GPs) (20 per cent of all encounters). In 2013, almost 2500 deaths were attributed to pneumonia and influenza, and 0.3 per cent of all deaths were asthma related. Asthma is one of Australia's National Health Priority Areas, and an estimated 2.5 million children and adults were diagnosed with this respiratory condition in 2014–15 (Australian Institute of Health and Welfare [AIHW], 2016).

People with asthma can experience reduced quality of life and require a wide range of health services, from primary and tertiary care consultations to Emergency Department visits and hospital inpatient care. Symptoms of asthma are usually reversible with treatment; however, severe exacerbations, or 'flare ups', of the disease can result in death. Whilst death rates from asthma in Australia have fallen over the years, they are still considered high by international standards. However, many asthma-related deaths are avoidable. Clinical reasoning skills are therefore imperative to prevent deterioration, adverse patient outcomes and death (AIHW, 2014).

KEY CONCEPTS

asthma
community-acquired
    pneumonia
hypoxia
oxygenation
respiratory distress

SUGGESTED READINGS

P. LeMone, K. Burke,
G. Bauldoff, P. Gubrud-Howe,
T. Levett-Jones,
T. Dwyer ... D. Raymond
(Eds). (2017). *Medical–Surgical Nursing: Critical Thinking in Person-Centred Care* (3rd edn). Melbourne: Pearson.

Chapter 33: A person-centred approach to assessing the respiratory system

Chapter 34: Assessing clients with upper respiratory disorders

Chapter 35: Nursing care of clients with ventilation disorders

Chapter 36: Nursing care of clients with gas exchange disorders

Caring for a person with hypoxia and hypoxaemia

SETTING THE SCENE

Research has identified new hope for asthma sufferers. Go to this National Health and Medical Research site for more information: <www.nhmrc.gov. au/_files_nhmrc/media_ releases/161014_ media_release_ asthma_0.pdf>.

Mr Trent Fulton, a normally fit and healthy 35-year-old gym instructor, had seen his GP complaining of shortness of breath, fever, headaches and a productive cough over the past week. The GP diagnosed Trent with a respiratory tract infection and prescribed roxithromycin (Rulide) 150 mg BD. After taking the antibiotic for two days, he returned to his GP feeling much worse. A chest X-ray showed bilateral pneumonia and Trent was admitted to hospital via the Emergency Department (ED).

Trent has a history of mild asthma which he has had since childhood. His symptoms often get worse with exercise and he takes salbutamol (Ventolin) via a metered dose inhaler (MDI) for symptom relief. Over the past few months, Trent and his partner, Ian, have been converting an old warehouse into a gym. During this time, both of them developed 'flu'-like symptoms, sore throats and chest infections. Trent has not had an influenza or pneumococcal vaccination as he says he 'doesn't believe in vaccinations'. He is immunocompetent and has not recently travelled to tropical Australia or overseas. When Trent arrives at the hospital with Ian, he appears anxious and breathless.

Trent and Ian at their gym

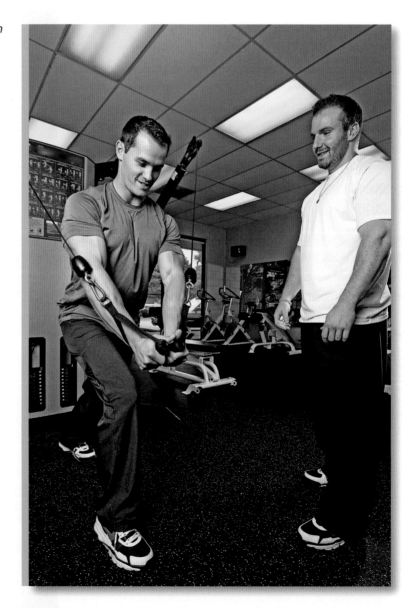

The epidemiology of pneumonia and asthma

In Australia, each year over 2000 people die from pneumonia, often as a complication of another respiratory disease. Aboriginal and Torres Strait Islander people are more likely to be hospitalised with pneumonia than non-Indigenous Australians (AIHW, 2014); the elderly and people who are immunocompromised are more likely to die as a result of this disease.

Australia has one of the highest rates of asthma in the world, with approximately 10 per cent of people affected. Rates of asthma are higher in Aboriginal and Torres Strait Islander people and people from lower socio-economic areas (AIHW, 2016).

> *The NSQHS Standards emphasise the importance of reducing the risk of patients acquiring preventable healthcare-associated infections, effectively managing infections if they occur and prudently using antimicrobial medications (ACSQHC, 2016).*

The aetiology and pathogenesis of pneumonia and asthma

Pneumonia is defined as inflammation of the lung parenchyma resulting from either infectious or non-infectious causes. Non-infectious causes include aspiration of gastric contents and inhalation of toxic gases (Hales, 2017). Infectious organisms include bacteria, viruses, fungi and protozoa. When infectious organisms colonise the alveoli of the lungs, inflammatory and immune responses occur. This in turn leads to vascular congestion and oedema as well as accumulation of infectious debris. Ventilation and gas exchange are impaired resulting in breathlessness and hypoxia. Pneumonia can be classified as either community-acquired or hospital-acquired (nosocomial). Community-acquired pneumonia is more common and results in approximately 1400 deaths per year. Hospital-acquired pneumonia results in 900 deaths per year (AIHW, 2014).

Asthma is a chronic inflammatory disorder of the airways characterised by variable episodes of wheezing, breathlessness, chest tightness and coughing, together with variable expiratory airflow limitation. These symptoms and the degree of airflow limitation usually vary in intensity and over time. Symptoms can reverse either spontaneously or with treatment (Hales, 2017); however, in some cases, particularly those complicated by infections and respiratory failure, acute asthma can result in death.

> *Access the NSW Health Community Acquired Pneumonia (CAP) Cheat Sheet at <http://cec.health.nsw.gov.au/__data/assets/pdf_file/0018/282114/CAP_Cheat_Sheet.pdf>.*

In asthma, airway narrowing can occur after a trigger initiates an inflammatory response leading to excess mucus production, bronchial oedema and airway hyper-responsiveness with broncho-constriction. Common triggers for asthma include household dust and allergens; environmental pollutants such as tobacco smoke, noxious gases and chemicals; respiratory infections; exercise; and emotional stress. Medications such as aspirin, non-steroidal anti-inflammatory drugs and beta-blockers can also trigger asthma (Hales, 2017).

Admission to the Emergency Department

On admission to the ED, Trent is sweating (diaphoretic) and flushed. He is alert and orientated but very breathless, with slight chest pain which he rates as 2 out of 10 on the numerical pain scale. Trent has a productive cough with green and malodorous sputum. The doctor examines Trent and notes decreased air entry and breath sounds and coarse rales (crackles) on the left side. His chest X-ray (CXR) shows consolidation in the middle left lobe but no pleural effusion. Trent says he has never smoked and drinks only socially. He is admitted to the medical ward accompanied by Ian, who helps him settle in and then goes home to look after their two dogs.

Admission observations

Temperature	38.8°C
Pulse rate	128 beats/min
Respiratory rate	31 breaths/min
Blood pressure	100/60 mmHg
SpO_2	92% on room air
ABGs	PaO_2 55, $PaCO_2$ 32, pH 7.48, bicarbonate 24 mEq/L

Co-morbidities

Asthma

Medical orders

Sputum cultures and sensitivities

Blood cultures

Serum for mycoplasma IgM

Influenza PCR nose and throat swab samples

MSU

Oxygen 4 L via nasal prongs

IV benzylpenicillin 1.2 g, every 6 hours

Oral doxycycline 200 µg day 1, then 100 µg daily for 5 days

Salbutamol (ventolin) via nebuliser, 5 mg in 1 mL normal saline (NS)

Chest physiotherapy

Q The decision to admit Trent was based on which parameters? (Select the three correct answers.)

    a Temperature: 38.8°C

    b Urine output: 40 mL/hr

    c Pain level: 2 out of 10

    d Blood pressure: 100/60 mmHg

    e Respiratory rate: 31 breaths/min

    f Pulse rate: 128 beats/min

    g Mental status: alert and orientated

> *Access the following resource and calculate Trent's risk of pneumonia using one of the pneumonia risk scores provided: <www.aci.health.nsw.gov.au/networks/eci/clinical/clinical-resources/clinical-tools/respiratory/pneumonia/pneumonia-scores>.*

Person-centred care

Trent was born in Tamworth where his parents and sister still live. At school, Trent excelled academically and in sport, despite having exercise-induced asthma. He moved to Sydney when he was 18 to undertake an accountancy degree. Ten years later, Trent completed a Certificate IV in fitness and qualified as a master trainer. With Ian, his partner of many years, he is now establishing his own gym. Trent has been working long hours and has also been training for an upcoming marathon.

1. CONSIDER THE PATIENT SITUATION

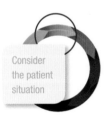

Morning handover report

Trent had a very disturbed evening after his partner left. At 2000 hours, we found him out of bed with his nasal prongs still in place but the tubing detached from the oxygen outlet. He was a bit confused and disorientated and it took us 25 minutes to settle him down. We eventually got him back to bed and put his oxygen on, but he was reluctant to lie down. At 0200 hours, his temperature was 39°C and his respirations were 33 per minute. It was difficult to monitor his saturations as he kept removing his finger probe but they varied between 80 and 92 per cent, so I changed him to a Hudson mask at 6 L/min.

After handover, you read through Trent's admission notes before going to his room.

QUICK QUIZ!

The admission notes and the handover report use a number of abbreviations and terminologies that you should be familiar with.

Q1 Match the terminology to the correct definition.

Diaphoretic	Increased respiratory rate
Febrile	A test of gases and pH in arterial blood
Tachycardic	Areas of density due to fluid, mucus and oedema on a chest X-ray

Tachypnoeic	Sweaty
Sats	High heart rate
ABGs	Coughing bloody sputum
Coarse rales	Bluish tinge around skin, nail beds and mucus due to lack of oxygen in blood
Haemoptysis	A series of short low popping sounds, also called 'crackles'
Cyanosis	High temperature
Consolidation	A test of the oxygen-saturated haemoglobin

Q2 Trent's oxygen flow rate with the Hudson mask was 6 L/min. What FiO_2% or percentage of oxygen was being delivered?

Q3 Trent's tachypnoea and cough are most likely due to which of the following?

   a His upper respiratory tract infection

   b His history of smoking

   c Early pulmonary oedema

   d None of the above

Q4 Pneumonia affects gas exchange in which of the following structures of the lungs?

   a Pleural space

   b Alveoli

   c Bronchi and bronchioles

   d Trachea

Access the Agency for Clinical Innovation web page for more information on pneumonia at <www.aci.health.nsw.gov.au/networks/eci/clinical/clinical-resources/clinical-tools/respiratory/pneumonia>.

2. COLLECT CUES/INFORMATION

(a) Review current information

While you are thinking about Trent's care, you look at his CXR.

Q You would expect a healthy patient to have areas of lung consolidation on chest X-ray.

   a True

   b False

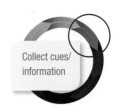

Collect cues/information

(b) Gather new information

You enter Trent's room and he appears to be more settled than he was overnight. His oxygen mask is still in place. You do another set of observations, with the following results:

Temperature	38.8°C
Pulse rate	110 beats/min
Respiratory rate	33 breaths/min
Blood pressure	100/55 mmHg
SpO_2	90%

You then repeat Trent's ABGs.

To help with this question, access <www.patient.info/doctor/chest-x-ray-systematic-approach>.

Q1 Which of the following should be included in an assessment for someone with suspected pneumonia? (Select the five most correct responses.)

   a Urine output

   b White cell count

c   Past cardiac history

d   ECG

e   Urinalysis

f   Mental status

g   Full blood count and serum electrolytes

h   Breath sounds

i   Assessment of pursed-lip breathing and/or use of accessory muscles

Q2   A person with pneumonia is likely to display rales (crackles) on auscultation.

a   True

b   False

Q3   A person with pneumonia is likely to display hyper-resonance on percussion.

a   True

b   False

Q4   Which two of the following is an abnormal finding on chest inspection?

a   Respiratory rate of 12–20 breaths/min in an adult

b   Abdominal movement

c   Mouth breathing

d   Inspiration lasting approximately twice as long as expiration

Q5   The body's respiratory centre is primarily stimulated by:

a   An increase in heart rate

b   A rise in blood carbon dioxide

c   A decrease in blood oxygen

d   All of the above

Q6   List four common causes of low arterial oxygen levels (hypoxaemia).

Q7   The inflammation of pneumonia is most likely to cause a change in:

a   Pulmonary circulation

b   Diffusion of gases

c   Work of breathing

d   Regulation of breathing

Q8   A person experiencing respiratory difficulties may be able to speak only one or two words between breaths.

a   True

b   False

Q9   When gathering information from a person who is very breathless, it is important to ask _____ ended questions.

> *To revise your knowledge of respiration and ventilation, access these web-based activities:*
>
> *<www.getbodysmart.com/ap/respiratorysystem/menu/menu.html>*
>
> *<www.khanacademy.org/science/health-and-medicine/respiratory-system-diseases>.*

> *Access these guidelines for acute oxygen use in adults: <www.thoracic.org.au/journal-publishing/command/download_file/id/34/filename/TSANZ-AcuteOxygen-Guidelines-2016-web.pdf>.*

(c) Recall knowledge

Care of a patient experiencing respiratory difficulties can be challenging because it requires analysis of the properties of gases and gaseous exchange, lung volumes and the mechanics of breathing, and the ability to apply this knowledge to clinical situations that are often complex and quickly changing.

QUICK QUIZ!

Test yourself with the following questions about pneumonia and hypoxia.

Q1 Select from the following, four groups of people most likely to be affected by pneumonia.

    a   Older people

    b   Sportsmen/women

    c   Those with alcoholism

    d   Immunocompromised people

    e   Indigenous Australians

    f   Those with a chronic illness

    g   Those with cancer

Q2 Match the following descriptions with the correct definition.

Build-up of fluid in the space between the lung and chest wall	Malaise
Pockets of pus in the space between the lung and chest wall	Bacteremia or septicaemia
Sputum material coughed up from the lungs	Lung abscess
Pockets of pus that form in the lung itself	Mucus production
Secondary bacterial lung infection after a viral infection	Pleural effusion
Bacteria in the bloodstream or throughout the body	Empyema
Clinical sign of hypoxia, manifested by a feeling of breathlessness	Secondary infection
Subjective sensation of a patient reporting loss of endurance	Dyspnoea
Generalised feeling of being unwell	Fatigue

> *Registered nurses require highly developed skills in patient assessment and, according to the NMBA's Registered Nurse Standards for Practice (2016), they must use a range of assessment techniques to systematically collect relevant and accurate information to inform their practice.*

3. PROCESS INFORMATION

(a) Interpret

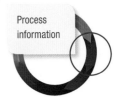

Process information

You review and interpret all the information you have about Trent's respiratory condition.

Q1 Trent's respiratory rate is 33 breaths/min. Is this described as tachypnoea or orthopnoea?

Q2 You review Trent's current ABGs. His PaO_2 is 50 mmHg. The normal PaO_2 for a healthy man of Trent's age would be between _____ and _____.

Q3 Trent's $PaCO_2$ is 37. A normal $PaCO_2$ for Trent would be between _____ and _____, while a normal pH would be between _____ and _____.

> *Access further information on arterial blood gases at <http://patient.info/doctor/arterial-blood-gases-indications-and-interpretation>.*

Q4 Trent's $PaCO_2$ is low and his pH of 7.45 indicates alkalosis. The most likely reason for this would be:

    a   Trent's respiratory rate is raised due to hypoxaemia and a low PaO_2 and he is retaining CO_2 which has raised his pH.

    b   Trent's respiratory rate is raised as he is hypoxic, he has a low PaO_2, and his rapid respiratory rate has caused him to 'blow off' CO_2 and raise his pH.

    c   Trent's respiratory rate is decreased, so he is retaining CO_2 and his pH is consequently raised.

    d   Trent's respiratory rate is faster and the low PaO_2 is causing a raised pH.

(b) Discriminate

From the cues and information you now have, you need to narrow down the information and identify what is most important.

To help you answer this question, access the Clinical Excellence Commission's Between the Flags: Standard Calling Criteria (2016): <www.cec.health.nsw. gov.au/patient-safety-programs/adult-patient-safety/between-the-flags/standard-calling-criteria>.

Q1 Select four cues that you believe are *most relevant* to the assessment of Trent's hypoxia.

a Blood pressure: 100/55 mmHg

b Respiratory rate: 33 breaths/min

c Temperature: 38.8°C

d Pulse rate: 110 beats/min

e Headache

f SpO_2: 90% on room air

g Appetite: decreased

h ABGs: PaO_2 50 mmHg, $PaCO_2$ 37 mmHg, pH 7.45

i Urine output: 40 mL/hr

Q2 When Trent complained of some pain in the chest during his initial assessment in the ED, the nurse asked him to describe the pain and whether it was travelling to his jaw or to his left arm. The nurse's question was asked to determine whether the chest pain could be due to:

a Myocardial infarction

b Congestive heart failure

c Bronchitis

d Pneumonia

(c) Relate

It is important to cluster the cues together and to identify relationships between them (based on the information you have collected so far).

Q1 Which of the following statements are true?

a Trent is tachypnoeic due to a high fever.

b Trent is hypoxic as mucus is partially blocking his airways and impeding gas exchange.

c Trent's pulse is faster as a compensatory mechanism to increase gas exchange.

Q2 Select the most important cue cluster for a patient with pneumonia.

a Purulent sputum, clubbing of the fingers, cyanosis, cough, hyper-resonance, excessive thirst

b Cough, low oxygen saturations, a high BGL, retention of fluid as evidenced by weight gain, hypo-resonance, tactile fremitus

c Tachypnea, fever, purulent sputum, a cough, coarse rales, oxygen saturation lower than normal

d Weight loss over a few weeks, fatigue, low oxygen saturations, frothy blood-tinged sputum

(d) Infer

It is time to think about all the cues you have collected about Trent's condition, and make inferences based on your analysis and interpretation of those cues.

Q1 In your opinion, and from what you know of Trent's history, signs and symptoms, Trent is (select two from the list below):

a Afebrile and tachypnoeic

b Hypertensive and tachycardic

c Tachypnoeic and tachycardic

d Hypertensive and afebrile

e Hypoxic and febrile

f Hypotensive and afebrile

Q2   Select five early signs of hypoxia from the list below.

   a   Tachypnoea or bradypnoea

   b   Dyspnoea

   c   Tachycardia or bradycardia

   d   Hypotension

   e   Fatigue

   f   Cyanosis

   g   Cardiac arrhythmias

   h PaO_2 50–60 mmHg

   i $PaCO_2$ 50–60 mmHg

   j   Confusion

Q3   From the list below, select the seven late signs of hypoxia.

   a   Dyspnoea

   b   Tachypnoea or bradypnoea

   c   Cyanosis

   d   Unresponsiveness to verbal command

   e   Tachycardia or bradycardia

   f   Hypertension

   g   Cardiac arrhythmias

   h   Fatigue

   i   Hypotension

   j PaO_2 <50 mmHg

   k $PaCO_2$ >60 mmHg

   l SpO_2 <90%

Q4   Trent's SpO_2 and PaO_2 are both abnormal, indicating hypoxia. What factors do you think have contributed to his hypoxia? (Select two.)

   a   Age

   b   Partial obstruction of his airways by mucus

   c   History of smoking

   d   Poor gas exchange due to mucus and fluid in the alveoli

   e   History of asthma

(e) Predict

Q1   If you do not take the appropriate actions at this time, what could happen to Trent if his hypoxia is not corrected? (Select two.)

   a   He will gradually improve over the next few days.

   b   He may become even more febrile and develop delirium.

   c   His chest pain could worsen leading to a cardiac arrest.

   d   His hypoxia will worsen and may lead to a respiratory arrest.

Q2   From the following list, choose the clinical indicator *most* indicative of impending respiratory arrest.

   a   Blood pressure: 100/55 mmHg

   b   Respiratory rate: 33 breaths/min

    c   Urine output: 40 mL/hr

    d   ABGs: PaO_2 50 mmHg, $PaCO_2$ 37 mmHg, pH 7.45

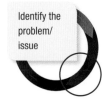

4. IDENTIFY THE PROBLEM/ISSUE

Q   Now bring together (synthesise) all of the facts you've collected and inferences you've made to identify the most correct nursing diagnosis for Trent.

    a   Risk of hypoxia due to confusion, low SpO_2 level, tachypnoea and abnormal ABGs

    b   Hypoxia related to ineffective breathing pattern as evidenced by confusion, low SpO_2, tachypnoea and abnormal ABGs

    c   Impaired gas exchange related to airway obstruction due to excessive secretions, bronchospasm and alveoli destruction

    d   Risk of oxygen toxicity related to the provision of high concentrations of oxygen over a prolonged period of time

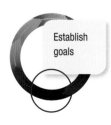

5. ESTABLISH GOALS

Before implementing any actions to improve Trent's condition, it is important to clearly specify what you want to happen and when.

Q   From the list below, choose the most important short-term goal for Trent's management at this time.

    a   For Trent to be afebrile and to have no pain within 20 minutes

    b   For Trent's infection to be resolved within 3–5 days

    c   For Trent to have a normal respiratory rate and an oxygen saturation level of >94%

    d   For Trent to be normotensive and euvolaemic

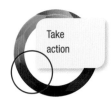

6. TAKE ACTION

Now you have a nursing diagnosis and short-term goals for Trent you need to identify appropriate nursing actions.

Q1   In the table below, match the rationales for care to the corresponding nursing action.

Nursing action	Rationale
Monitor oxygen saturations and ABGs regularly	Anxiety and restlessness may indicate worsening hypoxia
Check cognitive status regularly	To maintain psychosocial wellbeing
Position in semi- or high Fowler's	Changes may indicate worsening hypoxia
Teach patient deep breathing and coughing	To aid in removal of secretions
Keep patient well hydrated	To reduce pain and increase comfort
Maintain oxygen therapy via nasal prongs or Hudson mask	To increase partial pressure of oxygen in alveoli and increase diffusion into capillaries
Reassure patient and reduce anxiety	To reduce oxygen demand
Give patient paracetamol	To reduce viscosity of secretions

Respiratory conditions can change rapidly. When you check on Trent 15 minutes later, you find him collapsed on the floor with his oxygen disconnected. He is cyanotic and does not answer your questions. You note that he now has stridor. You do another set of observations, with the following results:

Respiratory rate	irregular and 5 breaths/min
Pulse rate	38 beats/min
Blood pressure	75/60 mmHg
SpO_2	85%

Q2 Identify three priority nursing actions from the list below:

  a Reassure patient.

  b Run to find another nurse to help you.

  c Initiate a rapid response or medical emergency team (MET) call.

  d Reconnect the oxygen.

  e Get ready to start CPR (cardiopulmonary resuscitation).

  f Check that Trent's fluids are running.

  g Monitor Trent's pain score.

  h Monitor Trent's vital signs and oxygen saturation level.

Q3 Identify three factors that may have caused deterioration in Trent's respiratory status, leading to severe hypoxia and acute respiratory failure.

> Members of the rapid response team typically include:
> ICU resident or registrar
> ICU ALS-trained RN
> Cardiology registrar or medical registrar.

  a Trent was given too much to drink as well as IV fluids, leading to fluid overload and pulmonary oedema.

  b The increase in Trent's mucus secretions led to decreased gas exchange.

  c Increasing confusion and continual removal of the oxygen mask led to increasing hypoxia.

  d Ventilation was reduced due to reduced chest wall expansion from increasing, untreated pain.

  e Decreased neurological status due to administering the central nervous system (CNS) depressant morphine, which affected the brain stem and reduced breathing rate.

  f Failure of the ward nurses to recognise Trent's increasing respiratory distress as evidenced by his increasing confusion and low SpO_2.

While waiting for the rapid response team/MET to arrive, a senior nurse comes to help and changes Trent's Hudson mask to a non-rebreather mask with a flow rate of 12 L/min. You are confused as you thought that nurses are only allowed to initiate oxygen using nasal prongs at 2 L/min. Access and read the article in the margin note, and decide what you would do in a similar situation.

> For further information, access Wong, M. & Elliott, M. (2009). The use of medical orders in acute care oxygen therapy. *British Journal of Nursing*, 18(8), 462–64.

Q4 Match the oxygen delivery devices to the appropriate flow rate and FiO_2:

Oxygen delivery device	Flow rate	FiO_2
Nasal prongs	6–15 L/min	0.24–0.36
Hudson mask	10–15 L/min	0.4–0.6
Non-rebreather mask	2–4 L/min	0.6–0.9

7. EVALUATE

Q1 With the correct treatment, you would expect Trent's SpO_2 to increase to ~97% and his respiratory rate decrease to between 12 and 18 if his condition resolves.

  a True

  b False

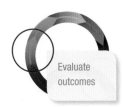

Evaluate outcomes

Q2 Match the expected outcome measures with the appropriate interventions:

Changing Hudson mask to a non-rebreather mask to increase available oxygen to improve Trent's oxygenation	Trent reports adequate sleep and rest
Position Trent in a high Fowler's to assist lung expansion	SpO$_2$ increases from 94% to 97%
Monitor Trent's vital signs every hour	Trent is able to expectorate secretions effectively
Promote adequate rest to support Trent's recovery	Changes in condition are identified early and associated actions initiated

Q3 What nursing actions may have prevented Trent's deterioration? (Choose three from the list below.)

    a A sedative should have been administered to help Trent settle.

    b More frequent observations of pulse oximetry and vital signs should have been conducted.

    c The significance of his ABGs should have been recognised.

    d A medical review should have been requested earlier.

    e Trent's fluids should have been increased.

    f Trent should have received more antibiotics to treat his infection.

Q4 The table below compares Trent's observations across his admission. Write one sentence that evaluates the trend.

Observations

On admission	0700	Now
Temperature 38.8°C	Temperature 38.8°C	Temperature 39°C
Pulse 128	Pulse 110	Pulse 38
Respiratory rate 31	Respiratory rate 33	Respiratory rate 5; stridor and cyanosis present
SpO$_2$ 92% on room air	SpO$_2$ 90% on 6 L/min via Hudson mask	SpO$_2$ 85% on 6 L/min via Hudson mask
Blood pressure 100/60 mmHg	Blood pressure 100/55 mmHg	Blood pressure 78/60 mmHg
ABGs PaO$_2$ 55, PaCO$_2$ 32, pH 7.48, bicarbonate 24 mEq/L	ABGs PaO$_2$ 50, PaCO$_2$ 37, pH 7.45, bicarbonate 24 mEq/L	

> The rapid response team uses the mnemonic DRABCD to assess and manage Trent:
> Danger
> Response
> Airway
> Breathing
> Circulation
> Defibrillation (not required)

    The rapid response team/MET quickly respond to your call. Trent is ventilated and transferred to the Intensive Care Unit (ICU) for further care. He remains in ICU for the next few days, until his condition improves and he returns to the ward.

8. REFLECT

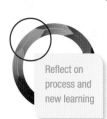

Reflect on process and new learning

Reflect on your learning from this scenario and consider the following questions.

Q1 What factors led to Trent's deterioration? Were they preventable?

Q2 What are three of the most important things that you have learnt from this scenario?

Q3 What actions will you take in clinical practice as a result of your learning from this scenario?

Q4 How would you respond to a colleague in the future if you believe that their clinical decision making is incorrect?

 SCENARIO 6.2 Caring for a person with respiratory distress

CHANGING THE SCENE

1. CONSIDER THE PATIENT SITUATION

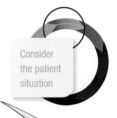

Consider the patient situation

Trent responds well to his treatment and, although he has been spiking temperatures during the last few days, he is now afebrile. Although he still feels fatigued at times, Trent wants to go home as the opening date for the gym is fast approaching and he and Ian need to finish the renovations. However, Trent confides in you that he is feeling anxious as he has had increasing episodes of what he describes as 'chest tightness' over the last two days.

Q1 Label the following as either objective or subjective clinical data.

    a Increased pulse rate

    b A nurse's assessment of a patient's temperature

    c A patient's report of breathlessness

    d Trent's complaint of chest tightness

In preparation for this scenario, access the Australian Asthma Handbook at <www.nationalasthma.org.au/health-professionals/australian-asthma-handbook>.

Q2 To further understand Trent's 'chest tightness', you would collect information about which of the following? (Select all you consider to be appropriate.)

    a Circulation

    b Respiration

    c Comfort

    d Skin

    e Pain

    f Sleep/rest pattern

    g Nutrition

    h Coping strategies

    i Musculoskeletal system

Q3 Which communication strategy would be most effective when assessing Trent's 'chest tightness'? (Select four correct responses.)

    a Using a calm tone of voice

    b Communicating to Trent what you think his problem is

    c Observing Trent's behaviours and respiratory effort

    d Assessing Trent's concerns while at the same time attending to other tasks and patients

    e Maintaining eye contact

    f Open-ended questions

    g Closed questions

2. COLLECT CUES/INFORMATION

(a) Review current information

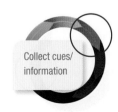

Collect cues/information

You review Trent's charts and note the following:

Temperature	37°C
Pulse rate	110 beats/min

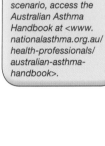

Respiratory rate	26 breaths/min
Blood pressure	140/85 mmHg
SpO_2	94% on room air
Hourly urine output (average)	40 mL/hr
Breath sounds	wheezing on auscultation
BGL	6.2 mmol/L

Q1 Which of these observations are not within normal limits?

Q2 While you are talking with Trent, he tells you that he had a vision when he was in ICU where an angel came and watched over him. From the following list, choose how you would respond.

   a Your vision probably occurred because you were hypoxic.

   b You were very ill at the time; it must be comforting to believe that someone was looking after you.

   c It was probably one of the nurses as angels don't exist.

   d Only a Catholic could believe that they saw an angel.

(b) Gather new information

Q You note that Trent is dyspnoeic. What respiratory assessments are required at this stage?

(c) Recall knowledge

QUICK QUIZ!

Q1 A wheeze is caused by:

   a Collapsed alveoli

   b Fluid in the alveoli

   c Narrowed airways

   d Collapsed lungs

Q2 An asthma exacerbation can be caused by substances released from mast cells which cause:

   a Smooth muscle dilation

   b Bronchodilation and capillary permeability

   c Broncho-constriction and inflammation

   d Decreased capillary permeability and fluid leakage

Q3 FEV_1 can be defined as:

   a The rate of gas exchange in the alveoli during normal respiration

   b The maximum amount of air a person is capable of blowing in one second

   c The amount of air left in the lungs at the end of maximal forced expiration

   d The amount of air that is breathed in and out during a single respiratory cycle

Q4 Expiration occurs when:

   a The intercostal muscles and diaphragm relax

   b The intercostal muscles and diaphragm contract

   c The diaphragm rises and the ribs move upward and outward

   d The air pressure inside the thorax decreases and becomes less than external air pressure

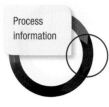

Process information

3. PROCESS INFORMATION

(a) Interpret, (b) Discriminate and (c) Relate

Q1 Which of the following is the *most* characteristic alteration in lung volume caused by air trapping in asthma?

    a   Tidal volume

    b   Inspiratory reserve volume

    c   Expiratory reserve volume

    d   Functional residual capacity

Q2 Which of the following is *necessary* to diagnose asthma?

    a   Reversibility of airflow limitation

    b   Reduced FEV_1

    c   Reduced FVC

    d   Irreversibility of airflow limitation

Q3 Which of the following is *not* suggestive of asthma?

    a   Chest tightness that recurs

    b   Cough that becomes worse at night

    c   Stridor

    d   Wheezing

Q4 Which of the following are characteristic of asthma? (Select four.)

    a   Clubbing of the fingers

    b   Shortness of breath

    c   Cough

    d   Blood pressure >140/90 mmHg

    e   Chest tightness

    f   Barrel chest

    g   Chest pain

    h   Wheeze

(d) Infer

Q   Which of the following factors might indicate asthma? (Select all you consider appropriate.)

    a   Presence of coarse rales (crackles)

    b   Worsening symptoms after taking aspirin or beta-blockers

    c   Worsening signs and symptoms after exposure to an identified allergy trigger

    d   A previous allergic reaction of any kind

(e) Predict

Q   Select four factors that would put Trent at an increased risk of deterioration.

    a   Previous ICU admissions

    b   Infrequent, mild asthma attacks

    c   Frequent prior hospitalisations

    d   Asthma requiring use of a reliever occasionally (once a month)

    e   Current or recent use of oral corticosteroids

    f   Previous severe exacerbations requiring hospitalisation

    g   No previous admissions to hospital

(f) Match

Q   Have you seen someone with the same signs and symptoms as Trent? If so, what was done to manage the situation?

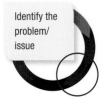

4. IDENTIFY THE PROBLEM/ISSUE

The current information that you have collected about Trent includes:

Temperature	37°C
Pulse rate	120
Respiratory rate	26
Blood pressure	140/85
Oxygen saturation level	93% on room air
Hourly urine output (average)	40 mL/hr
BGL	6.2 mmol/L
Breath sounds	wheezing on auscultation
Cough	productive
Spirometry	airflow limitation
Chest tightness	
Fatigue	

Q   Use this information to complete the following nursing diagnoses for Trent.

   a   Ineffective breathing pattern related to _____ and respiratory muscle fatigue, evidenced by restlessness, _____, tachypnoea, _____ and chest tightness.

   b   _____ related to bronchospasm and excess secretion, and retention of mucus, evidenced by _____, chest tightness, _____ and dyspnoea.

   c   Impaired gas exchange related to _____, and decreased amount of air exchanged during inspiration and expiration, evidenced by low _____ dyspnoea, _____, anxiety and coughing.

5. ESTABLISH GOALS

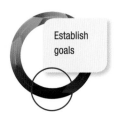

Q1   In relation to the nursing identified diagnoses, what are the three *most* appropriate short-term goals of management for Trent.

   a   For Trent to have normal food and fluid intake

   b   For Trent to feel calm and relaxed without chest tightness or discomfort, and for his respiratory rate to be within normal limits

   c   For Trent to have clear lung sounds and a reduced amount of secretions

   d   For Trent to be able to resume his normal exercise regime

   e   For Trent to have effective gas exchange, without dyspnoea or tachypnoea and with normal SpO$_2$ level

Q2   Side effects of bronchodilators that Trent may experience are:

   a   Insomnia and restless legs

   b   Dry mouth and furry tongue

   c   Palpitations, tachycardia and tremors

   d   Eye-watering and runny nose

6. TAKE ACTION

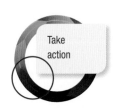

Q   In the table below, match the nursing interventions you would take to the appropriate rationale, in order to achieve the above goals.

Place in high Fowler's position	To detect increasing tachypnoea, tachycardia and increasing respiratory distress
Administer oxygen	To aid in bronchodilation
Administer nebuliser/spacer treatments as ordered	To conserve energy and reduce fatigue
Assess level of understanding of asthma and management	To promote rest
Monitor vital signs and laboratory results	To promote self-management in the recovery and rehabilitation phase
Assist with ADLs as needed	To reduce hypoxaemia
Provide rest between scheduled activities and reduce excessive environmental stimulus	To reduce the work of breathing and increase lung expansion

Trent is reviewed by the doctor who starts him on a preventer medication—fluticasone and salmeterol (Seretide), an inhaled corticosteroid—with a spacer, and long-acting β_2-agonist combination therapy. He is continued on the short-acting β_2-agonist, salbutamol (Ventolin), as a reliever therapy and commenced on home monitoring of his peak expiratory flow rate. He is also referred to the asthma physician and educator for review of his asthma management plan in preparation for discharge.

7. EVALUATE

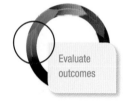

Evaluate outcomes

Q1 List five signs and symptoms you will observe Trent for, to determine whether his condition improves following clinical review and initiation of appropriate actions.

Q2 From the list below, select the four *most appropriate* interventions for long-term management of Trent's asthma.

  a Provide written or verbal instructions of correct techniques for use of inhalers.

  b Provide supplemental oxygen.

  c Teach the correct use of a PEFR meter.

  d Teach the importance of continuing his preventer medication, even if he feels well.

  e Discuss lifestyle changes, such as premedicating with his reliever therapy and warming up slowly before exercising.

  f Discuss dietary changes such as a low-fat, low-salt diet.

  g Discuss weight reduction strategies.

8. REFLECT

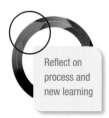

Reflect on process and new learning

Reflect on what happened to Trent and the care he received. Answer the following questions.

Q1 How could Trent's deterioration have been prevented?

Q2 What have you learnt from the scenario that you can apply to your future practice?

Q3 Why do some people with asthma develop a worsening of their symptoms after and during an acute respiratory infection?

Q4 Based on what you have learnt from this scenario, what advice would you give to people with asthma?

EPILOGUE

The gym opening had to be delayed for a few weeks while Trent recovered, but it was successfully launched two months later. Trent has remained well with no further respiratory infections. He visited his GP, respiratory physician and asthma educator and, with their help, developed a written asthma management plan, and optimised his asthma management knowledge and skills (National Asthma Council Australia, 2016). He continues to take his preventer medication as prescribed and regularly monitors his peak flow rate. He has also implemented some changes to his lifestyle: spending more time warming up before running, and taking his reliever before exercising. He decided not to participate in the marathon but plans to compete in next year's City to Surf race.

Trent has his asthma reviewed by his GP every six months and whenever his symptoms start to flare up.

FURTHER READING

Flenady, T., Dwyer, T. & Applegarth, J. (2017). Accurate respiratory rates count: So should you! *Australasian Emergency Nursing Journal, 20*(1), 45–47. doi: 10.1016/j.aenj.2016.12.003

Parkes, R. (2011). Rate of respiration: The forgotten vital sign. *Emergency Nurse, 19*(2), 12–18.

Pruitt, B. & Lawson, R. (2011). Assessing and managing asthma: A global initiative for asthma update. *Nursing, 41*(5), 46–52.

REFERENCES

Australian Commission on Safety and Quality in Health Care (ACSQHC). (2016). *National Safety and Quality Health Service Standards Version 2*. Draft, Sydney, Australia.

Australian Institute of Health and Welfare (AIHW). (2016). *Australia's Health 2016*. Australia's Health Series No. 15. Cat. No. AUS 199. Canberra: AIHW. Accessed March 2017 at <www.aihw.gov.au/WorkArea/DownloadAsset.aspx?id=60129555788>.

AIHW: Poulos, L. M., Cooper, S. J., Ampon, R., Redell, H. K. & Marks, G. B. (2014). *Mortality from Asthma and COPD in Australia*. Cat. No. ACM 30. Canberra: AIHW.

Clinical Excellence Commission. (2016). *Between the Flags: Standard Calling Criteria*. Accessed December 2016 at <www.cec.health.nsw.gov.au/patient-safety-programs/adult-patient-safety/between-the-flags/standard-calling-criteria>.

Hales, M. (2017). A person-centred approach to assessing the respiratory system. In P. LeMone, K. Burke, G. Bauldoff, P. Gubrud-Howe, T. Levett-Jones, T. Dwyer, ... D. Raymond (Eds), *Medical–Surgical Nursing: Critical Thinking in Person-Centred Care* (3rd edn). Melbourne: Pearson.

National Asthma Council Australia. (2016). *Asthma Action Plan*. Accessed December 2016 at <www.nationalasthma.org.au/health-professionals/asthma-action-plans>.

Nursing and Midwifery Board of Australia (NMBA). (2016). *Registered Nurse Standards for Practice*. Accessed at <www.nursingmidwiferyboard.gov.au/Codes-Guidelines-Statements/Professional-standards.aspx>.

Wong, M. & Elliott, M. (2009). The use of medical orders in acute care oxygen therapy. *British Journal of Nursing, 18*(8), 462–64.

PHOTO CREDIT

98 © Mat Hayward—Fotolia.com.

CHAPTER 7

CARING FOR A PERSON WITH A CARDIAC CONDITION

KERRY HOFFMAN AND AMANDA WILSON

LEARNING OUTCOMES

Completion of the activities in this chapter will enable you to:

○ explain why an understanding of ischaemia and arrhythmias is essential to competent practice (**recall** and **application**)

○ identify the clinical manifestations of chest pain that will guide the collection and interpretation of cues (**gather**, **review**, **interpret**, **discriminate**, **relate** and **infer**)

○ identify risk factors for cardiac conditions (**match** and **predict**)

○ review clinical information to identify the main nursing diagnoses for a person with cardiac conditions (**synthesise**)

○ describe the priorities of care for a person with a cardiac condition (**goal setting** and **taking action**)

○ identify clinical criteria for determining the effectiveness of nursing actions when managing chest pain and arrhythmias (**evaluate**)

○ apply what you have learnt about cardiac conditions and ischaemia to new clinical situations with different patients (**reflection** and **translation**).

INTRODUCTION

This chapter focuses on the care of Mr David Parker, a 55-year-old man who experiences a prolonged episode of chest pain and is admitted to the regional hospital near where he lives. Early presentation to health services in the event of chest pain is a key factor that can influence positive clinical outcomes (National Heart Foundation of Australia, 2011a). Accurate assessment of a person presenting with chest pain requires well-developed clinical reasoning skills and a sound knowledge base.

Although 66 per cent of people who present to hospital with chest pain are admitted, only 15 per cent are confirmed to have had an acute myocardial infarction (AMI). However, rates of mortality for those who are not admitted are up to four times higher than those who are admitted, as up to 5 per cent will have had a missed AMI. Geographical location also impacts clinical outcomes, with mortality rates following AMI significantly worse for those in remote areas—10 per cent higher than in urban areas and 30 per cent higher in very remote areas of Australia. Outcomes from acute cardiac events are influenced by geographical location, delayed presentation to hospital, capabilities of the rural or remote health services and knowledge of the person experiencing the cardiac event (Baker et al., 2011).

KEY CONCEPTS

chest pain
arrhythmias
ischaemia
cardiac arrest
heart failure
rehabilitation

SUGGESTED READINGS

P. LeMone, K. Burke, G. Bauldoff, P. Gubrud-Howe, T. Levett-Jones, T. Dwyer ... D. Raymond (Eds). (2017). *Medical–Surgical Nursing: Critical Thinking in Person-Centred Care* (3rd edn). Melbourne: Pearson.

Chapter 28: A person-centred approach to assessing the cardiac and lymphatic systems

Chapter 29: Nursing care of people with coronary heart disease

Chapter 30: Nursing care of people with cardiac disorders

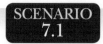

Caring for a person with ischaemic chest pain

SETTING THE SCENE

You are a registered nurse (RN) working in the Emergency Department of a regional hospital in the Snowy Mountains area when David Parker, a middle-aged man, is brought in by ambulance. His wife, Sophie, arrives at the same time through the main entrance. The man is sitting upright on the ambulance trolley with an oxygen mask over his ashen-grey face. He is diaphoretic and gripping the trolley with his right hand while his left hand is held close to his body holding an emesis bowl. He looks frightened. His wife rushes forward, telling him, 'Everything will be alright. You'll be fine.' She turns to you and asks, 'Won't he?'

The ambulance officer tells you that David was repairing fences on his property and the chest pain started when lifting heavy fence posts. He returned to the farmhouse and took some antacids but the pain continued. He had about two hours of central chest pain prior to his collapse at 1200 hours. He did not lose consciousness. Sophie called the ambulance against his wishes, as he had 'a lot of things to do'. The ambulance officer estimated the chest pain started at 1000 hours and it took the ambulance 90 minutes to get to the property and back. David's chest pain is centrally located and described as crushing. The pain is radiating to his left arm, neck and teeth. He is anxious and worried about his farm, where he runs large mobs of merino sheep. David is tachycardic and hypertensive. He has a history of hypertension but it is usually well controlled.

David Parker's farm in the Snowy Mountains, New South Wales

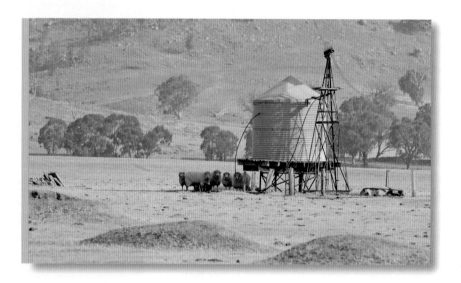

The epidemiology of ischaemic chest pain and heart failure

View this link for cardiovascular disease (CVD) mortality and trends at different ages: <www.aihw.gov.au/ cardiovascular-disease/ deaths>.

Coronary heart disease (CHD), also known as ischaemic heart disease (IHD), is the most common form of heart disease. There are two major clinical forms of CHD: (1) 'heart attack', clinically known as acute myocardial infarction (AMI); and (2) angina. CHD is responsible for 14 per cent of all deaths in Australia. In 2012, over 20 000 deaths were attributed to CHD, more than any other single disease; and of these, approximately half were from an acute AMI. Death rates from CHD have fallen steadily since the 1970s, not because there are fewer heart attacks, but because of better survival rates (AIHW, 2015a). CHD occurs more frequently in older people (2 per cent in those aged 45–54, rising to 17 per cent in Australians aged 75 years or over [AIHW, 2015b]). Men experience CHD more than women, and CHD is twice as common in Aboriginal people compared to non-Indigenous Australians (AIHW, 2015b).

The aetiology and pathogenesis of ischaemic chest pain and heart failure

The main cause of CHD is atherosclerosis, where lipids accumulate in the arteries forming a build-up called plaque. Blood flow through the coronary arteries becomes impaired by plaque as it reduces the lumen of these vessels. Plaque lesions may ulcerate, leading to clot (thrombus) formation that may completely block or occlude the vessel. The manifestations of CHD are angina pectoris, acute coronary syndrome and/or myocardial infarction. Chest pain precipitated by exercise (which increases oxygen demand) and relieved by rest (when oxygen meets myocardial demand) is the main characteristic of angina (LeMone et al., 2017).

If a coronary artery becomes completely occluded, blood supply to the myocardium is interrupted and the affected muscle tissue becomes ischaemic (acute coronary syndrome). These ischaemic tissues will eventually die if blood supply is not restored (myocardial infarction). Risk factors for CHD may be modifiable or non-modifiable and include age, heredity, hypertension, high serum cholesterol, diabetes mellitus and lifestyle factors, such as smoking, obesity and lack of exercise. Some of these risk factors are more common in Aboriginal and Torres Strait Islander people, with diabetes being four times as high as non-Indigenous people, and smoking and obesity twice as common in this population.

Heart failure is the most common disorder of cardiac function. It occurs as a result of impaired myocardial contraction. The heart cannot fill or contract with sufficient strength, so its ability to act as a pump is compromised. This 'pump failure' means there is less blood leaving the heart (cardiac output) and less oxygen reaching the body tissues (tissue perfusion). Hypertension is the leading cause of heart failure and the most common risk factor is CHD.

Admission to the Emergency Department

On admission to the Emergency Department (ED), David is diaphoretic and pale. He is alert and orientated but very anxious with central chest pain. The doctor examines him and orders a stat dose of IV morphine. David's ECG is attended and shows ischaemic injury (ST elevation) in the anterior leads. As ST elevation indicates a coronary artery blockage, treatment is aimed at unblocking the vessel.

The doctor asks David if he has any history of head injuries, malignancies, stroke or gastric bleeding to ensure there are no contraindications for thrombolytic treatment. No risk factors are identified and David is given thrombolytic therapy.

Admission observations

Temperature	36.8°C
Pulse rate	108 beats/min
Respiratory rate	24 breaths/min
Blood pressure	150/90 mmHg
SpO$_2$	95% on room air
BGL	14.1 mmol/L
Pain score	8
GCS	15

Co-morbidities

Osteoarthritis
Hypertension
Hyperlipidaemia
Type 2 diabetes mellitus

Medical orders

Full blood count (FBC)
Urea, electrolytes and creatinine (UECs)
Arterial blood gases (ABGs)
Troponin levels

> More information on risk prevention for CVD can be obtained from <https://heartfoundation.org.au/your-heart/know-your-risks>.

> The best treatment option for an AMI is percutaneous coronary intervention (PCI), provided an angiography laboratory is available. When this is not available, thrombolytic treatment is used to try to dissolve the clot. For more information, access the Acute Coronary Syndrome Clinical Care Standard at <https://safetyandquality.gov.au/wp-content/uploads/2014/12/Acute-Coronary-Syndromes-Clinical-Care-Standard.pdf>.

> Nurse Administered Thrombolysis (NAT) is a model of care for rural and remote hospitals that do not have 24-hour onsite doctors. The fact sheet for NAT (ACI, 2016) can be accessed at <www.aci.health.nsw.gov.au/__data/assets/pdf_file/0011/319196/NAT-clinican.pdf>.

Start GTN infusion and titrate to blood pressure and pain; maintain diastolic >60 mmHg

Morphine 2.5 mg IV PRN

Start rTPA

QUICK QUIZ!

Q1 The _____ has the thickest walls as it pumps blood to _____. Choose the correct response from the options below.

    a Right atrium, systemic circulation

    b Right ventricle, pulmonary circulation

    c Left atrium, pulmonary circulation

    d Left ventricle, systemic circulation

Q2 Freshly oxygenated blood enters the heart through the _____, and is pumped out into the _____. Choose the correct response from the options below.

    a Right atrium, aorta

    b Left atrium, aorta

    c Right ventricle, pulmonary arteries

    d Left ventricle, pulmonary arteries

Q3 Why do you think the ambulance officer was so precise in his estimation of times in David's admission story?

Person-centred care

Awareness of David's life story will assist you in understanding his responses to his situation, and in providing person-centred care. David is an Aboriginal man who was part of the 'stolen generation'. He was raised in a foster home in the region where he now lives. His childhood and adolescent life were difficult, although he managed to complete his schooling. He has no contact with any biological family members and does not know his family history. He believes that the past should remain 'where it can't hurt'.

David's foster family had a large property where he developed skills in animal husbandry, including breeding fine wool merino sheep. After school, he worked as a farm hand and, later, as a manager on the property where he now lives. David has a very strong work ethic and sense of responsibility. He married a local woman, Sophie, who is a teacher at the local high school and they have two teenage children. David's family describe him as 'driven' and as having difficulty relaxing. David smokes but he drinks alcohol only occasionally.

1. CONSIDER THE PATIENT SITUATION

Consider the patient situation

It is now eight hours since confirmation that David has had an acute myocardial infarction (AMI). He has been increasingly agitated since his admission, wanting to call the farm and check with his employees as it is lambing season. He has been rudely ordering his wife, Sophie, to bring his mobile phone and he has been increasingly abrupt with the staff.

1400 hours—Handover report

This is David Parker, a 55-year-old man with ACS, brought in by ambulance earlier today with chest pain. He's a type 2 diabetic, diet controlled, and his hypertension and cholesterol are managed and monitored by his GP. On admission, his pain was 7/10, central with some radiation into his jaw, associated with nausea and breathlessness. This was initially treated in ED with anginine and morphine, but the IV GTN is continuing to manage his pain. He's a STEMI and had rTPA in ED. He was supposed to have had a cardiology review last month but couldn't get away from work to attend. He manages a sheep farm and his wife works here in town. His troponin's back and it's pretty high at 0.25 µg/L. I'm a bit worried. He's been anxious this afternoon and I've asked his wife and children to leave so he can rest. I don't think he's being honest about his pain as all he wants to do is get back to work.

QUICK QUIZ!

Test your understanding of abbreviations and terminologies used in this handover report by selecting the correct response for each of the following.

Q1   What does ACS mean?

    a   Acute cardiac syndrome

    b   Actual coronary sickness

    c   Acute coronary syndrome

    d   Acute cardiac sickness

Q2   What does GTN mean?

    a   Glycerol trinitrate

    b   Glycerine tartrate

    c   Glycerol tartrate

    d   Glycerine trinitrate

Q3   What are the two signs of a myocardial infarction that may be seen on an ECG?

    a   ST depression

    b   ST elevation

    c   Abnormal Q wave development

    d   Abnormal P wave development

Q4   What does STEMI mean?

    a   Standard Total Emergency Myocardial Infarction

    b   ST Elevation Myocardial Infarction

    c   ST Emergency Myocardial Infarction

    d   Standard Total Evolving Myocardial Infarction

Q5   Normal troponin T level is less than 0.14 µg/L.

    a   True

    b   False

2. COLLECT CUES/INFORMATION

Q1   From the list below, identify the five cues that are *most relevant* to your assessment of David at this time.

    a   12-lead ECG

    b   Potassium level

    c   Blood pressure

    d   Sodium level

    e   Pain score

    f   Alcohol withdrawal score

Q2   As soon as David is stable, you plan to collect the following information to complete your assessment of his risk factors. Which cue will you *not* be able to collect?

    a   Weight

    b   Smoking history

    c   Alcohol consumption history

    d   Family history of cardiac conditions

    e   History of depression

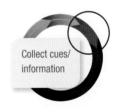

Collect cues/information

Access the National Heart Foundation (2016) site to review your risk of having a heart attack: <www.heartfoundation.org.au/your-heart/know-your-risks>.

Q3 The normal ST segment on an ECG is usually iso-electric.

   a True

   b False

(a) Review current information

Towards the end of the day, you are outside David's room preparing his medications and you hear him speaking to his wife, Sophie, saying, 'Where is my mobile phone? I told you to bring it hours ago. Why are the kids here? They don't need a day off school just because I'm stuck in here! I'm alright, I tell you. Why is everyone carrying on so much?' David pauses and then Sophie calls out, 'David? Nurse! Quickly! Something's wrong with David!' You enter the room to find him slumped in the bed with the following heart rhythm on the continuous cardiac monitor:

> Visit this resource for assistance in understanding cardiac rhythms: <www.rnceus. com/course_frame.asp? exam_id=16&directory= ekg>.

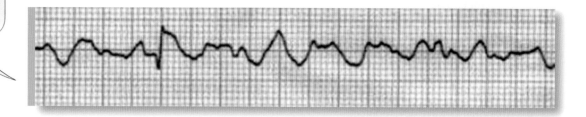

(b) Gather new information

Q1 What does the T wave on the ECG indicate is happening in the heart?

   a The atria have depolarised.

   b The ventricles are depolarising.

   c The ventricles have repolarised.

   d The atria are repolarising.

Q2 Cardiac output is calculated by:

   a Heart rate minus stroke volume

   b Stroke volume divided by heart rate

   c Heart rate plus stroke volume

   d Heart rate multiplied by stroke volume

Q3 David is in cardiopulmonary arrest.

   a True

   b False

> The chart at the following link provides information on managing coronary conditions: <www. heartfoundation.org. au/images/uploads/ publications/ACS_ therapy_algorithm-printable.pdf>.

(c) Recall knowledge

Caring for patients with coronary conditions requires knowledge and understanding of cardiac physiology, pathophysiology, pharmacology, epidemiology and therapeutics.

QUICK QUIZ!

Test your understanding of risk factors for coronary conditions by answering the following question.

Q Select from the following list, the five groups of people most likely to be affected by coronary disease.

   a People over 55 years of age

   b Sportsmen/women

c Alcoholics

d Men

e Obese people

f Healthy middle-aged women

g Aboriginal and Torres Strait Islander people

h People with diabetes mellitus

i People with cancer

3. PROCESS INFORMATION

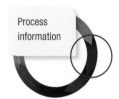

Process information

(a) Interpret

You review and interpret all the information you have about David's condition.

Q1 The monitor is showing ventricular fibrillation.

a True

b False

Q2 What is the most likely cause for this rhythm?

a He is experiencing a reperfusion arrhythmia due to the GTN infusion.

b He is experiencing an allergic reaction to repeated doses of morphine.

c He is experiencing a reperfusion arrhythmia following the dose of rTPA.

d He is experiencing an arrhythmia due to hypoxia from his AMI.

Q3 The rapid response team arrives and takes over the CPR that you have started. Reorder the following list to reflect the recommended order of actions.

a Check monitor and assess rhythm as shockable or non-shockable.

b Deliver shock.

c Continue CPR.

d Attach defibrillator pads.

Q4 The ratio of breaths to compressions in basic life support is:

a 15:1

b 15:2

c 30:2

d 40:2

Q5 Which of the following rhythms is a 'shockable' rhythm?

a Asystole

b Ventricular tachycardia with a pulse

c Ventricular tachycardia without a pulse

d Pulseless electrical activity

(b) Discriminate

From the cues and information you now have, you need to narrow down the information to what is most important.

Q1 What information do you think is *not* particularly important at this time?

a Impaired cardiac conduction due to a reperfusion arrhythmia

b Hypoxia due to impaired circulation

Access Grantham and Narendranathan (2012) for help in answering this question: <www.racgp. org.au/afp/2012/june/ basic-and-advanced-cardiac-life-support>.

   c   Impaired cardiac output

   d   Impaired glucose metabolism

Q2   In the list above, what is the *most* important information at this time?

(c) Relate

It is important to understand and cluster the cues you have collected so far.

Q1   Label the following 'true' or 'false'.

   a   Ventricular fibrillation causes ineffective quivering of the ventricles.

   b   Ventricular fibrillation has a regular pattern.

   c   Ventricular fibrillation has a rate exceeding 300 beats/min.

   d   Ventricular fibrillation has identifiable R waves.

Q2   Select the most important cue cluster for a patient with ventricular fibrillation:

   a   Audible heartbeat, no palpable pulse, normal respirations, non-responsiveness

   b   No audible heartbeat, a weak thready pulse, no respirations, diminishing responsiveness

   c   No audible heartbeat, no palpable pulse, no respirations, normal responsiveness

   d   No audible heartbeat, no palpable pulse, no respirations, non-responsiveness

(d) Infer

Think about all the cues that you have collected about David's condition, and make inferences based on your analysis and interpretation of those cues.

Q   Consider the following two statements and choose the one that is *most* correct.

   a   David is experiencing a cardiac arrest and will be defibrillated to deliver an electric current to the left ventricle so that it can re-establish the heart's pumping action and increase cardiac output.

   b   David is experiencing a cardiac arrest and will be defibrillated to deliver an electric current to depolarise a critical mass of cardiac cells so that, when the cells repolarise, the sinus node can recapture its role as the heart's pacemaker.

David is successfully defibrillated and his rhythm is re-established as sinus rhythm. You obtain another set of observations with the following results:

Pulse rate	65 beats/min
Respiratory rate	24 breaths/min
Blood pressure	100/60 mmHg
SpO$_2$	100% on 15 L/m with a non-rebreather mask

The rapid response team hand over care to the treating medical team and leave. You go with the doctor to speak to Mrs Parker. The doctor tells her that David is now stable. Initially, he had ischaemic changes in his anterior leads on ECG, indicating a blockage in his left anterior descending artery. This has damaged his heart muscle, as indicated by the troponin level. It appears the thrombolytic has unblocked this; however, this treatment may also have caused the change in his heart rhythm. You explain that more time is needed to determine the extent of the damage to the heart.

(e) Predict and (f) Match

At this stage, you need to consider the potential outcomes for David, as this will guide your actions.

Q   David may experience the following as a result of the AMI and episode of ventricular fibrillation. Match the possible outcome with the appropriate condition from the following list.

Outcome	Condition
David's condition may gradually improve over the next few days and he may have no adverse effects	… if he has suffered considerable myocardial damage and the pumping ability of the left ventricle is compromised
David's vital signs may continue within normal parameters	… unless his family can identify a management strategy to address his concerns
David may experience signs of heart failure	… if he experiences no further arrhythmias
David may experience more chest pain as a result of his anxiety about his farm	… if his myocardial demand can be reduced through oxygen supply, medication and bed rest

4. IDENTIFY THE PROBLEM/ISSUE

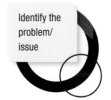

Identify the problem/ issue

Q   Now bring together (synthesise) all of the facts you've collected and inferences you've made to determine David's nursing diagnoses. Which of the following are correct nursing diagnoses?

   a   Chronic pain related to tissue ischemia, evidenced by facial grimacing, restlessness, changes in level of consciousness, changes in pulse rate and/or blood pressure

   b   Acute pain related to tissue ischemia, evidenced by further reports of chest pain with/without radiation, facial grimacing, restlessness, changes in level of consciousness, changes in pulse rate and/or blood pressure

   c   Risk of fluid volume deficit (hypovolaemia) related to decreased sodium/water retention

   d   Risk of fluid volume excess (hypervolaemia) related to increased sodium/water retention

   e   Risk of decreased cardiac output related to changes in rate, rhythm and electrical conduction

5. ESTABLISH GOALS

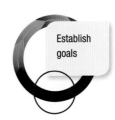

Establish goals

Before implementing any actions to improve David's condition, it is important to clearly specify what you want to happen and when.

Q   From the following list of goals for David's management at this time, choose the five most important *short-term* goals.

   a   For David to have no chest pain within 20 minutes

   b   For David's daily fluid restriction to be maintained during his admission

   c   For David to have no evidence of impaired gas exchange within one hour

   d   For David to participate in education and adhere to a self-care program following discharge

   e   For David to be normotensive and have a pulse rate in acceptable parameters within two hours

   f   For David to be free from anxiety by using stress reduction techniques within five days

   g   For David's ECG to show no signs of ischaemia on his next ECG

   h   For David to understand the reason for each of his medications prior to discharge

The NMBA's Registered Nurse Standards for Practice (2016) state that RNs must provide support, and direct people to resources to optimise their health-related decisions.

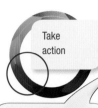

6. TAKE ACTION

You now need to decide which nursing actions take priority, and who should be notified and when.

Q   Using the *short-term* nursing goals identified above, create a care plan for David. Construct your care plan using the table below by matching the goals for care to the corresponding nursing action.

You may find this resource helpful in answering this question: <www.heartfoundation.org.au/information-for-professionals/Clinical-Information/Pages/acute-coronary-syndrome.aspx>.

Nursing goal	Nursing action

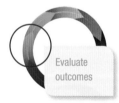

7. EVALUATE

Q   Using the following table, identify the trends in David's signs and symptoms that would indicate clinical improvement.

Sign or symptom	Desired observation
e.g. Blood pressure	Within normal range with no postural drop
Pulse	
Respirations	
Temperature	
Oxygen saturations	
Level of consciousness	
Chest pain level	
Urine output	

8. REFLECT

Reflect on your learning from this scenario and consider the following questions.

Q1 What factors led to David's deterioration? Were they predictable and preventable?

Q2 What are three important things you have learnt from this scenario?

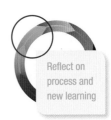

Reflect on process and new learning

SCENARIO 7.2 Caring for a person with heart failure

CHANGING THE SCENE

1. CONSIDER THE PATIENT SITUATION

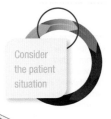

Consider the patient situation

David Parker recovered and was discharged with referrals to an outpatient cardiac rehabilitation program, his GP and a cardiologist. After returning home, David recommenced working on the farm almost immediately as lambing season had begun. He did not attend the cardiac rehabilitation program, saying that driving all the way into town and back would take up too much time. David soon began to experience breathlessness which was worse when lying down and not relieved by rest. He also developed a cough and increasing fatigue.

David made an appointment with the cardiologist who organised an echocardiogram, 12-lead ECG, chest X-ray, full blood count, urea, creatinine and electrolytes. The echocardiogram identified that his left ventricular ejection fraction was 38 per cent. The cardiologist diagnosed heart failure and started David on a number of new medications. He emphasised that David should attend the cardiac rehabilitation program so that he could learn to manage his heart failure as independently as possible.

The NSQHS Standards highlight the importance of comprehensive and coordinated healthcare that is aligned with an individual's expressed goals of care and healthcare needs, considers the impact of health issues on their life and wellbeing, and is clinically appropriate (ACSQHC, 2016).

QUICK QUIZ!

Q1 Remembering the difference between a sign and a symptom, which of the following is a sign of heart failure?

   a The person says he/she feels breathless.

   b The nurse notes the person's weight has increased by 2 kg.

   c The person says he has swollen lower legs in the evening.

   d The person feels increasingly tired.

Visit the following resource to learn more about how ejection fractions are determined: <www.hrsonline.org/Patient-Resources/The-Normal-Heart/Ejection-Fraction>.

Q2 Which of the following is *not* true of heart failure?

   a Myocardial failure leads to an increase in circulating volume.

   b Ischaemic heart disease and hypertension are common causes of heart failure.

   c One of the compensatory mechanisms activated in heart failure is the rennin-angiotension system.

   d Ventricular remodeling can occur as the myocardium adapts to increases in fluid volume and pressure.

Q3 Left ventricular ejection fraction is best described as the fraction of blood pumped out of the left ventricle during each heartbeat and it is equal to the stroke volume divided by the end-diastolic volume.

   a True

   b False

Q4 A normal left ventricular ejection fraction is an ejection fraction >50%.

   a True

   b False

To learn more about heart failure and cardiac rehabilitation, access <www.heartfoundation.org.au/for-professionals/clinical-information/chronic-heart-failure>.

Q5 The most informative test in determining heart failure is:

   a Chest X-ray

   b Blood tests

   c Echocardiogram

   d Electrocardiogram

Q6 Identify all of the statements below that are true.

   a Heart failure often develops at an earlier age in Aboriginal and Torres Strait Islander people.

   b Mortality from heart failure is higher in Aboriginal and Torres Strait Islander people.

   c Heart failure progresses more rapidly in Aboriginal and Torres Strait Islander people.

   d Aboriginal and Torres Strait Islander people generally have fewer hospital visits from heart failure than non-Indigenous people.

   e People living in remote and rural areas have less access to cardiac rehabilitation services.

   f Aboriginal and Torres Strait Islander people may feel more comfortable if an Aboriginal Liason Officer accompanied them to cardiac rehabilitation.

> *Hint: Read the recommended framework for cardiac rehabilitation: <www.heartfoundation.org.au/images/uploads/publications/Recommended-framework.pdf>.*

On his first visit to cardiac rehabilitation where you work, David is subdued and contemplative. He tells you that being diagnosed with heart failure has been a big shock, but he wants to improve his condition so he can get back to running the farm as quickly as possible. He asks you if the program will 'cure' his heart failure.

Q7 Write a short response to David's question.

2. COLLECT CUES/INFORMATION

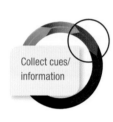

Collect cues/information

(a) Review current information

Q Review David's previous history and identify from the list below the three risk factors he has for heart failure.

   a Aged over 65

   b History of hypertension

   c Previous myocardial infarction

   d Damaged heart valves

   e History of a heart murmur

   f An enlarged heart

   g Family history of enlarged heart

   h Diabetes type 2

David's visit to his cardiologist and subsequent tests revealed the following:

Temperature	37°C
Pulse rate	68 beats/min
Respiratory rate	24 breaths/min
Blood pressure	140/85 mmHg
SpO$_2$	95% on room air
BGL	14.1 mmol/L
Breath sounds	inspiratory crackles (rales) on auscultation
Left ventricular ejection fraction	38%
Chest X-ray	some diffuse pulmonary infiltrates
Haemoglobin	150 g/L
White cell count	9.2×10^9
Urea	5 mmol/L

> *Visit this National Heart Foundation site for information on heart failure: <www.heartfoundation.org.au/information-for-professionals/Clinical-Information/Pages/heart-failure.aspx>.*

Creatinine   0.7 mg/dL
Potassium   4.0 mmol/L
Sodium   128 mmol/L

Medical orders

Ramipril 10 mg daily

Metoprolol 12.5 mg twice daily

Frusemide 40 mg mane

Aspirin 150 mg daily

Simvastatin 40 mg daily

Daily fluid restriction of 1500 mL

Yearly influenza and pneumococcal vaccination

Visit the following Heart Foundation site for a reference guide on the diagnosis and management of heart failure: <www.heartfoundation.org.au/images/uploads/publications/CHF-QRG-updated-2014.pdf>.

NYHA class	Symptoms
I	Cardiac disease, but no symptoms and no limitation in ordinary physical activity, e.g. no shortness of breath when walking, climbing stairs, etc.
II	Mild symptoms (mild shortness of breath and/or angina) and slight limitation during ordinary activity.
III	Marked limitation in activity due to symptoms, even during less-than-ordinary activity, e.g. walking short distances (20–100 m). Comfortable only at rest.
IV	Severe limitations. Experiences symptoms even while *at rest*.

(b) Gather new information

On David's presentation to the outpatient Cardiac Rehabilitation Unit, he is assessed prior to commencing the program.

Q From the following list, select the assessment that would *not* be appropriate.

a   Activity tolerance

b   Mood/depression

c   Health literacy (knowledge and understanding of disease process, management and treatment)

d   Patterns of rest and sleep

e   Cognitive functioning

f   Full neurological examination

g   Knowledge of appropriate diet

h   Medical history, including cardiovascular history

i   Cardiovascular risk assessment history, including smoking, alcohol intake, hyperliperdaemia

j   BMI and weight

k   Blood sugar level

l   Stressors and stress management techniques

m   Social factors (family and personal relationships, occupation)

n   Functional capacity (six-minute walking test and NHYA class)

Access National Heart Foundation of Australia's Multidisciplinary Care for People with Chronic Heart Failure (2011b) at </www.heartfoundation.org.au/images/uploads/publications/Multidisciplinary-care-for-people-with-CHF.pdf>.

(c) Recall knowledge

QUICK QUIZ!

Q1 People who have heart failure may think they have the 'flu', as:

    a They have a fever

    b They have a cough

    c They have a headache

    d They are sweating and nauseated

Q2 Congestive cardiac failure is a condition where excessive fluid builds up in the lungs due to inadequate pumping of the heart.

    a True

    b False

Q3 Pulmonary oedema is more likely to occur with:

    a Hypotension

    b Right-sided heart failure

    c Atrial fibrillation

    d Left-sided heart failure

Q4 Systemic oedema is more likely with:

    a Hypotension

    b Right-sided heart failure

    c Atrial fibrillation

    d Left-sided heart failure

Q5 Which of these statements are true regarding heart failure?

    a It causes simultaneous depolarisation.

    b It is caused mainly by obesity.

    c Failure of the left ventricle can lead to failure of the right ventricle.

    d Defibrillation is necessary when the patient in heart failure becomes more breathless.

Q6 Cardiac rehabilitation programs are an important part of recovery as they:

    a Provide education for the first few days

    b Help the person return to an active and satisfying life

    c Make people comply with treatments

    d All of the above

Q7 In left-sided heart failure, pressure builds up in the _____.

Q8 In right-sided heart failure, pressure builds up in the _____.

3. PROCESS INFORMATION

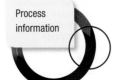

Process information

During his assessment by the multi-disciplinary team at the nurse-led Cardiac Rehabilitation Unit, it is identified that David is cognitively competent and has good support from his wife. However, he has continued to smoke, as he says it helps relieve the stress associated with running of the farm and financial issues. He has the occasional alcoholic drink, usually on Friday night at the 'local' with friends. His knowledge of the correct dietary management of his diabetes and heart disease is low, and he says that Sophie does all the cooking and buying of food. He does not do any particular exercise, as he says running the farm is exercise enough. David states he is not depressed and that he is motivated to improve his health, as 'the farm does not look after itself'. His knowledge of his medications is limited and he is not aware of what he should do if his condition worsens. David says that he finds it hard to stick to his fluid restriction, especially when he is working out in the fields, and he admits to having problems with his sexual function.

(a) Interpret, (b) Discriminate and (c) Relate

Q1 It is most likely that David did not attend the cardiac rehabilitation program initially as:

a He was busy with the farm and had little or no time

b He did not realise the seriousness of his condition and the possibility of it worsening

c The Cardiac Rehabilitation Unit was too far from his home

d All of the above

Q2 From the following list, identify the signs and symptoms you would expect if David developed subsequent right-sided heart failure:

a Orthopnea

b Distended neck veins

c Dependent area oedema

d Cyanosis

e Nausea and anorexia

f Right upper quadrant pain from liver engorgement

g Nocturia

h Crackles on auscultation

Q3 David is taking ramipril, an ACE inhibitor. Because of this, he needs to have blood tests regularly to monitor his:

a INR

b Potassium levels and renal function

c White cell count

d Blood sugar level and glycosylated haemoglobin

Q4 David should be taught which of the following, in relation to his diet and lifestyle?

a To make sure that he eats fatty foods to help put on weight.

b To ensure that he continues to smoke cigarettes as it will help to relax him.

c To ensure he reduces his salt intake.

d That engaging in high-intensity aerobic exercise is not advised for him.

Q5 David should be taught to _____ himself daily to be able to detect fluid retention and help prevent further deterioration.

Q6 Infection can lead to a worsening of David's heart failure. He should therefore be taught the signs and symptoms of infection. Circle the three from the following list that apply.

a Increased temperature

b Increased weight gain

c Swollen ankles

d Pain on urination

e Sore throat and cough

f Reduced bowel sounds

(d) Infer

Q   David's heart failure may have been exacerbated by not adhering to which elements of his cardiac rehabilitation program:

  a   Cessation of smoking

  b   Maintenance of a low-salt diet

  c   Appropriate activity and rest periods

  d   A decrease in stress through stress management programs

  e   Compliance with diabetic and healthy heart diet

(e) Predict

Q   Select three signs or symptoms from the list below that David would need to recognise in order to pre-empt a deterioration in his condition:

  a   New and increasing chest pain

  b   Improvement in activity tolerance

  c   Slow and steady weight loss

  d   Increasing shortness of breath

  e   Rapid weight gain

(f) Match

Q   Have you ever seen someone with the same signs and symptoms as David? If so, what was done to manage the situation and what was the outcome?

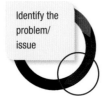

4. IDENTIFY THE PROBLEM/ISSUE

Q   Re-examine the information you have about David in both his medical examination and test results, as well as the cardiac rehabilitation assessment. From this information, identify three correct nursing diagnoses for David.

  a   Risk of impaired health maintenance due to lack of knowledge about diet, exercise and medications

  b   Risk of hyperglycaemia related to impaired kidney function

  c   Anxiety related to changing health status, resulting in inability to manage feelings of uncertainty and apprehension regarding the lifestyle changes

  d   Fluid volume deficit (hypovolaemia) related to increased cardiac output and glomerular filtration rate, evidenced by peripheral and pulmonary oedema

  e   Excess fluid volume (hypervolaemia) related to decreased cardiac output and reduced glomerular filtration rate, evidenced by peripheral and pulmonary oedema

  f   Activity intolerance related to muscular degeneration

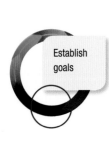

5. ESTABLISH GOALS

Q   With reference to the nursing diagnoses identified above, select five *long-term* goals for David:

  a   For David to have no pain within 20 minutes

  b   For David to maintain his daily fluid restriction

  c   For David to have no evidence of impaired gas exchange d For David to participate in education and adhere to a self-care program

e For David to be normotensive and have a pulse rate within acceptable parameters

f For David to be free from anxiety, using stress reduction techniques

g For David's next ECG to show no signs of ischaemia

h For David to understand what each of his medications do

i For David to significantly increase his aerobic exercise program

j For David and his family to obtain support from the community

Refer to the National Heart Foundation of Australia's Guidelines for the Prevention, Detection and Management of Chronic Heart Failure in Australia *(2011a) <www. heartfoundation.org.au/ images/uploads/ publications/Chronic_ Heart_Failure_Guidelines_ 2011.pdf>.*

6. TAKE ACTION

Q Using the correct *long-term* nursing goals from the list above, create a plan for David's care. Your care plan should include actions to achieve each of the nursing goals.

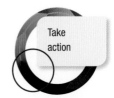

Take action

7. EVALUATE

Q List five outcomes you will assess to determine whether David's condition improves following cardiac rehabilitation.

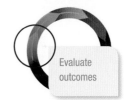

Evaluate outcomes

8. REFLECT

Reflect on what happened to David and the care that he received. Respond to the following questions.

Q1 What factors influence the success of discharge education and planning for someone who has had a heart attack?

Q2 How could David's deterioration after his heart attack have been prevented?

Q3 What have you learnt from the scenario that you can apply to your future practice?

Q4 What factors influence how people adapt to chronic and life-limiting conditions?

Q5 What strategies would you use to help people who find the transition to chronic illness particularly challenging?

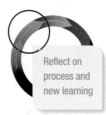

Reflect on process and new learning

EPILOGUE

David continued to recover from his heart attack and learnt to manage his heart failure with support from his family. During a visit to his GP, he expressed his gratitude at having the opportunity to re-evaluate his life and his priorities. He feels in the right frame of mind to find out more about his heritage and is making inquiries about how to trace members of his family. He has become a member of the local 'heart support' group and helps by visiting other farmers who are hospitalised with a cardiac condition, including other Aboriginal men. Although he delegates many of the heavier tasks in managing the farm to his employees, he continues with his sheep-breeding program and recently won the major title for a fine wool merino ram at the Royal Easter Show.

FURTHER READING

Agency for Clinical Innovation (ACI). (2013). *NSW Chronic Disease Management Program—Connecting Care in the Community*. Chatswood, NSW: Agency for Clinical Innovation.

Australian Commission on Safety and Quality in Health Care (ACSQHC). (2014). *Acute Coronary Syndromes Clinical Care Standards*. Sydney: ACSQHC.

Baker, T., McCoombe, S., Mercer-Grant, C. & Brumby, S. (2011). Chest pain in rural communities: Balancing decisions and distance. *Emergency Medicine Australia, 23*, 337–45.

Cooper, D. (2015). The use of primary PCI for the treatment of STEMI. *Bristish Journal of Cardiac Nursing, 10*(7), 354–60.

Driscoll, A., Parkerson, P., Clark, R., Huang, N. & Ahod, Z. (2009). Tailoring consumer resources to enhance self-care in chronic heart failure. *Australian Critical Care, 22*, 133–40. Accessed October 2011 at <www.heartfoundation.org.au/SiteCollectionDocuments/Tailoring-consumer-resources.pdf>.

Leung, Y. W., Brual, J., McPherson, A. & Grace, S. L. (2010). Geographical issues in cardiac rehabilitation utilisation: A narrative review. *Health & Space, 16*, 1196–205. Accessed November 2016 at <http://uhn.academia.edu/YvonneLeung/Papers/351489/Geographic_Issues_in_Cardiac_Rehabilitation_Use_A_Narrative_Review>.

Rolley, J. X., Davidson, P. M., Salmonson, Y., Fernandez, R. & Dennison, C. R. (2009). Review of nursing care for patients undergoing percutaneous coronary intervention: A patient journey approach. *Journal of Clinical Nursing, 18*, 2394–405.

REFERENCES

Agency for Clinical Innovation (ACI). (2016). *Nurse Administered Thrombolysis (NAT) for ST Elevation Myocardial Infarction (STEMI)*. Clinical Fact Sheet. Accessed November 2016 at <www.aci.health.nsw.gov.au/_data/assets/pdf_file/0011/319196/NAT-clinican.pdf>.

Australian Commission on Safety and Quality in Health Care (ACSQHC). (2016). *National Safety and Quality Health Service Standards Version 2*. Draft, Sydney, Australia.

Australian Institute of Health and Welfare (AIHW). (2015a). *Deaths from Cardiovascular Disease*. Accessed November 2016 at <www.aihw.gov.au/cardiovascular-disease/deaths/>.

Australian Institute of Health and Welfare (AIHW). (2015b). *How Many Australians Have Cardiovascular Disease*. Accessed November 2016 at <www.aihw.gov.au/cardiovascular-disease/prevalence/>.

Grantham, H. & Narendranathan, R. (2012). Basic and advanced cardiac life support. *Emergency Care, 41*(6), 386–90. Accessed November 2016 at <www.racgp.org.au/afp/2012/june/basic-and-advanced-cardiac-life-support>.

LeMone, P., Burke, K., Bauldoff, G., Gubrud-Howe, P., Levett-Jones, T., Dwyer, T., ... Raymond, D. (Eds). (2017). *Medical–Surgical Nursing: Critical Thinking in Person-Centred Care* (3rd edn). Melbourne: Pearson.

National Heart Foundation of Australia. (2016). *Know Your Heart Risks*. Accessed November 2016 at <www.heartfoundation.org.au/your-heart/know-your-risks>.

National Heart Foundation of Australia. (2011a). *Guidelines for the Prevention, Detection and Management of Chronic Heart Failure in Australia*. Accessed November 2016 at <www.heartfoundation.org.au/images/uploads/publications/Chronic_Heart_Failure_Guidelines_2011.pdf>.

National Heart Foundation of Australia. (2011b). *Multidisciplinary Care for People with Chronic Heart Failure: Principles and Recommendations for Best Practice*. Accessed November 2016 at <www.heartfoundation.org.au/images/uploads/publications/Multidisciplinary-care-for-people-with-CHF.pdf>.

Nursing and Midwifery Board of Australia (NMBA). (2016). *Registered Nurse Standards for Practice*. Retrieved from <www.nursingmidwiferyboard.gov.au/Codes-Guidelines-Statements/Professional-standards.aspx>.

PHOTO CREDIT

118 © Chris Burt/123RF.

CHAPTER 8

CARING FOR A PERSON WITH AN ACQUIRED BRAIN INJURY

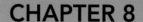

KERRY HOFFMAN, NATHAN HAINING AND AMANDA WILSON

LEARNING OUTCOMES

Completion of the activities in this chapter will enable you to:

○ explain why an understanding of neurological deterioration is essential to competent practice (**recall** and **application**)

○ identify the clinical manifestations of altered level of consciousness and deteriorating neurological status that will guide the collection and interpretation of cues (**gather, review, interpret, discriminate, relate** and **infer**)

○ identify patients at risk of increasing intracranial pressure (**match** and **predict**)

○ review clinical information to identify the main nursing diagnoses for a patient with an acquired brain injury, altered consciousness and disability (**synthesise**)

○ describe the priorities of care for a patient with an acquired brain injury, altered consciousness and disability (**goal setting** and **taking action**)

○ identify clinical criteria for determining the effectiveness of nursing actions taken to manage an acquired brain injury, altered consciousness and disability (**evaluate**)

○ apply what you have learnt about acquired brain injury, altered level of consciousness and disability to new situations involving different patients (**reflection** and **translation**).

INTRODUCTION

This chapter focuses on the care of a person who experiences a stroke. You will meet Mr Iosefa Apulu and follow his healthcare journey through acute care and into rehabilitation. Stroke is a medical emergency; recognition of the signs and symptoms, and early presentation to acute care are critical (National Stroke Foundation, 2016). Neurological deterioration following a stroke can occur rapidly and lead to serious complications; however, early intervention may prevent mortality and reduce the severity of long-term disability (National Stroke Foundation, 2016). Well-developed clinical reasoning skills will help you to recognise and manage people at risk of neurological deterioration, thus preventing or reducing adverse patient outcomes.

KEY CONCEPTS

stroke
acquired brain injury
altered level of consciousness
neurological deterioration
raised intracranial pressure
disability

SUGGESTED READINGS

P. LeMone, K. Burke, G. Bauldoff, P. Gubrud-Howe, T. Levett-Jones, T. Dwyer ... D. Raymond (Eds). (2017). *Medical–Surgical Nursing: Critical Thinking in Person-Centred Care* (3rd edn). Melbourne: Pearson.
Unit 11: Responses to altered neurological function

SCENARIO 8.1 — Caring for a person with an acquired brain injury and altered level of consciousness

SETTING THE SCENE

Mr Iosefa Apulu is a 52-year-old Samoan man who presented to his GP with dizziness and headaches. After clinical review, a CT scan was ordered. The results were normal but the GP told Mr Apulu that he had suffered a transient ischaemic attack (TIA). Mr Apulu was started on Cardiprin (aspirin), 100 mg once daily. However, his dizziness persisted, and he was started on prochlorperazine (Stemetil). Because of his history of high blood pressure and obesity, the GP also prescribed Avapro HCT (irbesartan plus hydrochlorothiazide) tablets 300/25 once daily, and amlodipine 5 mg once daily.

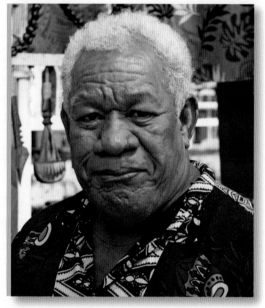

Mr Iosefa Apulu

A week after his review by the GP, Mr Apulu rose early to help his sons get ready for work. By 0500 he had developed a left-sided headache; by 1100 it was severe and intolerable so he went to the Emergency Department (ED) at his local hospital.

On admission to the ED, Mr Apulu's pain score was 8/10 and he had some transient weakness of his left side, face and arm. He stated that he had intermittent double vision, felt like he was spinning, but had no nausea or vomiting.

A neurological assessment identified that Mr Apulu had left upper limb weakness and atonia. He had some dysarthria and sensory disturbance, and decreased temperature on the left side. His uvula was deviated to the left. A basilar occlusion was suspected and a CT angiography was ordered.

The epidemiology of stroke

The acronym **FAST** has been introduced to educate the public on recognition of symptoms of stroke and the importance of timely access to care. It stands for:

Face—Has their mouth drooped?

Arms—Can they lift both arms?

Speech—Is their speech slurred? Do they understand you?

Time—Is critical. If you see any of these signs, call 000 straightaway.

Stroke death rates fell by 25 per cent between 1997 and 2009; however, as of 2009, strokes still accounted for 6 per cent of all deaths in Australia (AIHW, 2016). Older Australians are more likely to have a stroke, with 75 per cent of patients aged over 65 (AIHW, 2016). More women than men die from strokes, and Aboriginal and Torres Strait Islander people are twice as likely to suffer a stroke as non-Indigenous Australians. The incidence of stroke is also higher in Pacific Islanders (AIHW, 2016).

Although the rate of disability caused by stroke has fallen over the last decade, many survivors still experience significant health issues that impact their quality of life. One in three people who have a stroke will have a resulting disability that interferes with everyday activities, and will require ongoing care and assistance (AIHW, 2016). Many stroke survivors with disability return home and the burden of care often falls on family members.

The aetiology and pathogenesis of stroke

Refer to this blog for an overview of what strokes are and the signs: <https://strokefoundation. org.au/Blog/2016/09/12/ A-stroke-is-a-medical-emergency-the-facts>.

Stroke (also known as cerebrovascular accident [CVA] or brain attack) is an acquired brain injury that occurs when the blood supply to the brain is suddenly disrupted by either a blocked artery (ischaemic stroke) or haemorrhage (haemorrhagic stroke). Disruption of blood supply to the brain starves brain cells of oxygen and glucose, resulting in ischaemia and infarction (Brainlink, 2016).

An ischaemic stroke can be caused by either an emboli or a thrombus and accounts for approximately 80 to 85 per cent of strokes. Haemorrhagic strokes occur when blood vessels rupture, often as a result of long-standing hypertension (Brainlink, 2016).

Risk factors for developing a stroke include hypertension, obesity, cigarette smoking, a diet high in cholesterol, alcohol, lack of exercise, diabetes and atrial fibrillation (Brainlink, 2016).

On admission to the ward

Mr Apulu was transferred from the ED to the Stroke Unit under the care of a neurologist. The CT angiography showed a vertebral artery occlusion with a thrombus present. No bleed was noted. Mr Apulu was not a candidate for thrombectomy or stenting and did not receive a thrombolytic such as tPA as he had presented to the ED more than four hours after symptom onset.

IV heparin was commenced and he was also started on statins. An ECG showed that Mr Apulu was in normal sinus rhythm and a series of blood tests were taken:

Blood test results:

Cholesterol	5.9 mmol/L
Triglycerides	1.35 mmol/L
PT	14 secs
APPT	29 secs
INR	1.0
Hb	170 g/L
Urea	8.7 mmol/L
eGFR	86 mmol/L
Potassium	4.0 mmol/L
Sodium	139 mmol/L
ABGs	PaO_2 = 75, $PaCO_2$ = 37, pH = 7.38

Admission observations:

Temperature	36.5°C
Pulse rate	73, regular
Respiratory rate	15 breaths/min
Blood pressure	170/90
SpO_2	94% on room air
BSL	6.5 mmol/L
Pupil reaction to light	brisk and equal in both left and right pupil
Pupil size	3 mm left and right pupil
Limbs	left arm and leg severe weakness, right arm and leg normal strength
Glasgow Coma Scale	15: eyes open = 4 (spontaneously), best verbal response = 5 (orientated), best motor response = 6 (obeys commands)
BMI	35 kg/m²

Co-morbidities:

Type 2 diabetes (diet controlled)

Hypertension

Recurrent cellulitis right leg (currently no cellulitis present)

Smoking

Obesity (weight 110 kg), height 1.70 m, BMI 35 kg/m²

Osteoarthritis (Mr Apulu takes over-the-counter (OTC) paracetamol PRN)

Medical orders:

Maintain systolic blood pressure between 160 and 180

Oxygen therapy to maintain SpO_2 above 95%

Continue aspirin

Continue on heparin infusion with a target APPT of 60–80 secs

Neurological observations

Nil by mouth

IV fluids

For review by speech pathologist

Access *Stroke and Its Management in Australia: An Update (AIHW, 2013)* for further information on the epidemiology of stroke in Australia: <www.aihw.gov.au/WorkArea/DownloadAsset.aspx?id=60129=43611>.

Access *Brainlink* for further information on acquired brain injury and stroke: <www.brainlink.org.au/>.

Access this news update from American Heart Association on stent retrieval for people who have had a severe stroke: <http://news.heart.org/stent-retrievers-revolutionize-treatment-for-severe-strokes>.

For further information, access the NSW Agency for Clinical Innovation's Adult Neurological Observation Chart *in this education package:* <www.aci.health.nsw.gov.au/__data/assets/pdf_file/0018/201753/AdultChartEdPackage.pdf>.

Q   Review Mr Apulu's health history and identify five risk factors from the list below that he had for the development of an ischaemic stroke.

    a   Age over 65

    b   History of hypertension

    c   Previous TIAs

    d   Smoking

    e   Family history of stroke

    f   Cardiac arrhythmias, AF (atrial fibrillation)

    g   Diabetes

    h   Obesity

Person-centred care

Mr Apulu was born in the Independent State of Samoa. He moved to Auckland, New Zealand, with his family when he was a boy and came to Australia in his late teens to work on a construction site. He has worked in construction, mainly in Sydney, ever since. He married an Australian girl, Susan, 26 years ago and became an Australian citizen. Mr Apulu met Susan at a local church group. Susan died two years ago after suffering with multiple sclerosis for many years. Mr Apulu now lives with his two sons, Jonah and Joshua, who also work in construction. Due to his recent illness, he has been on sick leave but still cares for his two 'boys', getting them up for work and cooking and cleaning for them. His wife's mother helps out when she can, but she is 76 and not in good health. Mr Apulu and his sons have a 'tinnie' which they often take out on the weekends for fishing. He has a large extended family and a strong and supportive network of friends from church. Mr Apulu asks people to call him Joe, as he says most 'Aussies' have trouble pronouncing his Samoan name.

Something to think about ...

People from culturally and linguistically diverse (CALD) backgrounds experience a higher incidence of medication errors, misdiagnosis, incorrect treatment and poor pain management than English-speaking, Caucasian people. Culturally unsafe care with misunderstandings and miscommunication are frequently reported (Johnstone & Kanitsaki, 2006), and CALD patients often describe feelings of powerlessness, vulnerability, loneliness and fear when undergoing healthcare (Garrett et al., 2008).

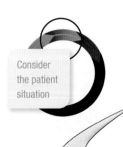

Consider the patient situation

1. CONSIDER THE PATIENT SITUATION

Mr Apulu has been on the stroke ward for 48 hours. You have just begun your shift and receive the following handover:

Morning handover report

We have Mr 'Joe' Apulu in room 10. He's 52 years old. He has had a vertebral artery stroke and is under Dr Isaacs. He has left-sided weakness and is NBM. He has had a speech pathology review and is for nasogastric feeds, waiting on a dietician review.

    Mr Apulu is a type 2 diabetic, diet controlled. He currently has an IV, normal saline at 84 mL/hr, IV heparin, and APPT to be kept between 60 and 80 seconds. His last APPT was 75, so he is due for further bloods and repeat APPT this am. He slept on and off overnight but seemed restless. He was a little confused when woken for 0600 observations; I am not sure if that is new or he was just sleepy. He has oxygen therapy at 4 L via nasal prongs and his sats are around 96%. His BGLs yesterday were stable and his 0600 BGL was 6.5 mmol/L. His obs are due again at 0800. He lives with his two sons; they will probably be in later today. His wife passed away a couple of years ago.

Patients with suspected stroke can be screened for swallowing difficulties using the ASSIST—Acute Screening of Swallow in Stroke/TIA (ACI, 2016) available at <www.aci.health.nsw.gov.au/__data/assets/pdf_file/0007/251089/ASSIST_screening_tool.pdf>.

QUICK QUIZ!

Q1 APPT is a clotting measure of blood and stands for:

   a Appointment time

   b Activated partial thromboplastin time

   c Advanced parallel processing time

Q2 A normal Glasgow Coma Score (GCS) would be:

   a 10

   b 12

   c 13

   d 15

Q3 Stroke should be considered a medical emergency, as:

   a Multi-disciplinary assessments need to be carried out within three hours of onset of symptoms to ensure the best chance of recovery.

   b Families are very distressed when a patient has a stroke and early attention to the stroke patient can relieve their distress.

   c Diagnosis and treatment with tPA needs to occur within four and a half hours from the onset of symptoms.

   d Stroke patients often deteriorate very rapidly and will need cardiopulmonary resuscitation.

Q4 A thrombus which has broken loose and is moving with the blood flow is called:

   a A thrombosis

   b An embolism

   c An occlusion

   d A clot

Q5 Atheroma is:

   a The blockage of a vein due to a clot

   b The blockage of an artery due to a clot

   c A weakness in an artery wall causing it to burst

   d Fatty plaque on the wall of an artery

Q6 Which of the following statements are *not true* regarding a TIA or 'mini stroke'?

   a A TIA is a stroke whose symptoms are milder and harder to detect.

   b A TIA is a brief period of localised ischaemia lasting less than 24 hours.

   c TIAs are often warning signs of an impending ischaemic stroke.

   d During a TIA, a person may experience signs and symptoms similar to a stroke.

Q7 A stroke-in-evolution is a thrombotic stroke that occurs rapidly but then progresses slowly over two to three days.

   a True

   b False

Q8 The immediate treatment for a stroke includes:

   a Taking an aspirin and calling an ambulance

   b Cardiopulmonary resuscitation

   c Receiving a thrombolytic in the Emergency Department once a CT scan has been done

   d All of the above

> *Strokes from a vertebral artery occlusion are not as common as strokes involving the middle cerebral artery. For information on the signs and symptoms of a vertebral artery stroke, see <http://patient.info/doctor/vertebrobasilar-occlusion-and-vertebral-artery-syndrome>.*

Q9 A patient who opens his eyes in response to pain, localises to pain and has incomprehensible speech has a GCS of:

a 7

b 9

c 11

d 15

Q10 In relation to obesity, mark each statement below as 'true' or 'false'.

a A body mass index of <30 kg/m² is considered as class 1 obesity.

b Obesity increases the likelihood of diseases such as diabetes, cardiac disease, sleep apnoea, cancer and osteoporosis.

c Obesity is one of the leading preventable diseases worldwide.

d People with central obesity (apple shape) have a greater risk of complications such as diabetes and heart disease.

e Peripheral obesity is more common in men.

Q11 The term 'cerebrovascular accident' (CVA) is currently less commonly used in relation to stroke. The term 'brain attack' has been adopted. Select the correct statements from the list below in relation to the reason for the adoption of the term 'brain attack'.

i A stroke is not really an 'accident'.

ii 'Cerebrovascular accident' is too long and hard to remember.

iii The term 'brain attack' stresses the urgency of a stroke, as does the term 'heart attack', and encourages people to access care quickly.

a i and ii

b i and iii

c ii and iii

d i, ii and iii

Q12 Which is the most important goal in the immediate phase of acute stroke care?

a Ensure the patient is comfortable and aware of what is happening.

b Maximise oxygen delivery to the patient and minimise oxygen demand.

c Test for a gag and cough reflex and instigate appropriate precautions.

d Minimise damage to the penumbra and re-establish perfusion as quickly as possible.

Q13 Write a short explanation for why tPA medication may be given for both a myocardial infarction and an ischaemic stroke, outlining its main mode of action and nursing implications.

2. COLLECT CUES/INFORMATION

(a) Review current information

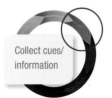

Collect cues/information

You go in to say good morning to Mr Apulu, who you had cared for the previous evening, and find that his confusion has worsened. You are concerned, so immediately take his vital signs and neurological observations:

Temperature	36.8°C
Pulse rate	68, regular
Respiratory rate	13
Blood pressure	175/85
SpO$_2$	97% on 4 L oxygen via nasal prongs
BGL	6.5 mmol/L
Pupil reaction to light	sluggish in left pupil

Pupil size	5 mm left pupil
Limbs	left arm and leg severe weakness, right arm and leg normal strength
GCS	12: eyes open = 3 (to command), best verbal response = 2 (inappropriate responses), best motor response = 6 (obeys commands)
Current APPT	75 secs

Q1 The difference between the systolic and diastolic pressures is called the:

    a Mean arterial blood pressure

    b Blood pressure

    c Pulse pressure

    d End-ventricular pressure

    e None of the above

Q2 Mr Apulu's pulse pressure on admission was:

    a 60

    b 70

    c 80

    d 90

Q3 Mr Apulu's pulse pressure is now:

    a 60

    b 70

    c 80

    d 90

Q4 Mr Apulu's GCS has changed by _____ points.

Q5 List any other changes you have noted since Mr Apulu's admission.

(b) Gather new information

What other clinical assessment information do you need to collect?

Something to think about . . .

Mr Apulu is from Samoa. A body of evidence has identified that health professionals who do not acknowledge and address cultural factors contribute significantly to adverse patient outcomes and health inequality (Johnstone & Kanitsaki, 2006). A practical strategy for enhancing culturally competent is to take a cultural assessment. Access this site to explore the ABCD mnemonic for taking a quick and easy cultural assessment (Kagawa-Singer & Backhall, 2001): <www.ausmed.com/articles/cultural-assessment>.

Q From the list below, identify the three cues that you believe are *most relevant* to your assessment of Mr Apulu at this time (that have not already been assessed).

    a Pattern of breathing

    b Temperature

    c Condition of oral mucosa

    d Headache

    e Nausea/vomiting

    f Colour

    g Increasing contra-lateral limb weakness

    h Level of thirst

(c) Recall knowledge

QUICK QUIZ!

To ensure that you have a good understanding of the key concepts related to stroke and deteriorating neurological status, test yourself with the following questions.

Q1 List three factors that can impair cerebral autoregulation.

Q2 What are the two major arteries supplying the brain?

Q3 Cushing's triad is associated with:

    a Tension pneumothorax

    b Cardiac tamponade

    c Massive haemothorax

    d Raised intracranial pressure

Q4 Identify three parameters from the list below that form Cushing's triad:

    a Raised temperature

    b Raised pulse pressure

    c Lowered pulse pressure

    d Decreased pulse

    e Normal breathing pattern

    f Abnormal breathing pattern

Q5 Mannitol is an osmotic diuretic. It would most likely be given for:

    a Cerebral oedema

    b Peripheral oedema

    c Pulmonary oedema

    d None of the above

Q6 The rigid cranial cavity contains three non-compressible elements, the _____ (80%), _____ (8%) and _____ (12%).

Q7 If the volume of any of these components increases, the volume of the others must decrease to maintain equilibrium. This is known as the M_____ hypothesis.

Q8 Normal intracranial pressure is:

    a 0–3 mmHg

    b 0–5 mmHg

    c 0–10 mmHg

    d 0–20 mmHg

3. PROCESS INFORMATION

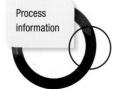

Process information

(a) Interpret

Q1 Which five of the following are considered to be within normal parameters for Mr Apulu?

    a Temperature   36.8°C

    b Pulse rate   68 beats/min, regular

    c Respiratory rate   13 breaths/min

    d GCS   12

    e SpO$_2$ 97% on 4 L oxygen

    f BGL   6.5 mmol/L

Q2 Mr Apulu appears to be hypertensive; however, his medical orders are to maintain his blood pressure at 160–180 systolic. Why might the medical team have decided to keep his blood pressure higher than normal.

Q3 The GCS is an important neurological observation. If a patient's GCS drops by more than 2 points, what action should a nurse take?

    a Lie the patient flat and raise their feet.

    b Sit the patient in a semi-Fowler's position.

    c Immediately contact the medical officer.

    d Continue monitoring GCS until it drops further.

(b) Discriminate

Q1 From the list below, select five cues that you believe are *most relevant* to Mr Apulu's neurological status *at this time*.

    a Blood pressure

    b Respiratory rate

    c Temperature

    d Pulse

    e Oxygen saturation

    f Condition of oral mucosa

    g Level of consciousness

    h Pupil size and reaction

    i Urine output

    j Pain

Q2 From the list below, identify the three conditions not usually causative of confusion and altered level of consciousness.

    a Pain

    b Hypoxia

    c Hypertension

    d Hypo/hyperkalemia

    e Hypoglycaemia

    f Seizures

    g Infection

    h Stroke

    i Tachycardia

    j Hyponatraemia

    k Drug withdrawal/drug overdose

    l Haemorrhage/head injury

Q3 List what can be done to determine the most likely cause of Mr Apulu's worsening confusion and altered level of consciousness.

(c) Relate

Mr Apulu's stroke is most likely to have been caused by atherosclerosis, which led to a thrombus in the vertebral artery.

Q   Which of the following is *not* a risk factor for developing atherosclerosis?

a   Male gender

b   Diabetes

c   Smoking

d   High HDL level

e   High dietary fat intake

(d) Infer

Q1   Early warning signs of an altered level of consciousness include which of the following? (Identify four.)

a   Increasing pulse pressure

b   GCS <12

c   A drop of GCS by 2 points

d   Unresponsiveness to verbal commands

e   BGL 1–2.9 mmol/L

f   Decreasing blood pressure

g   Any seizure

Q2   Late warning signs of an altered consciousness state are:

a   Increasing pulse pressure

b   GCS ≤8

c   Unresponsive to verbal command

d   Incomprehensible speech

e   Respiratory rate <9

f   BGL <1 mmol/L

Q3   Of most concern for Mr Apulu currently is the fact that:

a   He is afebrile and normotensive

b   He is hypertensive and afebrile

c   He has a decreasing GCS and pupillary changes

d   He is hypertensive with a normal heart rate

(e) Predict

Q   If you do not take the appropriate actions at this time, what might happen if Mr Apulu's altered level of consciousness is not addressed?

Identify the problem/ issue

4. IDENTIFY THE PROBLEM/ISSUE

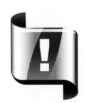

Something to think about …

Note: Mr Apulu's altered level of consciousness may be a warning sign that he is developing raised intracranial pressure (ICP) subsequent to cerebral oedema from his stroke. Cerebral oedema is an excess accumulation of fluid in the intra- or extracellular spaces of the brain. Strokes can cause cerebral ischaemia, resulting in cerebral oedema and raised intracranial pressure. If not attended to, rising intracranial pressure can have very serious consequences (including death) as pressure is exerted downward on the brainstem (Mellish, 2017).

Bring together (synthesise) all of the facts you've collected and inferences you've made to come to your nursing diagnoses.

Q   The nursing diagnoses below are all correct. From this list, identify the three *priority* nursing diagnoses for Mr Apulu.

a   Risk of impaired nutrition related to increased metabolic demands and inadequate intake

b   Risk of ineffective cerebral tissue perfusion related to increased ICP

c   Risk of ineffective airway clearance related to altered level of consciousness and diminished protective reflexes (cough, gag)

d   Risk of impaired skin integrity related to bed rest and hemiparesis

e   Risk of injury related to decreased level of consciousness

f   Risk of disturbed thought processes related to raised ICP and confusion

g   Risk of seizures related to increased ICP and hypoxaemia

h   Risk of impaired verbal communication related to confusion

5. ESTABLISH GOALS

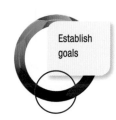

Q   From the list below, choose the three most important *short-term* goals for Mr Apulu's management at this time:

a   For Mr Apulu's GCS to improve within the next 24 hours

b   For Mr Apulu to be normovolaemic within the next 24 hours

c   For Mr Apulu's confusion to begin to resolve within 24 hours

d   For Mr Apulu to be normotensive within the next 24 hours

e   For Mr Apulu's pupil size to be 3 mm and reaction brisk within 24 hours

f   For Mr Apulu's oxygen saturations to be >95% within half an hour

6. TAKE ACTION

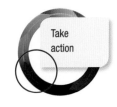

The medical officer reviews Mr Apulu and orders an urgent CT. A diagnosis of cerebral oedema and consequent neurological deterioration is determined. The medical officer orders IV mannitol stat, and for Mr Apulu to be transferred to ICU for ventilation if he continues to deteriorate or his airway and breathing become compromised.

Q   In the table below, match the rationales for care to the corresponding nursing actions.

Nursing action	Rationale
Notify Mr Apulu's doctor or rapid response team if his condition worsens	Establish baseline observations; sudden changes in neurological condition can indicate deterioration
Reassure Mr Apulu	This osmotic diuretic draws fluid out of the brain cells by increasing the osmolality of the blood
Check that the IV cannula is not kinked or blocked	To ensure patient is not retaining more fluid and or dehydrating after the osmotic diuretic, aim for normovolaemia
Administer IV mannitol as ordered	Emotional distress can raise ICP

(continues)

(continued)

Raise the head of Mr Apulu's bed to 30° and keep his head in midline	Patients experiencing raised ICP can suffer from seizures and need to be kept safe from injuring themselves if they have a seizure
Maintain a quiet environment	Constipation and bladder distension can raise ICP and impair venous drainage
Strictly monitor Mr Apulu's input and maintain hourly urine measures	The medical officer should be notified immediately of a change of 2 points in the GCS; the rapid response team (if available) can also be called
Monitor Mr Apulu's level of consciousness	Vital signs and changes in behaviour can indicate a further rise in ICP and further deterioration
Monitor Mr Apulu's pain score	Facilitates venous drainage, and prevents obstruction of the jugular veins which could raise ICP
Monitor Mr Apulu's vital signs, oxygen saturation level and behaviour	ICP can be elevated by noxious stimuli, including noise and emotional upset
Monitor Mr Apulu's ABGs and electrolytes	Severe headache can indicate worsening condition and can also cause anxiety, raising ICP
Instigate seizure precautions	Excess carbon dioxide and hypoxaemia can cause vasodilation and further raise ICP
Monitor bladder distention and bowel constipation	To ensure patency and delivery of IV medications and fluids

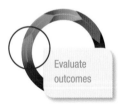

Evaluate outcomes

7. EVALUATE

It is now two hours since Mr Apulu was given a mannitol infusion. Each of Mr Apulu's signs and symptoms provide you with data to make a determination of whether or not these interventions have been effective and whether his condition is improving.

Q   Rate each of the following signs and symptoms as 'unchanged', 'improving' or 'deteriorating'.

   a   Cognitive status: patient confused and restless

   b   GCS: 13

   c   Pulse: 70

   d   Urine output: 60 mL/hr

   e   Left pupil size: 4 mm

   f   Pupil reaction: brisk both sides

   g   Blood pressure: 175/85

   h   Speech: inappropriate words

   i   Oxygen saturation level: 97% on 4 L

8. REFLECT

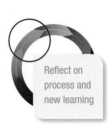

Reflect on your learning from this scenario and consider the following questions:

Q1 Might the outcome for Mr Apulu have been different if he and his family had been made aware of the early signs and symptoms of stoke? Why?

Q2 How could you promote understanding and use of the acronym FAST in your community?

Q3 What factors led to Mr Apulu's neurological deterioration following admission? Were they preventable?

Q4 What are three of the most important things that you have learnt from this scenario?

Q5 What actions will you take in clinical practice as a result of your learning from this scenario?

SCENARIO 8.2 Caring for a person recovering from a stroke

CHANGING THE SCENE

1. CONSIDER THE PATIENT SITUATION

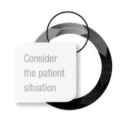

It is now 48 hours since Mr Apulu's condition deteriorated as a result of cerebral oedema and raised ICP. Although his condition is now stable, some expressive and receptive dysphasia remains, as does limb weakness and visual problems. Mr Apulu has also been a little impulsive at times and had a fall when trying to stand unaided to go to the bathroom. His IV fluids and IV heparin have been discontinued, but he continues on aspirin 100 mg daily via the nasogastric tube and is having diabetic nasogastric feeds.

Mr Apulu's sons think their father may be depressed, as he cries easily and does not seem interested in what is happening to him or around him. They are distressed that he had a fall and want to know what can be done to prevent further accidents from occurring. They are also distressed about how difficult it is to communicate with their father. Although Mr Apulu's sons helped look after their mother in the final stages of her illness, and have some understanding of what it is like to care for someone with a disability, they are not sure how they will manage their father's care at home.

Q What would you say to Mr Apulu's sons about their concerns? Who else might you bring into this discussion and why?

2. COLLECT CUES/INFORMATION

(a) Review current information

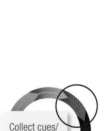

You review Mr Apulu's charts and identify the following:

Temperature	37°C
Pulse rate	67 (regular)
Respiratory rate	16
Blood pressure	150/95
Oxygen saturation level	96% on room air
GCS	13
Hourly urine output (average)	40–50 L/hr
BGL	6.1 mmol/L
Serum potassium	3.8 mmol/L
Serum sodium	130 mol/L

Q1 Complete the table below by matching the term to the definition.

Term		Definition	
1	Hemiplegia	a	The inability to recognise previously familiar objects
2	Aphasia/dysphasia	b	Unilateral or bilateral double vision
3	Dysarthria	c	Unaware of and inattentive to one side of the body
4	Hemianopia	d	Difficulty speaking/pronouncing words
5	Unilateral neglect	e	Paralysis of the left or right half of the body
6	Agnosia	f	Difficulty swallowing
7	Diplopia	g	Difficulty speaking/incomprehensible speech or inability to understand speech
8	Dysphagia	h	Loss of half of the visual field of one or both eyes

Q2 Stroke can affect many different body systems, leaving patients with a range of disabilities depending on which areas of the brain were damaged. The disabilities can be temporary but are more often permanent. Identify the deficits that Mr Apulu is currently displaying (accessing both current and previous information).

a Agnosia

b Dysphasia

c Dysarthria

d Diplopia

e Hemianopia

f Memory loss

g Short attention span

h Poor judgment

i Emotional lability

j Depression

k Dysphagia

l Hemiplegia

For further information about rehabilitation following a stroke, review Chapter 6 of the Clinical Guidelines for Stroke Management: <www.nhmrc.gov.au/_files_nhmrc/publications/attachments/cp126.pdf>.

   You are caring for Mr Apulu on a busy morning shift and when you walk into his room you find him trying to stand on his own. He is agitated and when you ask him what he needs you have difficulty understanding his answer. The nurse who is making beds in the same room repeats your questions to Mr Apulu slowly and in a very loud voice. You motion to a urinary bottle and Mr Apulu nods his head.

Q3 What assumption(s) did the nurse who shouted at Mr Apulu make? Which clinical reasoning error is this an example of?

(b) Gather new information

Q From the following list, select the eight assessments that are *most appropriate* at this stage:

a Glasgow Coma Scale: 13

b Pupillary response: PEARL (pupils equal and reactive to light)

c Falls risk (Ontario Modified Stratify): high

d   Pain score: 1

e   Waterlow score: high risk

f   Mental health assessment: emotionally labile

g   BGL: 6.1 mmol/L

h   Bladder scan: residual 130 mL

i   Temperature: 37°C

j   Oxygen saturation level: 96% room air

k   Limb strength: severe weakness left side

l   Respiratory rate: 16

m   Mobility assessment: assist with two persons

(c) Recall knowledge

QUICK QUIZ!

Q1   A stroke patient is the most likely to develop a deep vein thrombosis (DVT) following a stroke when:

a   He/she is a smoker or an ex-smoker

b   He/she has hypertension

c   He/she has decreased mobility

d   He/she is overweight

Q2   When monitoring for thrombophlebitis, limbs should be assessed for:

a   Decreased warmth, increased redness and decreased calf circumference

b   Increased warmth, increased redness and decreased calf circumference

c   Increased warmth, increased redness and increased calf circumference

d   Decreased warmth, decreased redness and increased calf circumference

Q3   Hyperthermia may develop in a stroke patient due to damage to the hypothalamus.

a   True

b   False

Q4   Mr Apulu had continuous cardiac monitoring in the acute phase following a stroke for what reason?

a   A stroke is likely to cause life-threatening ventricular fibrillation.

b   A stroke may directly cause cardiac damage.

c   A stroke may cause cardiac arrhythmias such as bradycardia and AV blocks.

d   A stroke may cause cardiomegaly and consequent changes on the ECG.

Q5   A stroke patient who has weakness in their dominant side will find it easier to learn to accomplish tasks with their non-dominant side after the stroke.

a   True

b   False

Q6   Indicate whether the following statements are 'true' or 'false'.

a   Supplemental oxygen should be given to all patients, even those who are not hypoxic.

b   Early BGL monitoring should be instigated for all stroke patients and patients kept euglycaemic if they are a known diabetic.

c   Antipyretics should routinely be used for stroke patients with a fever.

d   Patients who have seizures after a stroke should not be given anti-convulsants.

e   All stroke patients should be screened for swallowing ability before being given oral food, fluids or medications.

f   The gag reflex is a valid screening tool for dysphagia.

Q7 When communicating with Mr Apulu, you should do all of the following *except*:

a   Treat him as an adult

b   Don't let him know that you do not understand him

c   Use short simple sentences

d   Try alternative methods of communication, including writing boards, picture boards and flash cards

Q8 If Mr Apulu became frustrated and angry when trying unsuccessfully to communicate, what strategies would you use to help him?

> *Effective communication is essential to safe and person-centred care. The NMBA's Registered Nurse Standards for Practice (2016) state that RNs must communicate effectively, and be respectful of each person's dignity, culture, values, beliefs and rights.*

3. PROCESS INFORMATION

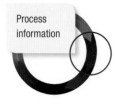

Process information

(a) Interpret

Indicate whether the following statements are 'true' or 'false'.

Q1 The deficits that Mr Apulu has have put him at risk of a fall.

Q2 Mr Apulu's loss of sensation and temperature in the affected limbs pose no risk of injury.

Q3 Mr Apulu's visual problems do not put him at risk of falls or injury.

Q4 Mr Apulu's limb weakness will make it difficult for him to mobilise.

Q5 It is common for patients post-stroke to display emotional lability.

(b) Discriminate, (c) Relate and (d) Infer

Q1 Mr Apulu's limb weakness makes him more prone to developing:

a   Joint dislocation

b   Foot drop

c   Sore feet

d   None of the above

Q2 Stroke patients who have dysphagia may become:

a   Overweight

b   Hungry

c   Malnourished

d   All of the above

> *The NSQHS Standards highlight the relationship between poor nutrition and pressure injuries, healthcare-associated infections and mortality in hospital, emphasising that strategies should be put in place to reduce these risks (ACSQHC, 2016).*

Q3 Stroke patients who are incontinent should have an indwelling catheter if:

a   They have urge incontinence

b   They have urinary retention

c   They are frequently incontinent

d   None of the above

Q4 Which of the two cues that Mr Apulu is displaying may indicate a mood disturbance?

a   Anxiety

b   Emotional lability

c   Aggression

d   Anger

e   Irritability/agitation

(e) Predict

Q Mr Apulu, like many people who have had a stroke, is at risk of serious complications. In the table below, indicate which complications he is most at risk of.

Complication	At risk	Not at risk
Shoulder dislocation		
Bleeding		
Aspiration pneumonia		
Seizures		
Pneumothorax		
DVT (deep vein thrombosis)		
Hepatic coma		
Pulmonary oedema		
Further stroke		

Something to think about …

People who have had a stroke are twice as likely to have a fall as other patients. They should be assessed for falls risk using a tool such as the Barthel's Index, and falls prevention should include exercises to strengthen muscles (Dean et al., 2011). Other interventions to prevent falls include easy access to the call bell, use of low-rise beds, avoidance of physical restraints, increased observation and surveillance, regular toileting, reduction of clutter, and observation when patients are walking and showering.

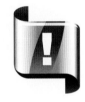

(f) Match

Q Have you ever cared for someone with the same or similar post-stroke signs and symptoms as Mr Apulu? If so, what was done to manage the situation?

4. IDENTIFY THE PROBLEM/ISSUE

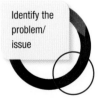

Identify the problem/issue

Q Complete the following nursing diagnoses for Mr Apulu.

    a Impaired verbal communication related to neuromuscular impairment, evidenced by dysarthria and _____.

    b Impaired physical mobility related to _____ and unilateral neglect, evidenced by _____, limited range of motion and decreased muscle strength/control.

    c Risk of impaired swallowing related to _____ _____.

    d Ineffective coping related to cognitive perceptual changes, evidenced by _____ _____.

    e Risk of falls related to hemiplegia, _____ and _____.

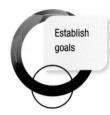

5. ESTABLISH GOALS

Q   From the list below, choose the eight most important *long-term* goals for Mr Apulu's management at this time.

    a   For Mr Apulu's pulse pressure to decrease within the next 24 hours

    b   For Mr Apulu to remain well nourished

    c   For Mr Apulu's GCS to improve within the next 24 hours

    d   For Mr Apulu to be able to communicate effectively

    e   For Mr Apulu's confusion to begin to resolve within 24 hours

    f   For Mr Apulu to be continent of urine and to have no constipation

    g   For Mr Apulu to be normotensive within the next 24 hours

    h   For Mr Apulu not to have any falls

    i   For Mr Apulu to mobilise safely

    j   For Mr Apulu to remain safe if a seizure occurs

    k   For Mr Apulu to remain free of further strokes

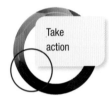

6. TAKE ACTION

Q1   In the following table, match the actions you would take in caring for Mr Apulu with the related rationales.

Nursing action	Rationale
Regular chest physiotherapy	Keep mouth clean and prevent infections and aspiration pneumonia
Anti-embolic stockings and early mobilisation	Maintain patient's dignity and decrease frustration with communication
Regular monitoring of vital signs and respiratory status	To help promote bladder tone and retraining
Assess for warmth, redness and increase in size of calves	To prevent chest infections such as aspiration pneumonia
Face patient, speak slowly and allow time for answers	Maintain and improve muscle strength and joint flexibility
Encourage fluids and high-fibre diet (high-fibre nasogastric feeds where appropriate)	Prevent thrombophlebitis and contractures
Mouth care, including suctioning on affected side	To assist in communication
Two-hourly position change	Monitor for development of thrombophlebitis

Nursing action	Rationale
Use picture boards, gestures, writing boards and computers	Detect early developing complications such as pneumonia or bleeding
Instigate range-of-motion exercises, and support joints and limbs at rest	To prevent constipation
Encourage patient to void on schedule, every two hours, using positive reinforcement	To prevent pressure areas developing

Key to quality care of people who have experienced a stroke is timely referral to appropriate members of the healthcare team during the acute and rehabilitation phases, and in the community. This requires you to be aware of the roles and responsibilities of team members, and to know when and how to coordinate referrals.

Q2 From the table below, match the allied health professional to their role in the care of Mr Apulu.

Health professional	Role and responsibilities
Social worker	Helps patients relearn how to carry out activities of daily living and educate patients about routine self-care
Psychologist	Helps patients with aphasia relearn how to communicate and assess ability to swallow
Dietician	Helps patients retrain motor and sensory impairments, and assess strength and endurance
Speech pathologist	Helps assess cognitive abilities of patients
Physiotherapist	Primary responsibility for managing and coordinating patient care
Occupational therapist	Helps determine right food choices for patients and also right food consistency
Physicians, neurologists, general practitioners	Helps improve motor skills and such things as grooming, preparing meals and house cleaning
Rehabilitation nurse	Helps patients organise such things as finances, vocational aspects and referrals

7. EVALUATE

Q Outline how you would determine the efficacy of each of the nursing actions in the table in the previous section.

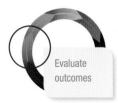

Evaluate
outcomes

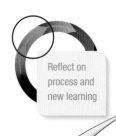

Caring for a family member who has had a stroke can be difficult. For more information read: Gillespie, D. & Campbell, F. (2011). Effect of stroke on family carers and family relationships. Nursing Standard, 26(2), 39–46.

8. REFLECT

Reflect on your learning from this scenario and consider the following questions.

Q1   How would you prepare Mr Apulu and his sons for eventual discharge?

Q2   How would you help Mr Apulu come to terms with the psychological distress caused by his disability and altered quality of life? Long term, what factors might indicate that he is not coming to terms with his condition?

Q3   What are three of the most important things that you have learnt from this scenario?

Q4   What actions will you take in clinical practice as a result of your learning from this scenario?

EPILOGUE

Mr Apulu remained on the acute stroke ward for two weeks, during which time he was assessed and managed by the multi-disciplinary stroke care team. He was then transferred to a rehabilitation unit.

While in rehabilitation, Mr Apulu's house was modified on the recommendation of the occupational therapist, and a raised toilet seat and shower chair were provided, as well as equipment to help him with activities of daily living. Two months later, Mr Apulu was discharged into the care of his sons and an aunt from New Zealand who stayed with them for a few months. A community nurse helps shower Mr Apulu in the morning and his sons assist with this on the weekends. Samoan friends from his church visit and help when they can.

Mr Apulu has mobilising splints for his arm and leg which his sons help him apply before they go to work so that he can mobilise independently if somewhat slowly. He still has some dysarthria, but his speech and comprehension have improved significantly. His vision problems remain, but he has learnt to cope with these and he borrows large-print books from the local library.

Mr Apulu now has a pureed diet and thickened fluids. He lost a lot of weight initially, as he did not enjoy this diet; however, he understands that it is important for him to maintain adequate nutrition. He has stopped smoking and his BGLs remain stable. He has continued on aspirin daily, as well as his blood pressure medications and statins.

Mr Apulu goes to hydrotherapy once a week and he attends a respite group where he enjoys participating in the activities. He is also a member of the local stroke support group and enjoys the outings they arrange. His friends pick him up on Friday nights to go to the local pub and, although he can no longer have a few beers, he enjoys getting out with his 'mates'. He has been fishing with his sons since his return home, but they now fish off the pier. Mr Apulu misses being able to go out in the 'tinnie' but it was too difficult for his sons to get him in and out of the small boat.

Mr Apulu still feels sad at the loss of his normal functioning but says he is learning to adapt to his disabilities. He has not been able to return to work and he finds it hard that his sons now need to care for him, as he feels he should still be caring for them. However, he is immensely proud of his 'boys' and what they do for him.

FURTHER READING

Australian Institute of Health and Welfare (AIHW). (2013). *Stroke and Its Management in Australia: An Update.* Cardiovascular Disease Series No. 37. Cat. No. CVD 61. Canberra: AIHW. Accessed March 2017 at <www.aihw.gov.au/WorkArea/DownloadAsset.aspx?id=60129543611>.

Considine, J. & McGillivray, B. (2010). An evidence-based practice approach to improving nursing care of acute stroke in an Australian emergency department. *Journal of Clinical Nursing, 19*(1–2), 138–44.

National Stroke Foundation. (2016). *Early Treatment After Stroke.* Accessed November 2016 at <https://strokefoundation.org.au/About-Stroke/Treatment-for-stroke/Early-treatment-after-a-stroke>.

REFERENCES

Agency for Clinical Innovation (ACI). (2016). *ASSIST—Acute Screening of Swallow in Stroke/TIA.* Accessed December 2016 at <www.aci.health.nsw.gov.au/_data/assets/pdf_file/0007/251089/ASSIST_screening_tool.pdf>.

Australian Commission on Safety and Quality in Health Care (ACSQHC). (2016). *National Safety and Quality Health Service Standards Version 2.* Draft, Sydney, Australia.

Australian Institute of Health and Welfare (AIHW). (2016). *Australia's Health 2016.* Australia's Health Series No. 15. Cat. No. AUS 199. Canberra: AIHW. Accessed November 2016 at <www.aihw.gov.au/WorkArea/DownloadAsset.aspx?id=60129555788>.

Brainlink. (2016). *Understanding Stroke.* Fact Sheet. Accessed November 2016 at <http://engonetbl.blob.core.windows.net/assets/uploads/files/factsheets/FS_Stroke.pdf>.

Dean, C., Rissel, C., Sharkey, M., Sherrington, C., Cumming, R., Barker, R., ... Kirkman, C. (2011). *Exercise Intervention to Prevent Falls and Enhance Mobility in Community Dwellers After Stroke: A Protocol for a Randomised Controlled Trial.* Sydney: NSW Ministry of Health. Accessed November 2016 at <www.health.nsw.gov.au/research/Publications/2006-exercise-for-falls.pdf>.

Johnstone, M. & Kanitsaki, O. (2006). Culture, language, and patient safety: Making the link. *International Journal for Quality in Health Care, 18*(5), 383–88.

Garrett, P., Dickson, H., Young, L., Whelan, A. & Forero, R. (2008). What do non-English-speaking patients value in acute care? Cultural competency from the patient's perspective: A qualitative study. *Ethnicity and Health, 13*(5), 479–96.

Kagawa-Singer, M. & Backhall, L. (2001). Negotiating cross-cultural issues at end of life. *Journal of American Medical Association, 286*(3001), 2993–99.

Mellish, L. (2017). Nursing care of people with intracranial disorders. In P. LeMone, K. Burke, G. Bauldoff, P. Gubrud-Howe, T. Levett-Jones, T. Dwyer, ... D. Raymond (Eds), *Medical–Surgical Nursing: Critical Thinking in Person-Centred Care* (3rd edn). Melbourne: Pearson.

National Stroke Foundation. (2016). *A Stroke Is a Medical Emergency: The Facts.* Accessed December 2016 at <https://strokefoundation.org.au/Blog/2016/09/12/A-stroke-is-a-medical-emergency-the-facts>.

Nursing and Midwifery Board of Australia (NMBA). (2016). *Registered Nurse Standards for Practice.* Accessed March 2017 at <www.nursingmidwiferyboard.gov.au/Codes-Guidelines-Statements/Professional-standards.aspx>.

PHOTO CREDIT

138 D. Smith/Travel-Images.com.

CHAPTER 9

CARING FOR A PERSON RECEIVING BLOOD COMPONENT THERAPIES

ELIZABETH NEWMAN AND KERRY HOFFMAN

LEARNING OUTCOMES

Completion of the activities in this chapter will enable you to:

○ explain why an understanding of blood components and their function is essential to competent practice (**recall** and **application**)

○ identify the clinical manifestations of anaemia, leucopenia, thrombocytopenia and transfusion reactions that will guide the collection and interpretation of appropriate cues (**gather information**, **interpret** and **discriminate**)

○ identify risk factors for patients receiving blood component therapies (**match** and **predict**)

○ review clinical information to identify the main nursing diagnoses for a person experiencing a transfusion reaction (**analyse**, **synthesise** and **evaluate**)

○ describe the priorities of care for a patient receiving blood component therapies and experiencing a transfusion reaction (**goal setting**)

○ identify clinical criteria for determining the effectiveness of nursing actions taken to manage transfusion reactions (**evaluate**)

○ apply what you have learnt to new situations (**reflection** and **translation**).

INTRODUCTION

In this chapter, you will follow the experiences of Mrs Aneesh Ayman as she undergoes treatment, initially for haemorrhage and later for leukaemia, across time and in different healthcare contexts. Managing the transfusion of blood cells, which are in fact live human tissues with significant risks, requires a depth of knowledge and sound clinical reasoning skills. However, there is added complexity when caring for someone who requires a transfusion because of leukaemia, as the person's own blood cells are affected by the disease process (Fleming, 2012). Therefore, excellent clinical reasoning skills are needed in order for you to recognise and respond to actual or potential problems that may arise from both the disease and the therapies provided.

Prior to seeking asylum in Australia, Mrs Ayman was exposed to prolonged periods of deprivation, human rights abuses, the loss of many members of her family and a perilous escape from her homeland. Learning about her story will help deepen your understanding of the importance of cultural empathy and cultural competence, and your role in promoting refugee health.

KEY CONCEPTS

blood component therapies
haematological diseases
transfusion reactions

SUGGESTED READINGS

P. LeMone, K. Burke, G. Bauldoff, P. Gubrud-Howe, T. Levett-Jones, T. Dwyer ... D. Raymond (Eds). (2017). *Medical–Surgical Nursing: Critical Thinking in Person-Centred Care* (3rd edn). Melbourne: Pearson.

Chapter 11: Nursing care of people with infection

Chapter 12: Nursing care of people with altered immunity

Chapter 13: Nursing care of people with cancer

Chapter 32: Nursing care of people with haematological disorders

T. Levett-Jones (Ed.), (2014). *Critical Conversations for Patient Safety: An Essential Guide for Health Professionals*. Sydney: Pearson.

Chapter 16: Communicating with people from culturally and linguistically diverse backgrounds

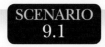

SCENARIO 9.1 Caring for a person requiring an emergency transfusion of packed red blood cells

SETTING THE SCENE

Mrs Aneesh Ayman, her husband and their 5-year-old daughter were among 82 asylum seekers aboard a barely seaworthy, wooden fishing boat. They had travelled from Indonesia and landed, despite rough seas, at Flying Fish Cove, Christmas Island. While disembarking, Mrs Ayman fell from the plank connecting the boat to the wharf and sustained a deep laceration to her thigh. She had considerable blood loss and was given first aid at the scene. Mrs Ayman was then transported to the medical facility at the detention centre.

> An 'asylum seeker' is a person who has fled their country and applies to the government of another country for protection as a refugee. A 'refugee' is a person who is outside their own country and is unable or unwilling to return due to a well-founded fear of being persecuted because of their race, religion, nationality or political opinion.

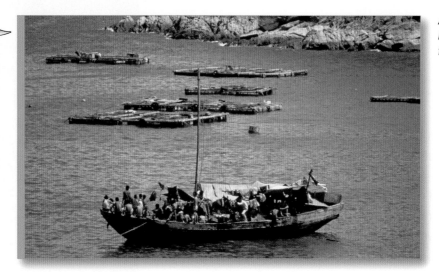

Aboard the fishing boat and destined for a 'safe place'

1. CONSIDER THE PATIENT SITUATION

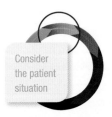

Consider the patient situation

You are a nurse working at the medical centre and will be responsible for Mrs Ayman's care while she undergoes treatment for blood loss and suturing of her wound. You receive the following handover from the emergency personnel who attended the scene.

Handover report

We have Mrs Aneesh Ayman from Iraq, who is 42 years old. She has a deep and dirty penetrating laceration to her left thigh that she received when she fell from the boat. We treated her at the scene and estimate at least 500 mL blood loss. The wound has been irrigated with normal saline and covered with a dressing and a pressure bandage. Her BP was initially 100/50 but she developed a postural drop and her MAP fell to 60, so we put in an 18 FG cannula and started some gelofusine running at 250 mL/hr. We started oxygen therapy on a Hudson mask and her sats are 95%. Her resps are 26, pulse 120 and she's afebrile. She is accompanied by her husband who can speak limited English. He is insisting on staying with her, saying that it's Sharia law. He couldn't tell us whether she has any allergies, but apparently she hasn't seen a doctor for years, so we haven't given any analgesia. Their daughter is also with them.

> Sharia is the code of conduct or religious law of Islam.

QUICK QUIZ!

To ensure that you have a good understanding of the terms used in this handover, try this quiz:

Q1 Normal saline is:

    a A sterile solution of water filtered to remove sodium chloride

    b A sterile solution that has the same tonicity as body fluids

    c A solution of 90 grams of sodium chloride in 1000 mL of water

Q2 FG means:

   a 'French gauge' and refers to the outside diameter of a cannula

   b 'Finish gauge' and refers to the number of lumens of a cannula

   c 'Finished grade' and refers to the quality of the cannula

Q3 Gelofusine is an intravenous solution used to replace:

   a Haemoglobin and red cells

   b Blood volume and white cells

   c Plasma and blood volume

Q4 MAP (mean arterial pressure) is a calculation that indicates:

   a Sufficient blood pressure to perfuse vital organs

   b Maximum blood volume

   c Sufficient blood pressure to perfuse the peripheries

> MAP is calculated using the following formula:
>
> $$MAP = \frac{(Diastolic\ BP \times 2) + Systolic\ BP}{3}$$

The doctor examines Mrs Ayman and orders a full blood count, group and cross-match. However, because of her extensive bleeding, he does not wait for cross-matched packed red blood cells (PRBCs) to be available, instead ordering an immediate transfusion of emergency PRBCs. He notes that Mrs Ayman appears dehydrated and exhausted, probably due to the unremitting sea-sickness she endured during the seven days she was on the boat. The doctor cleans, sutures and dresses the wound. He observes several bruises of various sizes and ages and assumes that Mrs Ayman has had other injuries while on the boat. The doctor then orders tests for tuberculosis (TB), human immunodeficiency virus (HIV), syphilis and malaria as part of the usual screening process.

Medical orders:

- One unit of PRBCs over 4 hours followed by 1000 mL of normal saline over 6 hours

- Morphine sulphate 5 mg IV

- Prophylactic tetanus injection

- Prophylactic antibiotics: penicillin 500 mg IV; ceftriaxone 2 g IV

> In providing safe blood management, the NSQHS Standards highlight the importance of actively involving patients and families in their own care, meeting the patient's needs for information and shared decision making (ACSQHC, 2016).

Something to think about ...

While reasons for blood component transfusions vary, the aim is to supplement depleted components within the blood, in order to relieve clinical signs and symptoms and prevent morbidity and mortality (Australian Red Cross Blood Service, 2016). For example, a person experiencing severe anaemia may require a transfusion of packed red blood cells (PRBCs); a person with a coagulopathy may need platelets; and if they also have a liver disorder or are about to undergo an invasive procedure, they may need fresh frozen plasma (Australian & New Zealand Society of Blood Transfusion Ltd, 2011).

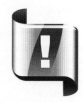

Person-centred care

The focus of Mrs Ayman's care so far has been the emergency management of her injury and bleeding, with the plan being to treat her injuries and return her to the detention centre where she will be processed for consideration as a refugee. However, you are concerned about Mrs Ayman and her husband as they seem to be confused, distressed and frightened. You contact the interpreter service as you want to help the Aymans understand what is happening, establish a culturally safe environment and develop a therapeutic relationship.

> The NMBA's Registered Nurse Standards for Practice (2016) state that RNs must work in partnership to determine factors that affect, or potentially affect, the health and wellbeing of people to determine priorities for action and/ or for referral.

The interpreter arrives and together you uncover the family's disturbing story … Mrs Ayman was born in the Kurdish section of Iraq and was present when the Kurdish people were attacked with toxic gases by the then Ba'athist regime led by Sadam Hussein. Most of Mr and Mrs Ayman's family, including their parents, were killed in the Iran–Iraq war of 1988. Mrs Ayman had five children, all delivered at home by the village midwife. Two died soon after they were born, and two were killed in the ethnic cleansing programs. Their remaining family members became part of the Kurdish diasporas seeking asylum in countries that accept refugees. Healthcare in Mrs Ayman's country of origin was extremely limited, but her husband tells you that she has not had any serious health issues.

> How much do you know about asylum seekers and refugees? Watch the SBS documentary, Go Back to Where You Came From, *then* access the related quiz.

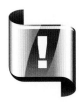

Something to think about …

Communication with people from a refugee background may be affected by language and cultural differences as well as different social, economic and political experiences. Read pages 31–43 of the following Foundation House (2012) resource to gain a deeper understanding of culturally competent communication and the use of interpreters: <http://refugeehealthnetwork.org.au/wp-content/uploads/ PRH-online-edition_July2012.pdf>.

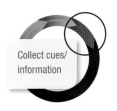

Collect cues/ information

2. COLLECT CUES/INFORMATION

The unit of blood arrives from the local hospital and you place it on the table behind the nurse's desk while you attend to another emergency situation. About an hour later, you are able to start the transfusion. You ask the translator to explain to Mr and Mrs Ayman the reason for the transfusion so that you can gain their consent. As the Aymans believe in Sharia law, you know that Mr Ayman must be involved in any decision to treat Mrs Ayman; however, you ask him to talk about the procedure with Mrs Ayman so that her consent can also be obtained. You complete a set of baseline observations and prepare to commence the transfusion.

To ensure that Mrs Ayman receives the right blood product, you undertake a number of checks at her bedside.

> How long can a unit of blood remain out of the blood fridge before commencing the transfusion?

Q1   Fill in the blanks in the following list of checks.

   a   The following checks must be undertaken at the _____ by two appropriate staff, one of whom must then connect and spike the bag.

   b   Blood pack label and _____ /paperwork are all identical/compatible and correct.

   c   The blood pack and _____ details are identical and correct.

   d   The _____ band(s) details are identical and correct.

   e   Ask the patient, if able, to state/spell their _____ and _____.

   f   Correct type of blood product including _____ provided (including CMV neg and irradiated products).

   g   _____ and time of blood pack (ensure cross-match specimen current).

> Hint: This transfusion checklist will help you answers this question: <http://resources. transfusion.com .au/cdm/singleitem/ collection/p16691coll1/ id/880>.

> The UR may be called something different —e.g. Medical Record Number (MRN), Hospital Record Number (HRN)— depending on which state you are in. It refers to the patient's unique identifying number.

Q2   Visual inspection of the blood pack:

   a   Bag intact. No _____ or evidence of tampering.

   b   No clots, unusual discolouration, _____ or _____.

   c   No significant _____ between tube segments and blood in bag.

Q3   Ensure _____ is completed and placed in the patient's medical record, with two nurses checking _____ and _____.

(a) Review current information

You review Mrs Ayman's baseline observations:

Temperature   36°C
Pulse rate   112
Respiratory rate   28
Blood pressure   90/50
Oxygen saturation level   95%

The blood is running quite slowly, so you open the IV to full so that it will go through on time. You then leave to attend to another patient.

How long should the nurse stay with the patient when a blood transfusion is started?

A few minutes later, Mr Ayman runs to you and tells you to come quickly. When you return, you observe that Mrs Ayman has started to shiver, and she is moaning and clutching her head with her hands. You stop the transfusion and immediately and check Mrs Ayman's vital signs.

(b) Gather new information

Q1 From the list below, identify the cues that you need to collect immediately.

    a Respiratory rate

    b Pain score

    c Level of consciousness

    d Skin colour

    e Temperature

    f Pulse rate

    g Blood pressure

    h Condition of the wound

Q2 What else would you check at this stage?

(c) Recall knowledge

QUICK QUIZ!

Caring for someone undergoing a blood transfusion and experiencing a possible reaction requires a sound knowledge base. Try this quiz to test your knowledge.

Revise your knowledge about blood transfusions by accessing the Clinical Transfusion e-learning package: <https://bloodsafelearning.org.au/course/clinical-transfusion-practice>.

Q1 The process of red blood cell destruction is called:

    a Erythrocytosis

    b Erythropoiesis

    c Haemocytosis

    d Haemolysis

Q2 If someone's blood agglutinates with both anti-A and anti-B antisera, what is their blood type?

    a B

    b AB

    c O

    d A

Q3 If someone's blood type is O and they have the RhD factor on the membrane of their red cells, their blood group is O+ve. What two blood groups are suitable for a transfusion for this person?

    a O–ve

    b O+ve

    c A+ve

d   A–ve

e   B+ve

f   B–ve

g   AB+ve

h   AB–ve

Q4   Blood with what blood group would be appropriate for Mrs Ayman's emergency transfusion?

    a   Type A (the most common group for Middle-Eastern people)

    b   Type B (least likely to be a mismatch)

    c   Type AB (universal recipient)

    d   Type O (universal donor)

Q5   Transfusion request forms in Australia should include a signed declaration verifying correct patient identification procedures have been followed. This declaration is designed:

    a   To confirm that the patient has consented to the blood transfusion

    b   To ensure the right blood is collected from the right patient and labelled correctly

    c   To document the collector's identity for the transfusion service provider's records

    d   To record the collector's details in case the transfusion service provider needs the specimen label amended

Q6   How often should transfusion observations be attended?

    a   During the transfusion of each unit according to hospital policy

    b   15 minutes after the transfusion commences

    c   Before the start of each unit of blood commences

    d   When the transfusion is complete

    e   All of the above

3. PROCESS INFORMATION

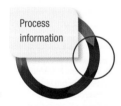

Process information

(a) Interpret and (b) Discriminate

You review and interpret Mrs Ayman's current observations:

Temperature	38.2°C
Pulse rate	118 beats/min
Respiratory rate	24 breaths/min
Blood pressure	100/60
Oxygen saturation level	95%

Q1   Which of the observations are within normal parameters for Mrs Ayman?

Q2   You identify that Mrs Ayman has been given Type O–ve blood. Is this of concern? Why or why not?

Access the following resources if you need help with this question: <http://resources .transfusion.com.au/ cdm/singleitem/ collection/p16691coll1/ id/643> and <www .transfusion.com.au/ blood_basics/antigens/ red_cell>.

(c) Relate and (d) Infer

Cluster the cues together to identify relationships between them and draw inferences based on what you know about Mrs Ayman's history and signs and symptoms.

Q   Which one of the following statements is true?

    a   Mrs Ayman could be hypertensive and tachycardic from a rapid IV rate.

    b   Mrs Ayman could be hypoxic and tachypnoeic as a result of pulmonary oedema.

    c   Mrs Ayman could be normotensive and bradycardic because she is anxious and frightened.

Further information on blood transfusion reactions can be revised using the following resource: <https://learn .transfusion.com.au/ course/view.php?id=54>.

d   Mrs Ayman could be hypotensive and tachycardic from the initial trauma and low blood volume.

e   Mrs Ayman could be febrile and tachycardic due to a transfusion reaction.

(e) Predict

Q   What could happen to Mrs Ayman if no action is taken and this situation is not corrected? Select the *incorrect* statement.

a   Mrs Ayman's condition will gradually improve over the next few days.

b   Mrs Ayman could develop acute kidney injury.

c   Mrs Ayman could develop circulatory overload.

d   Mrs Ayman could lose consciousness.

e   Mrs Ayman could die.

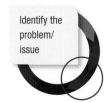

When answering this question, think about the causes and consequences of transfusion reactions. Access <http://cec .health.nsw.gov .au/patient-safety-programs/assurance-governance/blood-watch>.

4. IDENTIFY THE PROBLEM/ISSUE

Identify the problem/ issue

At this stage, you bring together (synthesise) all of the facts you've collected and inferences you've made to make a nursing diagnosis of Mrs Ayman's main problems or issues.

Q   Select from the following list two most likely nursing diagnoses for Mrs Ayman.

a   Acute lung injury (TRALI) related to fluid overload, evidenced by hypoxia and tachypnoea

b   A febrile transfusion reaction related to possible bacterial contamination, evidenced by chills, tachycardia, fever and hypotension

c   An anaphylactic reaction to an incompatible blood transfusion, evidenced by headache, chills, tachycardia, fever, urticaria and itching

d   A hypotensive episode related to a possible antibody/antigen reaction to morphine

e   Hypervolaemia related to a fluid overload, evidenced by tachycardia, headache and hypertension

f   A febrile non-haemolytic transfusion reaction related to possible antibody/antigen reaction, evidenced by headache, chills, tachycardia, fever and hypotension

5. ESTABLISH GOALS

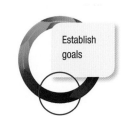

Establish goals

Q   Before implementing any actions to improve Mrs Ayman's condition, it is important to clearly specify what you want to happen and when. Which of the following are correct goals?

a   For Mrs Ayman to be afebrile and without shivering, headache, tachycardia or hypotension within 2 hours (and over the next week)

b   For Mrs Ayman to be afebrile and without headache, tachycardia or hypertension within 24 hours (and over the next month)

c   For Mrs Ayman to be febrile and without dark urine or urticaria within 4 hours (and over the next day)

d   For Mrs Ayman to be normotensive and without headache, tachycardia or urticaria within 48 hours (and over the next week)

6. TAKE ACTION

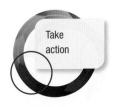

Take action

Q1 From the list below, choose the five *most immediate actions* you should take at this stage.

a   Reassure Mrs Ayman.

b   Maintain IV access.

c   Flush the existing IV line.

   d   Notify the doctor immediately.

   e   Re-perform steps 1 to 4 of the pre-transfusion check.

   f   Monitor Mrs Ayman's pain score.

   g   Monitor Mrs Ayman's vital signs and oxygen saturation level.

   h   Notify the transfusion service provider.

   i   Send blood pack to the transfusion service provider for culture and Gram stain.

A medical review is conducted and the doctor agrees with your nursing diagnoses. He believes Mrs Ayman is most likely experiencing a febrile non-haemolytic transfusion reaction, probably due to an antibody/antigen interaction. However, he does not rule out bacterial contamination, especially when you tell him that the blood sat on the nurse's desk for over an hour before being administered.

The doctor orders paracetamol and asks you to restart Mrs Ayman's transfusion if her symptoms resolve when the paracetamol takes effect. He wants you to monitor Mrs Ayman's condition very closely for the remainder of the transfusion and if there is any reoccurrence of her symptoms, the transfusion is to be ceased completely. However, the doctor specifies that if another unit of blood is required, cross-matching with full antibody screening will be necessary. Once Mrs Ayman's transfusion is completed, the doctor wants the normal saline started, as he is still concerned about her dehydration and hypovolaemia.

Q2   In the table below, match the rationales for care to the corresponding nursing action.

Nursing action	Rationale
Document all nursing observations and actions accurately and contemporaneously	Anxiety and restlessness may indicate worsening antigen/antibody reaction
Check cognitive status regularly	To maintain psychosocial wellbeing
Monitor haemodynamic status closely	Dark-coloured urine may indicate haemolysis
Examine skin regularly	To ensure adequate oxygen delivery; deterioration may indicate laryngeal oedema, bronchospasm or TRANI
Maintain patent IV access and monitor IV site regularly	To identify improvement or deterioration in Mrs Ayman's condition
Maintain oxygen therapy via nasal prongs and hourly oxygen saturations	To ensure clear, accurate and timely communication between all health professionals caring for Mrs Ayman
Reassure patient	To immediately identify an urticarial rash and any abnormal, unexplained bleeding
Check colour in each specimen of urine	To ensure cannula is patent as pain along the IV line may indicate haemolysis

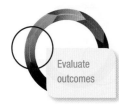

Evaluate outcomes

7. EVALUATE

Q   It is now two hours since Mrs Ayman's blood transfusion was completed and her normal saline IV commenced. Review the following signs and symptoms to determine whether Mrs Ayman's condition has improved. Label them as 'unchanged', 'improving' or 'deteriorating'.

Cognitive status	patient restless and anxious
Pulse rate	105
Blood pressure	100/55 lying; 90/50 sitting
Respirations	26
Oxygen saturation level	95%
Skin	no rash evident
Shivering	ceased
Temperature	37.2°C

8. REFLECT

Reflect on your learning from this scenario and consider the following questions.

Q1 What are three of the most important things that you have learnt from this scenario?

Q2 Could anything have prevented Mrs Ayman's transfusion reaction?

Q3 What actions will you take in clinical practice as a result of your learning from this scenario?

Q4 How do you think that your own cultural beliefs and values influence your ability to provide culturally competent care for your patients?

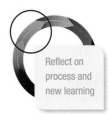

Reflect on process and new learning

SCENARIO 9.2   Caring for a person undergoing a transfusion of platelets and fresh frozen plasma

CHANGING THE SCENE

In Scenario 9.1, Mrs Ayman experienced a febrile non-haemolytic blood transfusion reaction. Despite the treatment provided, her haemoglobin remained low and her symptoms continued, so a second unit of cross-matched PRBCs was transfused without complications. Following treatment in the medical centre, Mrs Ayman returned to the accommodation section of the detention facility and waited for the processing of her refugee application. Mr and Mrs Ayman and their daughter were granted refugee status and six months later were settled in the Western Downs, about 350 kilometres from Brisbane, Queensland.

Over the ensuing 12 months, Mrs Ayman's fatigue did not resolve and she continued to experience bruising unrelated to trauma. Her gums also bled repeatedly, despite paying strict attention to her oral hygiene. Eventually, Mrs Ayman presented to the Emergency Department (ED) of the local hospital. A full blood count was ordered and it revealed that she had severe anaemia and thrombocytopenia. She was also diagnosed with acute myeloid leukaemia.

The epidemiology of leukaemia

In Australia, leukaemia is the ninth most commonly diagnosed cancer. There were 3624 people diagnosed with leukaemia in 2016, 2159 males and 1465 females. Survival rates from leukaemia have increased markedly over the past 20 years and the five-year survival rate is now 58 per cent (AIHW, 2017).

The aetiology and pathogenesis of leukaemia

Leukaemia is a disease in which malignant white blood cells (WBCs) proliferate in the bone marrow and peripheral blood supply, replacing normal cells. The aetiology of leukaemia is unknown; however, there are several predisposing factors associated with the development of the disease. These include high doses of radiation, exposure to benzenes and some viruses. There are also some genetic conditions that have been identified as risk factors, such as Down syndrome and Klinefelter's syndrome. A family history of leukaemia is also a risk factor (Fleming, 2012).

Person-centred care

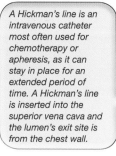

Why would these particular blood components be ordered?

Mrs Ayman was admitted to the Oncology Unit, and her initial treatment included three units of packed red blood cells (PRBCs) and a platelet infusion. Her husband told the team about her previous experience in the detention medical centre.

Chemotherapy was then organised for Mrs Ayman. As she was to have many transfusions and intravenous therapies, Mrs Ayman had a Hickman's line inserted in the operating theatre. She was then discharged and attended the outpatient oncology clinic for an aggressive regimen of chemotherapeutic agents.

Figure 9.1
Hickman's line

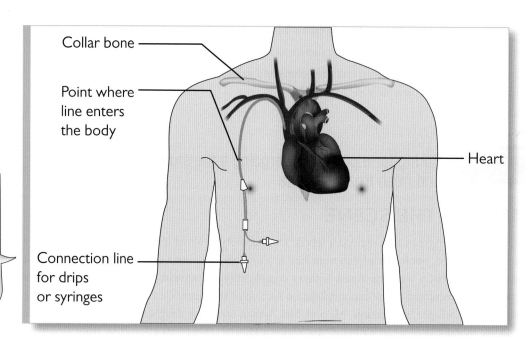

A Hickman's line is an intravenous catheter most often used for chemotherapy or apheresis, as it can stay in place for an extended period of time. A Hickman's line is inserted into the superior vena cava and the lumen's exit site is from the chest wall.

Collar bone

Point where line enters the body

Heart

Connection line for drips or syringes

1. CONSIDER THE PATIENT SITUATION

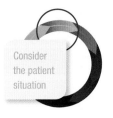

Consider the patient situation

On one of the days that Mrs Ayman attends the oncology clinic, she tells the nurse on arrival that she 'feels strange and not very well'. She is assessed and immediately admitted to the oncology ward. When you arrive for your shift, you are given the following handover:

Handover report

What are pancytopenia and neutropenia?

Mrs Ayman has acute myeloid leukaemia and is on her third round of chemo. Today she told the clinic staff she felt unwell. Her gums are bleeding slightly and she is pancytopenic and neutropenic, probably from her chemo. She is febrile—38.3°C; other obs OK. She needs a septic work-up for the source of infection and three units of packed cells. She is ordered penicillin 500 mg IV and ceftriaxone 2 g IV.

The doctor visits Mrs Ayman to discuss her pathology results, which show that she might have an underlying liver abnormality. He explains that this may account for some of her coagulopathies (bleeding tendencies). The doctor asks Mrs Ayman about her exposure to toxic gases in Iraq and explains that this may have led to her current liver problems and leukaemia. Mrs Ayman becomes very upset by the memories raised in this discussion and a counsellor from the local migrant and refugee resource centre is asked to come and support her.

Something to think about ...

Most people from refugee backgrounds will have been exposed to traumatic events such as prolonged periods of deprivation, human rights abuses, the loss of loved ones or a perilous escape from their homelands. Read pages 24–28 and 45–75 of the Foundation House (2012) resource to understand more about trauma and torture experiences, and the role of health professions in promoting refugee health: <http://refugeehealthnetwork.org.au/wp-content/uploads/PRH-online-edition_July2012.pdf>.

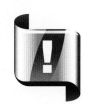

Mrs Ayman completed her PRBC transfusion without any incidents. She also had an MSSU, CXR, stool culture and a blood culture attended as part of her septic work-up.

2. COLLECT CUES/INFORMATION

(a) Review current information

The following day you are caring for Mrs Ayman again. Most of the results from her investigations are available so you begin to review them and think about Mrs Ayman's septic work-up:

- CXR: No collapse or consolidation is detected. No pleural effusion seen. No rib fractures seen.
- Stool culture: No significant growth.
- MSSU (MC & S): Anti-bacterial activity—not detected. Culture—no significant growth.
- Blood culture: No growth to date. A further report will follow if growth occurs.

Access the ECU video, 'He's not from here', at this site to examine the impact of cultural insensitivity towards people from a refugee background: <www. ecu.edu.au/community-engagement/health-advancement/ interprofessional-learning-resources/ resources/hes-not-from-here>.

(b) Gather new information

What other clinical assessment information do you need to collect?

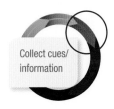

Collect cues/information

Q1 From the list below, identify the two cues that you believe are *most* relevant to your assessment of Mrs Ayman at this time.

    a Respiratory rate

    b Sputum culture

    c Pain

    d Cognitive state

    e Swab of the catheter site

    f Mobility

Hint: Check the approved abbreviations on this site: <http:// nursing.flinders.edu .au/students/studyaids/ clinicalcommunication/ page_glossary .php?id=13>.

Q2 One of your colleagues says in passing, 'I bet the infection is because of where she lives. "They" always live in dirty, overcrowded places.' Which clinical reasoning error is this nurse's comment an example of?

    a Racism

    b Pattern matching

    c Diagnostic momentum

    d Fundamental attribution error

Something to think about ...

The notion of cultural competence being integral to safe and effective clinical practice, and a key attribute of professional competence, is undisputed (NMBA, 2016). Yet cultural empathy, a driving motivation for culturally competent practice, is not well understood. Cultural empathy refers to the ability to perceive and share experiences through the unique lens of values, beliefs and perspectives of people from cultural backgrounds different to one's own (Wang et al., 2003). To what extent do you think your practice is informed by cultural empathy?

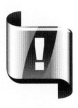

(c) Recall knowledge

QUICK QUIZ!

To ensure that you have a good understanding of the key concepts related to sepsis, immunity and allergic reactions, test yourself with the following questions.

Q1 Which of the following is *not* a type of leucocyte?

    a Macrophage

    b Eosoniphil

    c Monocyte

    d Keracyte

Q2 Malaise, fever, heat, swelling, pain and pus are all signs of infection. Currently, the only sign exhibited by Mrs Ayman is fever. Which statement is correct?

    a Mrs Ayman is neutropenic, so her total white cell count is compromised.

    b Mrs Ayman is neutropenic and she does not have enough neutrophils to produce the classic signs of infection.

    c Mrs Ayman is neutropenic, so her lack of thrombocytes prevent redness and swelling.

    d Mrs Ayman is pancytopaenic, so her lack of erythrocytes prevent redness and swelling.

Q3 A normal leucocyte count is $4.9–11.0 \times 10^9$/L.

    a True

    b False

Q4 A differential count is the percentage of each cell type in the blood. The differential for neutrophils is:

    a 2–8%

    b 0.5%

    c 55%

    d 20–40%

Q5 Which of the following does *not* constitute a risk for a neutropenic patient?

    a Presence of chronic illness

    b Altered immune response

    c Skin breakdown

    d Presence of invasive or indwelling medical device

    e Non-refrigerated food

Q6 Symptoms of an anaphylactic reaction include:

    a Hypovolaemia and hypertension

    b Bradycardia and hypotension

    c Broncho-constriction and bronchospasm

    d Urticaria and flushed skin

Q7 The first drug to be administered in anaphylactic shock should be:

    a Adrenaline

    b Oxygen

    c Corticosteroids

    d None of the above

Q8 The first phase of haemostasis is:

    a Separation of globin and haeme

    b Activation of prothrombinase

    c Platelet aggregation

    d Vascular spasm

Q9 When a wound occurs in humans, the platelets in the blood activate a substance that starts the clotting process. What is that substance?

    a Adenosine

    b Histamine

    c Lecithin

    d Thrombin

The source of Mrs Ayman's infection is found to be her Hickman's line and she is scheduled to return to the operating theatre to have it replaced. In view of her coagulopathy and her impending surgery, she is ordered a platelet infusion which she has without incident. This is to be followed by a transfusion of four units of fresh frozen plasma (FFP).

Q10 What process should be followed when commencing a platelet transfusion?

    a The same process as red blood cells but without the need to do vital signs as a baseline

    b The same process as red blood cells

    c The same process as red blood cells but non-ABO identical platelets are not uncommon

    d The same process as red blood cells but without the need to check expiry date

> *Visit Australian Red Cross Blood Service resource* Flippin' Blood *(2012, pp. 24–27) to revise your knowledge of platelet transfusions: <http://resources .transfusion.com.au/ cdm/ref/collection/ p16691coll1/id/20>.*

Q11 The storage of a platelet transfusion is different from the storage of red blood cells, in that they must not be refrigerated.

    a True

    b False

Q12 Which of the following statements is the *most* correct?

    a One unit of FFP is the plasma taken from a unit of whole blood.

    b FFP is frozen within eight hours of collection.

    c FFP contains all coagulation factors in normal concentrations.

    d FFP may be transfused up to five days after thawing.

    e FFP may have two expiry dates to be checked (one for collection and one for thawing).

    f All of the above are correct.

> *Why would FFP be ordered?*

3. PROCESS INFORMATION

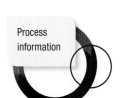

Process information

The FFP may be delivered to the ward frozen and must be thawed, although this is usually performed by the transfusion service provider. The process takes approximately 30 minutes using a water bath. *Never* improvise by using other methods such as hot water or a microwave, as this could damage the product and make it unsafe.

You do another set of baseline observations before giving the FFP and review Mrs Ayman's pathology results. Her results are as follows:

Temperature	38.0°C
Pulse rate	98 beats/min
Respiratory rate	20 breaths/min
Blood pressure	110/60
Oxygen saturation level	95%

Haemoglobin	120 g/dL
Total white cell count	3.0×10^9/L
Blood group	O+ve

You then begin the checking procedure for the transfusion of the FFP. You notice that the FFP is from a number of different ABO groups.

(a) Interpret

Q   Which of the following units are considered to be appropriate for Mrs Ayman's FFP transfusion?

   a   Unit labelled A

   b   Unit labelled AB

   c   Unit labelled B

   d   Unit labelled O

   e   All of the above

> Why can FFP come from different blood groups? Access Australian Red Cross Blood Service resource Flippin' Blood (2012, pp. 28–31) for more information about FFP transfusions: <http://resources.transfusion.com.au/cdm/ref/collection/p16691coll1/id/20>.

(b) Discriminate and (c) Relate

Q   After the first 15 minutes, you do a second set of observations. Which of the following are considered to be within normal parameters for Mrs Ayman while she is receiving this blood transfusion?

   a   Temperature: 37.5°C

   b   Pulse rate: 122 beats/min

   c   Respiratory rate: 28 breaths/min

   d   Blood pressure: 112/60

   e   Oxygen saturation level: 95%

Mrs Ayman is restless and scratching her arms. She says she is very thirsty and is having trouble breathing. She reaches for a glass of water and you observe that she has a weakness in her hands. When you intervene to prevent her dropping the glass, she tells you that she has a terrible headache and a pain in her right leg.

(d) Infer

Q   From what you have observed and from what you have learnt about blood transfusions, what are four signs or symptoms that may indicate a transfusion reaction to FFP?

(e) Predict

Q   What might happen if Mrs Ayman's FFP transfusion is not stopped and appropriate actions taken at this time? Choose the response that is *most* correct for this new situation.

   a   Mrs Ayman could go into shock and cardiac arrest.

   b   Mrs Ayman's condition will gradually improve over the next few days.

   c   Mrs Ayman could develop acute kidney injury.

   d   Mrs Ayman could lose consciousness.

   e   Mrs Ayman could die.

   f   Mrs Ayman could become hypoxic by developing a compromised airway.

Warning signs of adverse reaction to blood component therapies

Nurses have the primary responsibility for monitoring blood transfusions and it is imperative that they recognise and respond immediately to deterioration in the patient's condition. Reactions can be categorised into:

1   Mild reaction

2   Moderately severe reaction

3   Life-threatening reaction

In Scenario 9.1, Mrs Ayman's transfusion reaction would have been categorised as 1, a mild reaction.

Q   The following list of 12 signs and symptoms may indicate a potential category 2 (moderately severe) transfusion reaction in Mrs Ayman. From the following list, enter the appropriate signs and symptoms for each type of reaction into the table below.

a   Flushing

b   Urticaria

c   Rigors

d   Fever

e   Restlessness

f   Tachycardia

g   Anxiety

h   Pruritus

i   Palpitations

j   Mild dyspnoea

k   Headaches

l   Tremor

Allergenic reaction: antibodies to proteins including IgA	Febrile non-haemolytic reaction: possible contamination with pyrogens and/or bacteria	Both
e.g. Palpitations	Fever	Tremor

(f) Match

Q   In what way is this transfusion reaction similar to, or different from, the transfusion reaction that occurred in Scenario 9.1?

4. IDENTIFY THE PROBLEM/ISSUE

Q1   At this stage, you bring together (synthesise) all of the facts you've collected and inferences you've made to make nursing diagnoses of Mrs Ayman's main problems or issues.

Q2   Select from the following most likely nursing diagnoses for Mrs Ayman.

a   Acute lung injury (TRALI) related to fluid overload, evidenced by hypoxia and tachypnoea

b   A febrile transfusion reaction related to possible bacterial contamination, evidenced by chills, tachycardia, fever and hypotension

c   An allergic response related to a possible antibody/antigen reaction from the transfusion, evidenced by tachycardia, tachypnoea, low-grade temperature, headache and urticaria

d   Hypervolaemia related to a fluid overload, evidenced by tachycardia, headache and hypertension

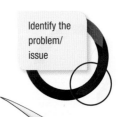

Identify the problem/ issue

Hint: Think about the causes and consequences of transfusion reactions. See <www.transfusion .com.au/adverse_ events/risks>.

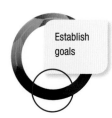

5. ESTABLISH GOALS

Q   From the list below, choose the most important *immediate* goal for Mrs Ayman's management at this time.

     a   For Mrs Ayman to be afebrile with respiratory distress, hypotension, headache or urticaria within the next 24 hours

     b   For Mrs Ayman to be afebrile with no respiratory distress, hypotension, chest tightness or headache, and with reducing urticaria, within the next 2 hours

     c   For Mrs Ayman to be afebrile with no shivering, respiratory distress, hypertension, headache or urticaria within the next 2–4 hours

     d   For Mrs Ayman to be afebrile with no shivering, respiratory distress, hypertension, headache or urticaria within the next 24 hours and for the following week

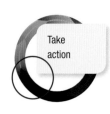

6. TAKE ACTION

Q   What are the 10 *most immediate* nursing actions required at this time?

     a   Consult a doctor for an order for an antihistamine.

     b   Complete transfusion reaction form and send to blood bank.

     c   Give adrenaline injection.

     d   Give diuretic.

     e   Arrange for repeat blood pathology.

     f   Administer 1 L of normal saline to flush cannula and line.

     g   Restart transfusion if reaction subsides.

     h   Reassure Mrs Ayman.

     i   Maintain IV access.

     j   Flush the existing IV line.

     k   Notify the doctor immediately.

     l   Raise the foot of Mrs Ayman's bed.

     m   Re-perform steps 1 to 4 of the pre-transfusion check.

     n   Monitor Mrs Ayman's level of consciousness.

     o   Monitor Mrs Ayman's pain score.

     p   Monitor Mrs Ayman's vital signs and oxygen saturation level.

     q   Notify the transfusion service provider.

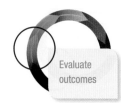

7. EVALUATE

Q   Use the following table to construct a list of the signs and symptoms you will monitor to evaluate whether Mrs Ayman's condition has improved and whether the transfusion should be recommenced.

Sign or symptom	Desired observation
e.g. Blood pressure	Stable with no postural drop

8. REFLECT

Reflect on your learning from this scenario and consider the following questions.

Q1 What are three of the most important things that you have learnt from this scenario?

Q2 What actions will you take in clinical practice as a result of your learning from this scenario?

Q3 If you had to teach another nurse about the key concepts related to the transfusion of red blood cells, platelets and fresh frozen plasma, what key areas would you target?

Q4 How has your understanding of cultural competence and cultural empathy developed as a result of completing this scenario?

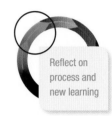

Reflect on process and new learning

EPILOGUE

Mrs Ayman recovered from her transfusion reaction, and all future transfusions were managed with careful monitoring. She had her Hickman's catheter replaced and she completed her cytotoxic chemotherapeutic regime. She then entered a period of remission. Unfortunately, six months later Mrs Ayman's symptoms returned. Her treatment using apheresis did not harvest enough antilogous stem cells, so a traditional bone marrow transplant was recommended. She was matched with a donor in the stem cell bank and had a successful allogeneic bone marrow transplant.

Over the next two years, Mrs Ayman's health improved and after the five-year waiting period Mr and Mrs Ayman and their daughter became proud Australian citizens. Mrs Ayman has learnt to speak English fluently and she now works as an interpreter and an assistant in nursing while she is studying to become a registered nurse. She attributes her commitment to nursing to the care she received during her many hospitalisations and to the empathetic and person-centred nurses she encountered.

For more information about stem cell transplantation, access the EdCaN learning resources at <http://edcan.org. au/edcan-learning-resources/supporting-resources/stem-cell-transplantation/ principles-of-transplantation/role-in-cancer-control>.

FURTHER READING

BloodSafe eLearning Australia. (2013). *Clinical Transfusion Practice.* Accessed January 2017 at <https://bloodsafelearning.org.au/course/clinical-transfusion-practice>.

Hurrell, K. (2014). Blood transfusion 3: Safe administration of blood components. *Nursing Times, 110*(38), 16–19.

Katz, E. A. (2009). Blood transfusion: Friend or foe. *AACN Advanced Critical Care, 20*(2), 155–63.

NSW Health. (2017). *Clinical Excellence Commission. Blood Watch—Every Drop Counts.* Accessed January 2017 at <www.cec.health.nsw.gov.au/patient-safety-programs/assurance-governance/blood-watch>.

REFERENCES

Australian Commission on Safety and Quality in Health Care. (2016). *National Safety and Quality Health Service Standards Version 2.* Draft, Sydney, Australia.

Australian Institute of Health and Welfare (AIHW). (2017). *Leukaemia in Australia.* Accessed January 2017 at <www.aihw.gov.au/cancer/leukaemia>.

Australian & New Zealand Society of Blood Transfusion Ltd. (2011). *Guidelines for the Administration of Blood Products* (2nd edn). Accessed January 2017 at <www.anzsbt.org.au/data/documents/guidlines/ANZSBT_Guidelines_Administration_Blood_Products_2ndEd_Dec_2011_Hyperlinks.pdf>.

Australian Red Cross Blood Service. (2016). *Transfusion Checklist.* Accessed January 2017 at <http://resources.transfusion.com.au/cdm/singleitem/collection/p16691coll1/id/880>.

Australian Red Cross Blood Service. (2012). *Flippin' Blood: A BloodSafe Flip Chart to Help Make Transfusion Straightforward.* Accessed January 2017 at <http://resources.transfusion.com.au/cdm/ref/collection/p16691coll1/id/20>.

Fleming, D. R. (2012). *Leukemia: Understanding Its Types and Treatments.* Accessed January 2017 at <www.oncologynurseadvisor.com/ce-courses/leukemia-understanding-its-types-and-treatments/article/232931>.

Foundation House. (2012). *Promoting Refugee Health: A Guide for Doctors, Nurses and Other Health Care Providers Caring for People from Refugee Backgrounds* (3rd edn). Brunswick, Vic.: Foundation House, Victorian Foundation for Survivors of Torture. Accessed March 2017 at <http://refugeehealthnetwork.org.au/wp-content/uploads/PRH-online-edition_July2012.pdf>.

Nursing and Midwifery Board of Australia (NMBA). (2016). *Registered Nurse Standards for Practice.* Retrieved from <www.nursingmidwiferyboard.gov.au/Codes-Guidelines-Statements/Professional-standards.aspx>.

Wang, Y. W., Davidson, M. M., Yakushko, O. F., Savoy, H. B., Tan, J. A. & Bleier, J. K. (2003). The scale of ethnocultural empathy: Development, validation, and reliability. *Journal of Counseling Psychology, 50*(2), 221.

PHOTO CREDIT

160 Peter Turnley/Corbis/VCG via Getty Images

CHAPTER 10

CARING FOR A PERSON WITH SEPSIS

NATALIE GOVIND AND MARCIA INGLES

LEARNING OUTCOMES

Completion of the activities in this chapter will enable you to:

- explain why an understanding of sepsis is essential to competent practice (**recall** and **application**)
- identify the clinical manifestations of sepsis and septic shock that are used to guide the collection and interpretation of appropriate cues (**gather**, **review**, **interpret**, **discriminate**, **relate** and **infer**)
- identify risk factors for sepsis and septic shock (**match** and **predict**)
- review clinical information to identify the main nursing diagnoses for a patient with sepsis and/or septic shock (**synthesise**)
- describe the priorities of care for a patient with sepsis and septic shock (**goal setting** and **taking action**)
- identify clinical criteria for determining the effectiveness of nursing actions taken to manage sepsis and septic shock (**evaluate**)
- apply what you have learnt about sepsis to new situations (**reflection** and **translation**).

INTRODUCTION

The scenario introduced in this chapter focuses on the care of a person who experiences sepsis. You will be introduced to Damien Arnold and follow his healthcare journey from admission to discharge. Sepsis is a time-critical emergency and one of the leading causes of morbidity and mortality in hospitalised patients worldwide (Fleischmann et al., 2016; Vincent et al., 2014). It affects more than 30 million people globally each year and is one of the most underestimated health risks (Reinhart et al., 2013). Each year in Australia, more than 3000 people die from sepsis and this figure translates to a greater burden of death than either breast, prostate or colorectal cancer (Kaukonen et al., 2014). A reduction in the incidence of sepsis could be achieved through improved adherence to hygiene standards, detection and early recognition of signs and symptoms, and accurate and time-critical clinical management. Excellent clinical reasoning skills will help you to identify and manage people with sepsis, with the aim of preventing deterioration and adverse patient outcomes.

KEY CONCEPTS

sepsis
septic shock
lactate
deterioration
rapid response

SUGGESTED READINGS

P. LeMone, K. Burke, G. Bauldoff, P. Gubrud-Howe, T. Levett-Jones, T. Dwyer . . . D. Raymond (Eds). (2017). *Medical–Surgical Nursing: Critical Thinking in Person-Centred Care* (3rd edn). Melbourne: Pearson. Chapter 10: Nursing care of people experiencing trauma and shock

J. Vaughan & A. Parry. (2016). Assessment and management of the septic patient: Part 1. *British Journal of Nursing, 25*(17), 958–64.

G. Casey. (2016). Could this be sepsis? *Kai Tiaki Nursing New Zealand, 22*(7), 20–24.

SETTING THE SCENE

Damien Arnold, an 18-year-old male, was brought to the Emergency Department (ED) of a regional hospital by his mother, Margaret. She was very worried and told the triage nurse that, 'Damien is never sick! He hasn't even been coming out of his room to eat … it's just not like him.'

Margaret gave the nurse a letter from the after-hours GP practice they had attended; it stated that 'Damien was playing football three days ago and sustained an abrasion on his left forearm, which is now cellulitic in appearance. He has been feeling unwell for the last two days with weakness, loss of appetite and thirst, but he assumed that it was due to alcohol consumption during post-game celebrations. Significant medical history is Wegener's granulomatosis (now in remission) resulting in a kidney transplant three years ago, which is currently managed with immunosuppressant medications.'

Damien was given an Australian Triage Score (ATS) of 2 and transferred to an acute bed.

> The NSQHS Standards emphasise that parents know their children best and can be acutely aware when their child is unwell or 'just not right', sometimes before the physiological parameters become abnormal. Concern on the part of a parent should be given appropriate consideration and may require escalation (ACSQHC, 2016).

The epidemiology of sepsis

Due to the ageing population, the greater number of invasive procedures being performed and the increase in disease survival, the incidence of sepsis is increasing worldwide (Singer et al., 2016). However, because of the complexities of the disease and the limited reporting within the Global Burden of Disease study, the true incidence of sepsis remains unknown (Fleischmann et al., 2016; Vincent et al., 2014). In Australia, there are approximately 16 000 people admitted to ICU with sepsis each year with a cost of nearly $40 000 per person; 18 per cent of these patients die from sepsis-related complications (Clinical Excellence Commission, 2015).

> Globally, someone dies from sepsis every 3.5 seconds. For more information about how sepsis impacts patients and families, go to <http://sepsistrust.org/professional/educational-tools> and <www.sepsis.org/resources/video-library>.

The aetiology and pathogenesis of sepsis and septic shock

In simple terms, sepsis is a life-threatening condition where the body's response to an infection causes injury to its own tissues and organs (Singer et al., 2016)—see Figure 10.1. In 2016, the definition of sepsis was revised by the Third International Consensus Definitions Task Force (Sepsis-3). Sepsis is now defined as 'a life-threatening organ dysfunction caused by a dysregulated host response to infection' (Singer et al., 2016, p. 804). Septic shock is defined as 'a subset of sepsis in which underlying circulatory and cellular/metabolic abnormalities are profound enough to substantially increase mortality' (Singer et al., 2016, p. 805).

> Watch the following video: Consensus Definitions for Sepsis and Septic Shock (2016): <https://youtu.be/1S8l5D2xr6w>.
>
> Watch this brief animation to gain an understanding of the pathophysiology of sepsis: <https://vimeo.com/63845243>.
>
> Watch this brief animation to gain an understanding of the pathophysiology of septic shock: <www.youtube.com/watch?v=bt-H5VQl5E>.

Person-centred care

Damien was born in Wamberal, a coastal town on the New South Wales Central Coast, and lives with his parents Margaret and David. He enjoys being physically active, surfs and plays basketball and football. When Damien was 14 years old, he was diagnosed with Wegener's granulomatosis, a rare type of inflammation that targets the arteries, veins and capillaries of the kidneys and the respiratory system. By the time he was diagnosed, Damien had sustained significant and irreversible damage to his right kidney, and his left kidney function was also deteriorating, so he was given a kidney transplant from an anonymous donor. Since then, Damien has been in remission and is taking immunosuppressant medications for maintenance therapy. Due to his illness, Damien was absent from school for long periods of time, so at the age of 17 he decided to leave school and take up an apprenticeship with his father's electrical business.

> Consider how a parent of a child who has had a transplant may feel if their child becomes unwell. How would you address their concerns?

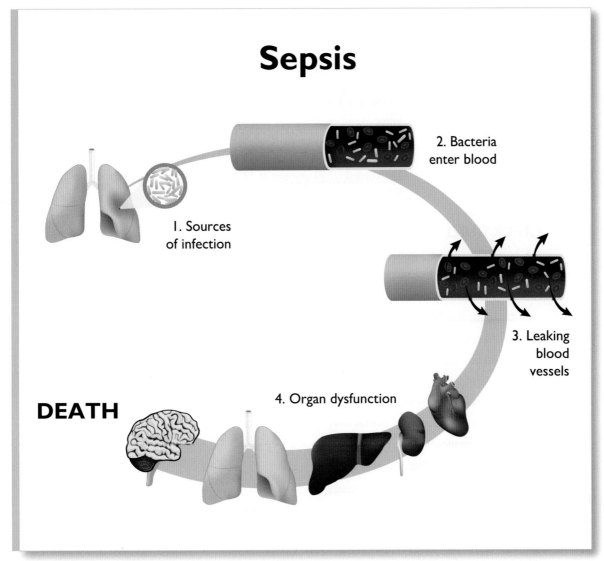

Sepsis

1. Sources of infection

2. Bacteria enter blood

3. Leaking blood vessels

4. Organ dysfunction

DEATH

Figure 10.1
Cascade of events in simulation

Source: © Designua/Shutterstock.com

1. CONSIDER THE PATIENT SITUATION

At 2100 hours, Damien is allocated to your care. He is pale and is lying in a supine position with his eyes closed. You receive the following handover from the triage nurse.

Handover report

This is Damien Arnold, an 18-year-old with suspected sepsis. He has a history of feeling unwell for the last two days with weakness, loss of appetite and thirst. There is a 3-day-old abrasion on his left forearm. Medical history includes Wegener's granulomatosis, which resulted in a kidney transplant three years ago; he is now in remission. His only medications are immunosuppressants.

Damien states that he has no pain in his arm or anywhere else in his body. He has an ATS 2 and I have commenced the adult sepsis pathway. The senior medical officer has been informed and is on his way to assess Damien. His mum, Margaret, has gone to call his father. I have asked the administration staff to send her straight through when she returns.

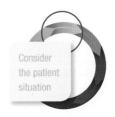

Consider the patient situation

Admission observations:

Airway	patent
Respiratory rate	26 breaths/min
SpO$_2$	97% on room air
Heart rate	110 beats/min
Blood pressure	135/90 mmHg
AVPU	voice
Temperature	38.6°C
Fluids in	last intake at 2000 hrs approximately 400 mL H$_2$O
Fluid out	last voided small amount at 1730 hrs, dark urine appearance
BGL	6.5 mmol/L

> *Refer to the article 'Could this be sepsis?' (Casey, 2016) for information about the development and risks of sepsis.*

QUICK QUIZ!

Q1 An ATS score of 2 indicates that the maximum waiting time for a person to receive medical assessment and treatment is:

   a 120 minutes

   b Immediately

   c 10 minutes

   d 20 minutes

Q2 The AVPU scale is a system by which a healthcare professional can measure and record a patient's responsiveness, indicating their level of consciousness. The acronym stands for:

   a Alert, Vision, Pain, Unconscious

   b Appearance, Verbal, Pain, Unresponsive

   c Alert, Voice, Pain, Unresponsive

   d Aware, Voice, Pain, Unconscious

Medical assessment of Damien

At 2110, the senior medical officer arrives to examine Damien. A trauma call is received so, after she completes her assessment, she asks the junior medical officer to insert two PIVC and collect two sets of blood cultures from two separate sites. Other bloods collected include VBG for lactate, FBC, EUC, CRP, LFTs and coags. The senior medical officer prescribes 2 g IV cephazolin 8-hourly and an IV fluid bolus of 20 mL/kg stat. She asks you to swab the wound to send to pathology, and to continue monitoring Damien's observations. She states that she will return as soon as possible to review his condition and that Damien is to stay in overnight.

Q1 Why might the senior medical officer have decided to hospitalise Damien overnight?

You assist the junior medical officer to prepare for cannula insertion but he appears hurried and you notice that he has forgotten gloves and alcohol-based swabs. You go and get the equipment but by the time you return the first cannula has been inserted. You suggest that he perform hand hygiene, don gloves and use the alcohol-based swabs before he inserts the second peripheral cannula, but he shakes his head saying, 'It's all good, I washed my hands before and gloves make it too difficult to find the vein. Don't worry, I have never had any issues.'

> *Preventing and controlling healthcare-associated infection is one of the NSQHS Standards. The purpose of this standard is to minimise risk and exposure to preventable infections, and if they do occur, to use evidence-based treatment approaches (ACSQHC, 2016).*

Q2 How would you respond if you were to encounter a similar situation in your future practice?

QUICK QUIZ!

The medical orders included a number of abbreviations. Before progressing to the next stage of the clinical reasoning cycle, test your understanding of these terms.

Q Match each abbreviation to the correct definition.

Peripheral intravenous cannula/catheter (PIVC)	Protein made by the liver and secreted into the blood. It is often the first evidence of inflammation or an infection in the body.
Full blood count (FBC)	From the Latin word *statim* meaning 'Immediately'.
Electrolytes, urea, creatinine (EUC)	This test is performed to determine the coagulation activity of a person to control the blood clotting process.
Liver function tests (LFT)	A device inserted into a small peripheral vein for therapeutic management such as administration of medications and fluids.
Stat	It is a screening panel that examines different components of the blood checking for conditions such as anaemia, infection and many other disorders.
C-reactive protein (CRP)	This test is performed to look at the basic chemical balance of the blood, as well as kidney function.
Venous blood gas (VBG)	This test is a screening panel that looks at ALT, AST, alkaline phosphatase, PT, INR, albumin and bilirubin.
Coags	An alternative technique of estimating lactate and pH levels that does not require arterial blood sampling.

Caring for an immunocompromised patient suspected of having sepsis is challenging. For further information, access the article by Donnelly et al. (2016).

2. COLLECT CUES/INFORMATION

The Sepsis Alliance (www.sepsis.org) developed SEPSIS as an acronym to aid in recognition of the signs and symptoms of this condition:

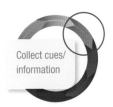

Collect cues/ information

S—Shivering, fever or feeling very cold
E—Extreme pain or general discomfort
P—Palor or discolouration of skin
S—Sleepiness, difficult to rouse, confusion
I—'I feel like I might die' (sense of impending doom)
S—Shortness of breath (dyspnoea)

(a) Review current information

The next stage of the clinical reasoning cycle is to collect relevant cues and information. Start by reviewing Damien's current observations:

Airway	patent
Respiratory rate	28 breaths/min
SpO$_2$	93% on room air
Heart rate	118 beats/min
Blood pressure	115/70 mmHg
Temperature	38.6°C
BGL	5.5 mmol/L
Lactate	2 mmol/L

Q The triage nurse stated that the adult sepsis pathway had been commenced. Using the information you now have, identify relevant risk factors for Damien.

For more information, refer to the NSW Health, Sepsis Kills: Adult Sepsis Pathway: <www.cec.health.nsw.gov.au/__data/assets/pdf_file/0005/291803/Adult-Sepsis-Pathway-Sept-2016-with-watermark.pdf>.

The NMBA's Registered Nurse Standards for Practice (2016) state that RNs must comply with legislation, regulations, policies, guidelines and other standards or requirements relevant to the context of practice when making decisions.

(b) Gather new information

Q   From the list below, identify the three additional cues that are *most* relevant to your assessment of Damien at this time.

    a   Weight (75 kg)

    b   Capillary return (<2 secs)

    c   Level of consciousness (voice)

    d   Pain 1/10

    e   Alcohol withdrawal score of 2

    f   Urine output (nil since presentation to ED)

(c) Recall knowledge

While cue collection involves reviewing current information and gathering new information, it also requires you to recall related knowledge.

QUICK QUIZ!

To build on your understanding of the key concepts related to sepsis, test yourself with the following questions.

Q1   Sepsis is a progressive condition that _____ capillary permeability due to a rise in _____ acid and _____ oxide. This triggers _____ and interrupts the body's ability to provide adequate _____, oxygen and nutrients to the _____ and cells.

Q2   What signs and symptoms are *most common* in patients presenting with sepsis? (Match the sign/symptom with the percentage.)

Acute oliguria	99%
Tachycardia	45%
Changes in mental status	54%
Fever >38.5°C	97%
Metabolic acidosis	70%
Tachypnoea	13%
Hypothermia <36°C	38%

3. PROCESS INFORMATION

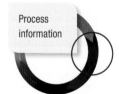

Process information

(a) Interpret

The next step of the clinical reasoning cycle is to interpret the data (cues) that you have collected by careful analysis and applying your knowledge of sepsis. By comparing normal versus abnormal, you will come to a more complete understanding of Damien's signs and symptoms.

Q1   Which of the following are considered to be within normal parameters for Damien?

    a   BGL: 5.5 mmol/L

    b   Heart rate: 118 beats/min

    c   Respiratory rate: 28 breaths/min

    d   Blood pressure: 115/70 mmHg

    e   Urine output: nil since presentation to ED

You review Damien's recent venous blood gas (VBG). His lactate is 2.0 mmol/L and his pH is 7.28, indicating metabolic acidosis.

Q2   What is the normal lactate level in both arterial and venous blood?

Q3 Damien's current observations indicate that he is tachypnoeic. Tachypnoea is the most common early detectable clinical sign of sepsis.

   a True

   b False

Q4 Tachypnoea is the respiratory system compensating for metabolic acidosis. Damien's brain is sending a message to stimulate an increase in respiratory rate in order to increase the carbon dioxide levels within his body.

   a True

   b False

Q5 Damien's current observations indicate that he is tachycardic. Unless a person has a cardiac conduction defect or is taking beta-blockers, tachycardia is an early detectable sign of sepsis. Tachycardia is a vital compensatory mechanism that aims to maintain _____ in response to _____ volume deficits, decreased cardiac contractility and _____.

(b) Discriminate

From the cues and information you now have, you need to narrow them down to the most important.

Q From the list below, select five cues that you believe are *most relevant* to Damien's condition *at this time*.

   a Blood pressure

   b Respiratory rate

   c Temperature

   d Heart rate

   e Condition of wound

   f Oxygen saturation

   h Level of consciousness

   i Appetite

   j Urine output

   k Pain

   l BGL

   m Lactate level

(c) Relate

It is important to cluster the cues together and to identify relationships between them (based on the information you have collected so far).

Q Label the following 'true' or 'false':

   a Damien is normotensive due to the beta-blocker medications he is prescribed.

   b Damien is febrile because his inflammatory response has been activated as a result of the invasion of pathogens.

   c Damien has an increased heart rate as a compensatory mechanism to increased cardiac output.

   d Damien has decreased oxygen saturations as a result of hypertension and tachypnoea.

   e Damien has a wound and is immunocompromised, which are two factors that increase his risk of developing sepsis.

   f Damien could be oliguric from hyperglycaemia.

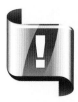

Something to think about ...

Following renal transplant, a regimen of immunosuppressive medications are prescribed to prevent organ rejection. However, these medications reduce the function of the naturally occurring immune system within the body, making patients more susceptible to infection. Some studies indicate that infections are responsible for the deaths of nearly 20 per cent of transplant recipients. Treatment of infections is complicated by the fact that drug interactions frequently occur between antibiotics and the immunosuppressive regimen (Silkensen, 2000).

(d) Infer

It is time to think about all the cues that you have collected about Damien's condition, and to make inferences based on your analysis and interpretation of those cues.

Q   From what you know about Damien's history, and signs and symptoms (as well as your knowledge about sepsis), identify which three of the following inferences are correct.

     a   Damien is normotensive and bradycardic.

     b   Damien is oliguric and tachycardic.

     c   Damien is hypertensive and tachycardic.

     d   Damien is febrile and normotensive.

     e   Damien is hypoxic and febrile.

     f   Damien is polyuric and hypotensive.

(e) Predict

At this stage, you begin to consider the consequences of your actions, or inaction, by predicting potential outcomes for your patient.

Q   If you do not take the appropriate actions at this time and Damien's condition is not managed correctly, what could happen? (Select the four that apply.)

     a   Damien could develop disseminated intravascular coagulation (DIC).

     b   Damien's condition will gradually improve over the next few days.

     c   Damien could develop acute kidney injury.

     d   Damien could develop acute respiratory distress syndrome.

     e   Damien could die.

     f   Damien could become hypertensive and hypoglycaemic.

     g   Damien could develop septic shock.

4. IDENTIFY THE PROBLEM/ISSUE

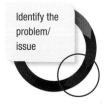

Identify the problem/issue

Now bring together (synthesise) all of the facts you've collected and inferences you've made to identify a *priority* nursing diagnosis for Damien.

Q   Select from the following list the four correct nursing diagnoses for Damien.

     a   Ineffective tissue perfusion related to an inflammatory response to infectious pathogens, as evidenced by decreased oxygen saturation level, tachypnoea, tachycardia, oliguria and increased lactate level

     b   Fluid volume overload related to damaged capillary walls and vasodilation, as evidenced by hypotension, oliguria and bradycardia

     c   Risk of decreased cardiac output related to decreased preload

     d   Impaired skin integrity related to poor hygiene, as evidenced by abrasion on left forearm, increased temperature and tachycardia

e   Acute pain related to cellulitic wound on left forearm, as evidenced by hyperthermia, tachypnoea, hyperglycaemia and hypertension

f   Hypovolaemia related to damaged capillary walls and vasodilation, as evidenced by hypotension, oliguria and bradycardia

g   Risk of septic shock related to inflammatory response to infectious pathogens, ineffective tissue perfusion and hypovolaemia

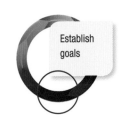

Remember, time is critical when caring for a person with sepsis, as early recognition and treatment improves patient outcomes.

5. ESTABLISH GOALS

Q   Before implementing any actions to improve Damien's condition, it is important to specify what you want to happen and when. From the list below, choose the *most important* short-term goals for Damien's management at this time.

a   Damien's wound will be cleaned and a sterile dressing applied within the next 15 minutes.

b   Damien will be discharged home from the ED within the next 3 hours.

c   Damien will have no evidence of further deterioration within the next 60 minutes.

d   Damien will be normotensive with urine output greater than 80–100 mL/hr within the next 24 hours.

6. TAKE ACTION

This stage of the clinical reasoning cycle requires knowledge, clinical skills, effective communication skills and sophisticated clinical reasoning ability. The nurse has to decide which actions take priority, who should be notified and who is best placed to undertake each nursing action.

Q   From the list below, choose the eight *most immediate* actions you should take at this stage.

a   Administer oxygen therapy to maintain saturations ≥95%.

b   Monitor Damien's pain score.

c   Continuous monitoring and documentation of Damien's vital signs and oxygen saturation level.

d   Monitor and document the condition of Damien's wound.

e   Administer IV antibiotics as ordered within 60 minutes.

f   Administer a normal saline fluid bolus as ordered (20 mL/kg stat).

g   Collect a venous blood sample for lactate and glucose levels.

h   Position Damien in a semi-Fowler's to high-Fowler's as tolerated.

i   Assess Damien's level of consciousness using AVPU every 30 minutes.

j   Reposition Damien to minimise pressure area development.

k   Strictly monitor and document Damien's fluid input/output and maintain hourly urine measures.

Something to think about …

Antimicrobial resistance is an ever-increasing threat to safe patient care. For further information about the use of antibiotics and microbial resistance, access

Responding to the threat of antimicrobial resistance *at*

<www.health.gov.au/internet/main/publishing.nsf/Content/1803C433C71415CACA257C8400121B1F/ $File/amr-strategy-2015-2019.pdf>

and

Antimicrobial stewardship. Why all the fuss? *at*

<www.cec.health.nsw.gov.au/__data/assets/pdf_file/0003/273045/AMS-Tool-Kit-Why-all-the-fuss-Clinician-handout.pdf>.

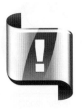

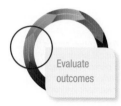

7. EVALUATE

It is now 2300, two hours since Damien presented to the ED. He has been given a 1500 mL fluid bolus (20 mL/75 kg) stat; broad-spectrum IV antibiotics have been administered as ordered; and he has oxygen therapy at 3 L/min via nasal prongs. Damien's signs and symptoms provide you with data to make a determination of whether or not the nursing and medical interventions have been effective, and whether his condition is improving.

Q1 Rate each of the following signs and symptoms as unchanged, improving or deteriorating.

   a   Oxygen saturations: 97%

   b   Heart rate: 90 beats/min

   c   AVPU: voice

   d   Respirations: 23 breaths/min

   e   Temperature: 38.0°C

   f   Lactate: 1.5 mmol/L

   g   Urine output: 20 mL/hr

   h   Blood pressure: 110/75

   i   Colour: pale

   j   BGL: 7.5 mmol/L

Q2 You now need to synthesise these parameters to decide whether Damien's condition has improved overall. Which of the following statements is the *most correct*?

   a   Damien's condition has improved significantly.

   b   Damien's condition has not improved and you need to call a rapid response.

   c   Damien's condition has improved but still requires careful monitoring and reassessment. You will need to contact the doctor again if further improvement is not seen in the next hour.

   e   Damien's condition has not improved but you will monitor his condition carefully for the next 24 hours.

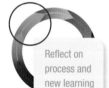

8. REFLECT

The final stage of the clinical reasoning cycle is 'reflection'. Reflect on your learning from this scenario and consider the following questions.

Q1 What are three of the most important things that you have learnt from this scenario?

Q2 What actions will you take in clinical practice as a result of your learning from this scenario?

SCENARIO 10.2   Caring for a person with septic shock

CHANGING THE SCENE

1. CONSIDER THE PATIENT SITUATION

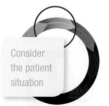

At 2330 hours, Damien's condition is stable and he is transferred to the short-stay ward for observation. He has IV fluids running at 100 mL/hr and is to have IV antibiotics as prescribed.

The following day you return for another night shift. It is quiet in the ED, so you are sent to the short-stay ward, which is busy and short staffed. By chance, you are allocated to the care of Damien and you look forward to seeing how he is progressing. The afternoon staff provide the following handover report:

Handover report

Damien Arnold, 18 years, was admitted last night via ED with sepsis, most likely due to a cellulitic wound on his left arm. His obs have been stable; they were last taken at 1800 hrs by one of the AINs. I presume they are OK as she hasn't voiced any concerns.

> The NMBA (2007) specifies that RNs can delegate nursing care activities only when the appropriate level of supervision can be provided. When an RN delegates care to an AIN, they must provide guidance, assistance, support and clinically focused supervision.

Damien's medications have been administered as charted, although his 1600 hrs IV antibiotic wasn't given until 1800 hrs because we've been so busy. He has an IV at 100 mL/hr via PIVC in the right cubical fossa; it's patent but a bit red. His mum keeps saying 'it should come out', but Damien is not complaining. The other PIVC is in the left hand and currently capped.

Damien is taking sips of water but has not eaten today; he says he is not hungry. He is passing small amounts of urine. He was getting up to the bathroom this morning but has been sleeping for most of the afternoon/evening. We've just let him sleep as we have been flat out. We are still waiting for results from his blood cultures and wound swab; I've asked the medical team to follow this up. Also, as per the sepsis pathway, another VBG was collected for lactate; I haven't had a chance to see if the results are back yet. Damien's mother has been here all day. She keeps saying to anyone who will listen that he is not getting better ... she requires lots of reassurance. I think because Damien had a kidney transplant three years ago, Margaret is overprotective.

> *Overdue doses (i.e. medications that are prescribed but not administered on time) are the second largest cause of reported medication incidents. Importantly, failure to administer antibiotics at the prescribed time can lead to serious patient harm (Coleman et al., 2013).*

Q1 Based on the handover report, what are your initial concerns about Damien's current situation?

Q2 The nurse's comment about Margaret being 'overprotective' is an example of which clinical reasoning error?

2. COLLECT CUES/INFORMATION

(a) Review current information

You review Damien's charts and identify that the following observations were documented at 1800:

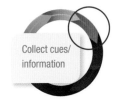

Collect cues/information

Respiratory rate	26
Oxygen saturation level	94% 3 L O_2 via NP
Heart rate	105 beats/min
Blood pressure	105/70 mmHg
AVPU	voice
Temperature	38°C
Fluids IN	100 mL/hr (total IN from midnight: 1900 mL)
Fluids OUT	380 mL (since midnight)
BGL	6.2 mmol/L

(b) Gather new information

When you enter Damien's room at 1920 hours, Margaret says, 'Oh, you're the nurse from ED; I am so glad to see you. He's not getting better; he can't keep his eyes open, his breathing sounds funny and no one will listen to me! Please help him.'

You note that Damien is lying on his left side with his eyes closed. You observe that his nasal prongs have slipped down to his chin and there is increased work of breathing. You touch his arm and it feels cool. When you ask, 'How are you feeling Damien?' he doesn't open his eyes, but quietly moans. You then conduct a head-to-toe assessment.

Q From the following list, select the seven cues that are *most relevant* at this stage.

   a Respiratory rate: 32 and observed increase work of breathing

   b Oxygen saturations: 90% 3 L O_2 via NP

   c Heart rate: 115 beats/min

   d Blood pressure: 90/55 mmHg

   e Glasgow Coma Scale: 11

   f Pupillary response: PEARL (Pupils Equal and Reactive to Light)

   h Mobility status: 1 × assistance

   i BGL: 7.8 mmol/L

   j Temperature: 38.0°C

k   Lactate: 4 mmol/L

l   Condition of wound to forearm: dressing dry and intact, no ooze

n   PIVC in right cubical fossa: redness and tracking along vein noted

o   Nil signs of pressure area development

(c) Recall knowledge

QUICK QUIZ!

Q1 Fill in the missing words in this paragraph:

Shock is a life-threatening condition related to the failure of the _____ system, characterised by _____ leading to poor oxygenation and nutrition delivery to the tissues. Due to the _____ _____ in the body, the effects of shock are initially _____. However, the person's condition will rapidly deteriorate without _____ appropriate management and the shock will become _____ resulting in _____ _____ _____ _____ (_____) and _____.

Q2 Septic shock is a form of:

a   Cardiogenic shock—reduction in cardiac output due to a primary cardiac disorder

b   Obstructive shock—interference with the mechanical mechanisms of the heart

c   Distributive shock—maldistribution of intravascular volume

d   Hypovolaemic shock—decreased intravascular volume

Q3 Lactate is an indicator of tissue hyperperfusion.

a   True

b   False

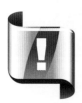

To learn more about lactate and sepsis, access the resource at <www.cec.health.nsw.gov.au/__data/assets/pdf_file/0007/259387/lactate-information-sheet-for-clinicians.pdf>.

Q4 What are the normal levels of serum lactate?

a   <1.0 mmol/L

b   1.0–2.0 mmol/L

c   2.0–4.0 mmol/L

d   4.0–6.0 mmol/L

Something to think about

Lactate is a normal product of anaerobic cell metabolism. It is released into the blood and metabolised by the liver when there is insufficient oxygen for cellular activity. Elevated lactate is typically present in patients with severe sepsis or septic shock. A lactate level above 4.0 mmol/L is associated with a 27 per cent mortality rate (Boschert, 2007) and should activate an immediate rapid response call.

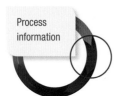

Process information

3. PROCESS INFORMATION

(a) Interpret, (b) Discriminate and (c) Relate

Q   Which seven of the following signs and symptoms is Damien displaying that are suggestive of septic shock?

a   Tachypnoea

b   High pain score

c   Hypertension

d   Decreased level of consciousness

    e   Hyperglycaemia

    f   Pupillary response: PEARL

    g   Hypotension

    h   ECG rhythm: sinus tachycardia

    i   Temperature: 38°C

    j   Lactate: 4 mmol/L

    k   Hypoglycaemia

    l   Hypoxia

    m Oliguria

(d) Infer

Q From what you know about sepsis and septic shock, what are four signs or symptoms that may be an early warning for a potential adverse outcome for Damien?

(e) Predict

Q What could happen to Damien if appropriate action is not taken at this time? (Select all that apply.)

    a   Damien could have a cardiac arrest.

    b   Damien could develop multi-organ dysfunction syndrome (MODS).

    c   Damien's condition will gradually improve over the next few days.

    d   Damien could develop pulmonary oedema.

    E   Damien could die.

    f   Damien could develop disseminated intravascular coagulation (DIC).

(f) Match

Q Have you ever seen someone with the same signs and symptoms as Damien? If so, what was done to manage the situation?

4. IDENTIFY THE PROBLEM/ISSUE

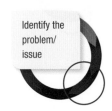

Identify the problem/ issue

Q1 From the information that you currently have, identify the *three correct* nursing diagnoses for Damien:

    a   Hypoxia related to increased airway secretions, as evidenced by coughing, tachypneoa and decreased saturations

    b   Ineffective tissue perfusion related to decreased cardiac output and massive vasodilation, as evidenced by hypotension, tachycardia, decreased level of consciousness and cool peripheries

    c   Fluid volume deficit related to maldistribution of intravascular volume to the interstitial spaces, as evidenced by tachypneoa, tachycardia, hypotension and oliguria

    d   Ineffective breathing pattern related to shallow respirations and increased work of breathing, as evidenced by decreased oxygen saturations, increased respirations and tachycardia

    e   Impaired gas exchange related to interference with oxygen delivery from endotoxin-induced damage to the cells and capillaries, as evidenced by tachypnoea, increased work of breathing and hypoxia.

Q2 Factors contributing to a failure to recognise and respond to a deteriorating patient are multifaceted. With reference to James Reason's 'Swiss Cheese Model' (2000), label Figure 10.2 with the factors that may have contributed to Damien's deterioration.

If you do not understand the analogy of the Swiss Cheese Model, read p. 18 in Chapter 2.

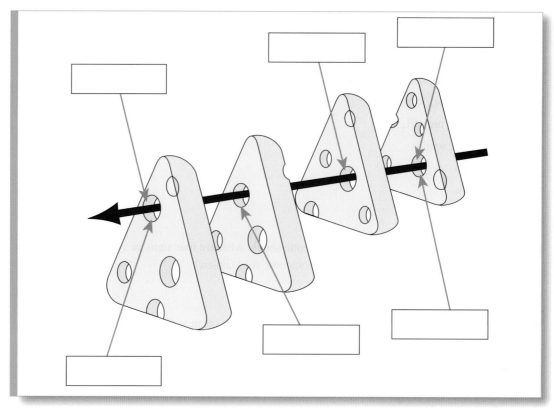

Figure 10.2
Reason's Swiss Cheese Model

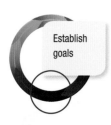

5. ESTABLISH GOALS

Before implementing any actions to improve Damien's condition, it is important to clearly specify what you want to happen and when.

Q   From the list below, choose the four *most important* goals for Damien's management at this time.

   a   Damien will be self-caring and ambulant within the next 24 hours.

   b   Damien will be haemodynamically stable with an adequate circulating blood volume within 4–6 hours.

   c   Oral food and fluid intake will be established within 60 minutes.

   d   The potential source of infection will be identified and/or removed within 15 minutes.

   e   Damien will maintain his airway and will achieve adequate oxygenation saturations (>95%) within 30 minutes.

   f   Damien's urine output will be at least 37.5 mL/hr (0.5 mL/kg/hr) within 4 hours.

   g   Damien will not display evidence of pressure area development within 30 minutes.

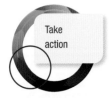

6. TAKE ACTION

Q1   From the list below, choose the eight most *immediate* actions you should take at this stage.

   a   Call a rapid response.

   b   Administer a diuretic.

   c   Continue to monitor haemodynamic status and vital signs closely.

   d   Administer oxygen therapy to maintain saturations >95%.

e Complete and document vital signs QID.

f Remove the PIVC from right cubical fossa and collect tip to send to pathology.

g Check weight each day.

h Decrease IV rate TKVO pending medical orders.

i Monitor cognitive status.

k Maintain patent IV access.

j Monitor for improvement in serum bloods including lactate.

k Lie Damien down and raise his legs above the level of his heart.

l Administer oxygen 2 L/min via nasal prongs.

m Assess and maintain patent airway.

n Prepare handover and remain with Damien until the rapid response team arrives.

Q2 Using ISBAR (Identity, Situation, Background, Assessment, Request/Recommendation), document how you would communicate with the rapid response team leader.

7. EVALUATE

Q List six signs and symptoms that will indicate to you that Damien's condition has improved following the rapid response call and initiation of appropriate actions.

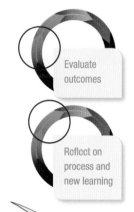

Evaluate outcomes

Reflect on process and new learning

8. REFLECT

Contemplate what you have learnt from this scenario and how this learning will inform your practice. Respond to the following three questions with reference to Scenario 10.2.

Q1 How could Damien's deterioration have been prevented?

Q2 What have you learnt from the scenario that you can apply to your future practice?

Access this video to gain a deeper understanding of the risk's associated with complacency when caring for a person with sepsis: <https://youtu.be/Ch-XuVY_T9M>.

EPILOGUE

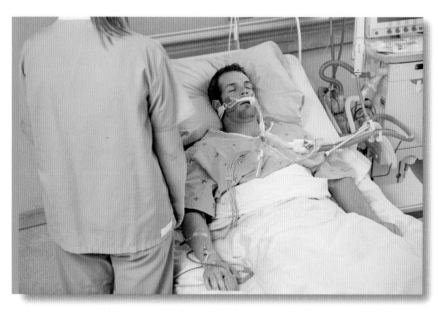

Damien being treated for septic shock in the ICU

Damien was assessed by the rapid response team and transferred to the Intensive Care Unit (ICU) for ongoing clinical management. A central line and arterial line were inserted and Damien was intubated and ventilated. Despite fluid resuscitation, his blood pressure remained low and a noradrenaline (vasopressor) infusion was commenced to maintain his blood pressure to the target of MAP >65 mmHg. Damien continued to deteriorate and he was diagnosed with acute kidney injury. On days 6–10, he required continuous renal replacement therapy (CRRT) (dialysis). He also required an insulin infusion as his BGLs were unstable due to his critical illness. Throughout this time, Damien remained sedated with morphine and midazolam infusions. On day 12, Damien displayed signs of respiratory and haemodynamic stabilisation and by day 14 he was extubated and the noradrenaline ceased. Damien remained in ICU for another three days and was then transferred to the High Dependency Unit (HDU).

Damien spent 35 days in hospital before being discharged. He still suffers from disabling fatigue, poor concentration, insomnia and nightmares. Fortunately, his kidneys did not suffer any further damage and, despite the insult on his body systems, his Wegener's granulomatosis remained in remission. Damien hopes to return to work, at least part-time, within two to three months. Margaret believes that it was the ED nurse who saved her son's life, as no one else would listen to her concerns.

FURTHER READING

Clinical Excellence Commission (CEC). (2011). *Sepsis Kills Program.* Accessed November 2016 at <www.cec.health.nsw.gov.au/patient-safety-programs/adult-patient-safety/sepsis-kills>.
Surviving Sepsis Campaign. (2016). Accessed March 2017 at <www.survivingsepsis.org>.
World Sepsis Day. Accessed March 2017 at <www.world-sepsis-day.org>.

REFERENCES

Australian Commission on Safety and Quality in Health Care (ACSQHC). (2016). *National Safety and Quality Health Service Standards Version 2.* Draft, Sydney, Australia.
Boschert, S. (2007). Is it septic shock? Check lactate level. *ACEP News.* Accessed March 2017 at <www.acep.org/content.aspx?id=33984>.
Casey, G. (2016). Could this be sepsis? *Kai Tiaki Nursing New Zealand, 22*(7), 20–24.
Clinical Excellence Commission (CEC). (2015). *Antimicrobial Stewardship: Why All the Fuss?* Accessed November 2016 at <www.cec.health.nsw.gov.au/__data/assets/pdf_file/0003/273045/AMS-Tool-Kit-Why-all-the-fuss-Clinician-handout.pdf>.
Coleman, J., Hodson, J., Brooks, H. & Rosser, D. (2013). Missed medication doses in hospitalised patients: A descriptive account of quality improvement measures and time series analysis. *International Journal for Quality in Health Care, 25*(5), 564–72.
Donnelly, J. P., Locke, J. E., MacLennan, P. A., McGwin, G., Jr., Mannon, R. B., Safford, M. M., … Wang, H. E. (2016). Inpatient mortality among solid organ transplant recipients hospitalized for sepsis and severe sepsis. *Clinical Infectious Diseases, 63*(2), 186–94.
Fleischmann, C., Scherag, A., Adhikari, N., Hartog, C., Tsaganos, T., Schlattmann, P., … Reinhart, K. (International Forum of Acute Care Trialists). (2016). Assessment of global incidence and mortality of hospital-treated sepsis: Current estimates and limitations. *American Journal of Respiratory Critical Care Medicine, 193*(3), 259–72.
Kaukonen, K., Bailey, M., Suzuki, S., Pilcher, D. & Bellomo, R. (2014). Mortality related to severe sepsis and septic shock among critically ill patients in Australia and New Zealand. *JAMA, 311*(8), 1308–16.
Nursing and Midwifery Board of Australia (NMBA). (2016). *Registered Nurse Standards for Practice.* Accessed March 2017 at <www.nursingmidwiferyboard.gov.au/Codes-Guidelines-Statements/Professional-standards.aspx>.
Nursing and Midwifery Board of Australia (NMBA). (2007). *A National Framework for the Development of Decision-Making Tools for Nursing and Midwifery Practice.* Australian Nursing and Midwifery Council.
Reinhart, K., Daniels, R., Kissoon, N., O'Brien, J., Machado, F. & Jimenez, E. (GSA Executive Board and WSD Executive Board). (2013). The burden of sepsis—A call to action in support of World Sepsis Day 2013. *Journal of Critical Care, 28*(4), 526–28.
Sepsis Alliance (2017). Accessed March 2017 at <www.sepsis.org>.
Silkensen, J. (2000). Long-term complications in renal transplantation. *American Society of Nephrology, 11*, 582–88.
Singer, M., Deutschman, C. S., Seymour, C. W., Shankar-Hari, M., Annane, D., Bauer, M., … Angus, D. C. (2016). The Third International Consensus Definitions for Sepsis and Septic Shock (Sepsis-3). *JAMA, 315*(8), 801–10.
Vincent, J. L., Marshall, J. C., Namendys-Silva, S. A., Francois, B., Martin-Loeches, I., Lipman, J., … ICON Investigators. (2014). Assessment of the worldwide burden of critical illness: The Intensive Care Over Nations (ICON) audit. *Lancet, Respiratory Medicine, 2*(5), 380–86.

PHOTO CREDIT

CHAPTER 11

CARING FOR A 'CHALLENGING' PATIENT WITH A DUAL DIAGNOSIS

TERESA STONE AND RACHEL ROSSITER

LEARNING OUTCOMES

Completion of the activities in this chapter will enable you to:

- define the terms 'substance use disorder' and 'dual diagnosis' (**gather information, interpret** and **discriminate**)
- explain why an understanding of substance use disorder and generalised anxiety disorder is essential to competent nursing practice (**recall** and **application**)
- outline the clinical manifestations of substance use disorder and generalised anxiety disorder that will guide your collection of appropriate cues (**gather information, interpret** and **discriminate**)
- identify risk factors for substance use disorder (**match** and **predict**)
- review clinical information to identify the main nursing diagnoses for a person experiencing agitation and anxiety (**synthesise**)
- describe the priorities of care for the management of a person experiencing agitation and anxiety (**goal setting** and **taking action**)
- consider how stigma may interfere with person-centred care (**reflection** and **translation**)
- reflect on personal reactions to people who abuse alcohol or other drugs and identify appropriate self-management strategies (**reflection** and **translation**).

We simply assume that the way we see things is the way they really are or the way they should be. And our attitudes and behaviours grow out of these assumptions. (Covey, 2004)

INTRODUCTION

The two scenarios introduced in this chapter focus on the care of a patient with a substance use disorder and dual diagnosis, who many nurses might find 'challenging'. Difficulties in relating to someone who behaves like Shawn Bolton may compromise care and lead to avoidance. Anyone can nurse a grateful and compliant patient. It takes an empathic and professional nurse to care for someone like Shawn. People who complain, swear and demand constant attention are too often seen as being undeserving of care, and nurses may find it difficult to establish and maintain a therapeutic alliance with them. Add to that some tattoos, a criminal record and a stigmatising condition such as substance use disorder or mental illness, and less than optimal nursing care may result (Stone, McMillan & Hazelton, 2010).

Patients with complex needs and 'challenging' behaviours may be perceived by health workers to be time consuming, difficult to manage and a waste of resources. Too often they are labelled as 'frequent flyers' because of recurrent relapses and repeated presentations to emergency departments (Althaus et al., 2011). As soon as we hear labels such as 'frequent flyer', we know that there may be stigmatisation occurring. Goffman (1986) conceptualised stigma as an attribute that is 'deeply discrediting' and makes the person carrying it 'different from others and of a less desirable kind' (p. 3). Stigma diminishes self-esteem and robs people of social opportunities because of stereotype, prejudice and discrimination (Corrigan, 2004).

This chapter illustrates the types of ethical problems and conflicts that nurses often encounter when dealing with people with complex psychosocial and pathophysiological needs. However, excellent clinical reasoning skills will help you to recognise and manage dilemmas such as those portrayed here, resulting in empathic, accurate, timely and person-centred care.

KEY CONCEPTS

anxiety
substance use
stigma

SUGGESTED READINGS

P. LeMone, K. Burke, G. Bauldoff, P. Gubrud-Howe, T. Levett-Jones, T. Dwyer ... D. Raymond (Eds). (2017). *Medical–Surgical Nursing: Critical Thinking in Person-Centred Care* (3rd edn). Melbourne: Pearson.
Chapter 5: Nursing care of clients with problems of substance misuse
Chapter 50: Mental healthcare in the Australian context

F. Althaus, S. Paraz, O. Hugli, W. A. Ghali, J. B. Daeppen, I. Peytremann-Bridevaux & P. Podenmann. (2011). Effectiveness of interventions targeting frequent users of emergency departments: A systematic review. *Annals of Emergency Medicine, 58*(1), 41–52.e42.

Australian Institute of Health and Welfare. (2014). *Australia's Health 2014*. Canberra: AIHW.

J. R. Hughes, S. T. Higgins & W. K. Bickel. (1994). Nicotine withdrawal versus other drug withdrawal syndromes: Similarities and dissimilarities. *Addiction, 89*(11), 1461–70. doi: 10.1111/j.1360-0443.1994.tb03744.x

National Health and Medical Research Council. (2009). *Australian Guidelines to Reduce Health Risks from Drinking Alcohol*. Canberra: Commonwealth of Australia.

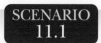

Caring for a person with a substance use disorder

SETTING THE SCENE

Mr Shawn Bolton is a 25-year-old man who was brought into hospital by ambulance following an accident on his motorbike. He underwent surgery for internal fixation of a fractured tibia and fibula. At the time of his accident, he had a blood alcohol level of 0.08 mmol/L and he has been charged with mid-range drink driving. This is not his first offence; he was also charged with assault when he was 15.

As a result of his accident and the charge against him, Shawn has been told by his boss that he no longer has a job. Since being in hospital, Shawn has complained incessantly about the no smoking policy, frequently using obscene language, and on two occasions he has been found smoking in the bathroom.

Shawn admits to drinking beer on a daily basis but denies using illicit drugs. Nurses have voiced their doubts about this, because a visitor apparently had marijuana on him when he was visiting Shawn, and there has been a lot of talk that this visitor is a drug dealer.

Shawn's fractures are healing. Although there are clinical concerns about his substance use, some of the nurses think the bed should be 'freed up' for a 'more deserving' patient.

The epidemiology of substance use disorder

In Australia, mental illnesses are one of the leading causes of disease burden, accounting for 13 per cent of the total burden of disease (AIHW, 2014). About 45 per cent of Australians aged 16–85 have experienced a mental disorder at some stage in their lifetime. Most commonly, these included anxiety disorders (14.4 per cent of the population), affective (mood) disorders (6.2 per cent) and substance use disorders (5.1 per cent) (AIHW, 2014).

The Diagnostic and Statistical Manual of Mental Disorders-V (DSM-V) (American Psychiatric Association, 2013) states that an essential feature of a substance use disorder is a cluster of cognitive, behavioural and physiological symptoms indicating that the individual continues using the substance despite significant substance-related problems. Alcohol use disorders are a subset of substance use disorders and refer to problematic patterns of alcohol use, leading to clinically significant impairment or distress (American Psychiatric Association, 2013).

Substance abuse and dependence are major problems in Western cultures and there has been a lot of concern raised about young people and 'binge drinking'. Although current guidelines for healthy people stipulate that drinking no more than four standard drinks on a single occasion will reduce the risk of alcohol-related injury on that occasion, to reduce lifetime risk, no more than two standard drinks per day should be consumed (National Health and Medical Research Council, 2009). However, one in five (18.2 per cent) Australians over the age of 14 drink at levels that put them at risk of alcohol-related harm over their lifetime, and around 1 in 6 people aged 12 years or older have consumed 11 or more standard drinks on a single occasion in the past 12 months. Alcohol abuse is a pattern of drinking that results in harm to one's health, interpersonal relationships or the ability to work. One of the questions you will need to ask yourself is whether Shawn has a substance use disorder or not.

About a third of Australians over the age of 14 have used marijuana at least once (AIHW, 2014) and its use has always been a hotly debated topic, with many arguing that it should be decriminalised because it is thought to be relatively harmless. However, long-term, cumulative and potentially permanent effects of chronic abuse can include addiction; bronchitis; emphysema; adverse effects on the immune system; increased risk of head, neck and lung cancer; and decreased testosterone levels, sperm counts and sperm motility.

In 2013, 13 per cent of Australians smoked daily in 2013, the lowest rate ever reported; 15 per cent of Australians had used an illicit drug in the previous 12 months; and 42 per cent had used an illicit drug in their lifetime. Cannabis, ecstasy, methamphetamine and cocaine were the most commonly used illicit drugs (AIHW, 2017).

To learn more about binge drinking, access <https://adf .org.au/wp-content/ uploads/2016/10/Binge-drinking.pdf>.

To find out how alcohol use by young people has changed, access Australian Psychological Society (2008), Substance use in the 21st century: Different or more of the same? at <www.psychology.org. au/inpsych/substance_ use>.

Access this site to examine the effects of substances on the brain: <http://learn.genetics .utah.edu/content/ addiction/mouse>.

Aboriginal and Torres Strait Islander people are more than twice as likely to smoke tobacco, with almost half being current smokers, which is more than double the rate of other Australians. Although Aboriginal and Torres Strait Islander people are more likely to abstain from drinking than other Australians, they are more likely to binge drink, with 17 per cent binge drinking compared with 8 per cent of other Australians (Australian Drug Foundation, 2011).

The aetiology and pathogenesis of substance use disorder

Factors that contribute to or affect patterns of substance use are many and varied, and include availability, genetic background, culture, family systems, social relationships, trauma, mental illness and medical illness (Johnson, 2003).

1. CONSIDER THE PATIENT SITUATION

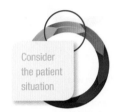

Consider the patient situation

It is now 0700 hours. You are allocated Shawn to care for on the morning shift and you are provided with the following handover report:

Handover report

Shawn Bolton is in room 4. He is day 2 post-op following internal fixation of a fractured tibia and fibula following an MVA. Self-caring, all obs stable, but he said he has a headache and sore throat—probably getting the flu as it's going around. He has been up all night demanding to go out for a smoke and agitated. He swore at me. I told him it was not appropriate, and walked out and have left him to his own devices. The only reason he is still here is that he has no discharge address; he has just found out that his flatmate has chucked out his stuff for non-payment of rent. The social worker should be in later today to sort out accommodation. Good luck to her. Watch him because he can be aggressive—he has a criminal record.

> The NSQHS Standards highlight the importance of structured effective clinical handovers for communication of critical patient information (ACSQHC, 2016).

Medical orders

Paracetamol 500 mg
Codeine phosphate 30 mg (Panadeine Forte) x ii PRN
Encourage mobilisation with physiotherapist
Observe for signs of alcohol withdrawal (refer to the Alcohol Withdrawal Scale)

Before proceeding to the next stage of the clinical reasoning cycle, consider the potential impact of this handover on Shawn's care.

Q1   How might the tone and content of this handover influence the care provided to Shawn during the next shift?

> Refer to the Alcohol Withdrawal Scale (AWS) (NSW Health, 2008, p. 84) at <www1.health .nsw.gov.au/pds/ ActivePDSDocuments/ GL2008_011.pdf>.

Q2   With reference to professional standards and codes of nursing practice, discuss whether the nurse who gave this handover displayed professional care.

Q3   If you were nursing Shawn overnight and his behaviour was as described, how might you care for him?

In response to unacceptable levels of aggression in the workplace, most health departments have introduced a zero tolerance to violence policy. NSW Health defines violence as 'any incident in which an individual is abused, threatened or assaulted and includes verbal, physical or psychological abuse, threats or other intimidating behaviours, intentional physical attacks, aggravated assault, threats with an offensive weapon, sexual harassment and sexual assault' (NSW Health, 2003, p. 7). This policy acknowledges other legislation such as the *Mental Health Act 2007* (NSW) and the *Anti-Discrimination Act 1977* (NSW), and states that 'consideration should always be given to the possible clinical aspects, [as behaviour] may be secondary to a number of medical conditions, physical or mental, and initial clinical assessment and prompt treatment should be of primary concern' (NSW Health, 2003, p. 29).

> The NMBA's Registered Nurse Standards for Practice (2016) state that RNs must practice care based on purposefully engaging in effective therapeutic and professional relationships, communicating effectively and being respectful of a person's dignity, culture, values, beliefs and rights.

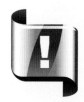

Something to think about …

Clear zero tolerance policies aim to ensure that service users are aware of their rights and responsibilities, and that they understand the consequences of initiating violence. However, the phrase 'no tolerance' suggests that there is no discretion which may invite an inflexible adherence to the rules and adversarial attitudes towards patients.

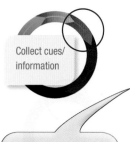

Collect cues/
information

If Shawn was
withdrawing from
alcohol, what else might
you notice about his
observations?

2. COLLECT CUES/INFORMATION

(a) Review current information

You realise that you are not really sure what is happening with Shawn, but based on the handover provided you are concerned about alcohol withdrawal. You decide to review his vital signs:

Temperature	36.7°C
Pulse rate	112
Respiratory rate	22
Blood pressure	125/80
Pain score	3/10 using a numerical rating scale where 10 is the worst pain ever experienced and 0 represents no pain

(b) Gather new information

Q1   Do you think that you have all the information you need at this stage? What other clinical assessment information do you need to collect?

Q2   You realise that there are some gaps in Shawn's drug and alcohol history. How would you approach this with Shawn in order to collect all the relevant information?

   a   'Shawn, I notice that there is some missing information in your file. Is this a good time to ask you some further questions?'

   b   'Shawn, can you give me some more information about how much alcohol you were using? Is it just a couple of drinks a night?'

   c   'You seem to be agitated and aggressive. Is there anything I need to know about how many drugs you were using?'

   d   'Hey Shawn. If I take you outside for a cigarette, would you give me some more info about your drug and alcohol intake?'

The aim of a drug and alcohol assessment is to obtain a relevant history and categorise a patient's readiness to change. This information is then used to formulate a management plan based on the individual's needs. In the past, confrontational approaches to dealing with substance use have been used, but assessment should be a therapeutic process and a chance to help patients to think about their substance use. Nurses should precede the drug and alcohol assessment by explaining why he or she is taking a history and establishing appropriate confidentiality.

To determine Shawn's current and past use of drugs and alcohol, the following questions should guide your thinking:

- What are the patterns of use and route of administration?
- Has the person experienced any physical and psychosocial consequences?
- What is their motivation for taking substances? What effect does it have?
- What is the frequency/duration/amount used?
- Have there been previous attempts at reduction or cessation of substance use and does your patient want to stop or cut down?

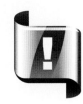

Something to think about ...

Tobacco is also an addictive substance and abrupt cessation of tobacco produces a withdrawal syndrome. Many of the symptoms of nicotine withdrawal are similar to those of other drug withdrawal syndromes: anxiety, awakening during sleep, depression, difficulty concentrating, impatience, irritability/anger and restlessness (Hughes, Higgins, & Bickel, 1994). For more information, refer to <www.tobaccoinaustralia.org.au/chapter-6-addiction/6-9nicotine-withdrawal-syndrome>.

Young people use alcohol and drugs for many different reasons, including as a reaction to disturbed backgrounds, broken schooling and the influence of peers and societal attitudes. There is a strong link between drug and alcohol use and criminal offending, with 70 per cent of youths being intoxicated at the time of their last offence (Prichard & Payne, 2005). However, it should be noted that most young people who appear in court do not reoffend (Prichard & Payne, 2005).

(c) Recall knowledge

QUICK QUIZ!

To ensure that you have a good understanding of the key concepts related to substance use, test yourself with the following questions.

> To find out whether red or white wine gives the worst hangover, try the Spinner Game: <http://yourroom.com.au/spinner-game>.

Q1 The mechanism of the action of alcohol on the brain is attributed to:

    a Release of GABA

    b Release of dopamine

    c Suppression of acetylcholine

    d Release of epinephrine

Q2 Fill in the missing words:

    a Thirty per cent of all suicides are attributed to this substance: _____

    b Forty per cent of all deaths due to accidental falls are attributed to this substance: _____

    c A chemical considered to be carcinogenic to humans: _____

    d Use of this substance is more closely associated with violent crime than any other substance: _____

    e Use of this substance leads to unprotected sex, with the increased risk of AIDS, other sexually transmitted diseases and pregnancy: _____

    f This substance causes more damage to the developing baby's brain than any other substance during pregnancy: _____

Q3 Smoking cigarettes results in which of the following changes?

    a The amount of a brain chemical (dopamine) that allows us to experience pleasure

    b Blood flow to the brain

    c The rate at which alcohol is absorbed

    d Blood flow to the liver

Q4 With regard to marijuana, indicate whether these statements are 'true' or 'false':

    a The tetrahydrocannabinol (THC) content of marijuana is several times higher than it was in the 1960s.

    b Higher THC levels mean lower potency, more likely to induce tolerance and addiction.

    c Higher THC levels mean higher potency, more likely to induce tolerance and addiction.

    d   It impairs coordination and balance (by affecting the cerebellum and basal ganglia).

    e   It impairs ability to store and retrieve learnt information but not memory.

    f   It increases heart rate (by affecting the hypothalamus and brain stem).

    g   It can cause anxiety and panic attacks (by affecting the amygdala).

Q5   Shawn's friend asks you whether it is safe to smoke marijuana. What would be the most appropriate reply?

    a   It depends whether it is hydroponic or naturally grown.

    b   Cannabis is an illegal substance and it is not appropriate that I answer your question.

    c   There is no safe level of drug use. Use of any drug always carries some risk.

    d   It is a safer drug than alcohol as long as you do not drive under the influence.

Q6   After a puff of a cigarette, nicotine is in the brain in how many seconds?

    a   8

    b   18

    c   28

    d   80

Q7   In the brain, nicotine locks into receptors on neurons making the smoker feel:

    a   Irritable

    b   Sleepy

    c   Alert and satisfied

    d   Anxious

Q8   Match the signs and symptoms of withdrawal and intoxication in column 1 with the related terms in column 2.

i	Drowsiness	a	Sedative withdrawal, or stimulant toxicity
ii	Agitation	b	Alcohol and opioid withdrawal
iii	Tremor	c	Alcohol, benzodiazepines, opiates
iv	Diaphoresis	d	Alcohol, benzodiazepine intoxication
v	Slurred speech, ataxia	e	Especially seen in opiates
vi	Pinpoint pupils	f	Alcohol, benzodiazepine withdrawal

Q9   With regard to Figure 11.1, indicate whether the following are 'true' or 'false':

    a   A standard drink of white wine has a lower alcohol content than a standard drink of fortified wine.

    b   Counting standard drinks is a more reliable measure of how much alcohol is consumed than counting glasses, bottles or cans.

    c   100 mL of wine = 1 standard drink.

    d   The number of standard drinks is depicted on the label of alcoholic beverages in Australia.

    e   In order to reduce the risk of alcohol-related injury arising from a single occasion, healthy men and women should drink no more than two standard drinks.

    f   For table wine, a standard drink corresponds to 100 mL, whereas a typical restaurant serve is 150 mL.

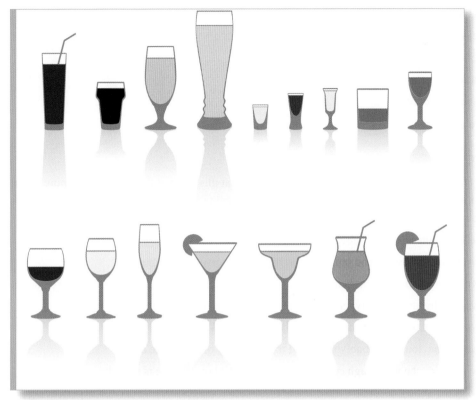

Figure 11.1
What is a standard drink?
Source: © grafistart/123RF.

3. PROCESS INFORMATION

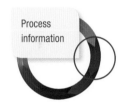

Process
information

(a) Interpret

The next step of the clinical reasoning cycle is to interpret the data (cues) that you have collected by careful analysis and by comparing normal versus abnormal.

Q Which of the following are considered to be within normal parameters for Shawn?

  a Temperature: 36.7°C

  b Pulse rate: 72

  c Respiratory rate: 22

  d Blood pressure: 125/80

  e Pain score: 3/10

(b) Discriminate

From the cues and information you now have, you need to narrow down the information to what is most important.

Q1 From the list below, identify the seven cues that would most concern you when assessing Shawn at this time.

  a Presence of visual or auditory hallucinations

  b Presence of a tremor

  c Dry mouth and oral mucosa

  d Low respiratory rate

  e High temperature

  f Low pulse rate

When 'discriminating', it is helpful to focus first on examination of any aberrations from normal.

  g Variable level of consciousness

  h Increasing level of agitation

  i Presence of a headache

  j Sweating and clamminess

  k Nausea and vomiting

Q2 Are there any gaps in the information that has been collected so far?

(c) Relate

What we currently have is a list of important cues. However, at this stage of the clinical reasoning cycle, you need to cluster the cues together to tell a coherent story and to find the patterns or interrelationships between the cues.

Q Label the following 'true' or 'false'.

  a Shawn's blood pressure and pulse are too high for a person of his age.

  b Shawn's history and current behaviour suggest that he has a long-standing personality disorder.

  c Shawn's tachycardia and hypertension are indicative of post-operative bleeding.

  d Shawn's agitation and behaviour are likely to be related to pain.

  e Shawn's behaviour is probably unrelated to his history of substance abuse.

  f Shawn's headache and cough could indicate the 'flu'; however, he is not febrile.

  g Shawn's irritability, insomnia and craving for nicotine suggest that he may be experiencing a type of substance withdrawal.

(d) Infer

It is time to think about all the cues that you have collected about Shawn and to make inferences based on your analysis and interpretation of those cues.

Q From what you know about Shawn, identify which of the following inferences are correct. (Select one correct answer.)

  a He has a diagnosis of antisocial personality disorder.

  b He is withdrawing from alcohol.

  c He is experiencing post-operative pain.

  d He is withdrawing from nicotine.

  e He is having an allergic reaction to the Panadeine Forte.

  f He is reacting badly to hospitalisation and rules because of his history.

(e) Match

Q Think back to your clinical placements or experience. Have you ever seen anyone presenting in a similar way? How were they managed? What were the key concerns of the health professionals involved?

(f) Predict

Now is the time to consider the consequences of your actions or inaction by predicting potential outcomes for your patient.

Q Shawn is likely to be discharged today. If you do nothing, what might be the consequences? Label the following as 'high likelihood', 'possible' or 'low likelihood'.

  a Shawn's alcohol problem will remain untreated.

  b Shawn's alcohol problem will get worse because of his social circumstances.

   c   With maturity Shawn will learn to manage his life better.

   d   Shawn will probably incur a more serious criminal conviction.

   e   Shawn's substance abuse issues will not be resolved.

   f   Shawn's psychosocial issues will not be resolved.

4. IDENTIFY THE PROBLEM/ISSUE

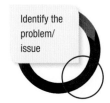

At this stage, you bring together (synthesise) all of the facts you've collected and inferences you've made to make a definitive nursing diagnosis of Shawn's main problems.

Q   Select from the following list the *most* correct nursing diagnoses for Shawn.

   a   Alcohol withdrawal related to sudden reduction in alcohol intake, evidenced by aggression, bradycardia and fever

   b   Acute pain related to recent surgery, evidenced by agitation and headache

   c   Allergic reaction related to Panadeine Forte, evidenced by tachypnoea and agitation

   d   Nicotine withdrawal related to limited access to cigarettes whilst hospitalised, evidenced by agitation, insomnia and headache

5. ESTABLISH GOALS

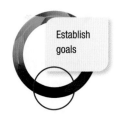

Before implementing any actions to improve Shawn's condition, it is important to clearly specify what you want to happen and when.

Q   From the list below, choose the three most important *short-term* goals for Shawn's management at this time.

   a   To be discharged as soon as possible so that he can smoke when and where he likes

   b   To have counselling for his substance abuse issues

   c   To minimise the effects of nicotine withdrawal

   d   To access psychosocial support for Shawn so that he will have suitable accommodation on discharge

   e   To ensure that Shawn understands that if his behaviour does not improve he will be in violation of the hospital's 'zero tolerance' policy

6. TAKE ACTION

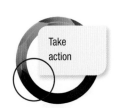

Q   Which of the following actions would be most helpful in caring for Shawn at this time? (Select six correct answers.)

   a   Do not confirm or deny any hallucinations that he may experience.

   b   Continue to monitor Shawn's condition and document it on an alcohol withdrawal chart.

   c   Remind Shawn firmly that the hospital has a 'zero tolerance' policy for physical and verbal aggression.

   d   Agree on a clear management plan with Shawn and the treatment team.

   e   Ensure that Shawn has no visitors so that he cannot receive illicit drugs or cigarettes.

   f   Respond to the person not the label.

   g   Try to make friends with Shawn so that you can help him with some of his problems.

   h   Set appropriate limits and boundaries about appropriate and inappropriate behaviour.

   i   Ask for a psychiatric review.

   j   Communicate with Shawn in a non-judgmental way to establish a therapeutic relationship.

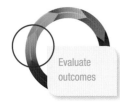

Evaluate
outcomes

7. EVALUATE

Q   You discuss with Shawn the option of trying nicotine patches while he is in hospital. How would you determine whether or not the patches have been effective? From the following assessment criteria, identify those that would demonstrate improvement in Shawn's condition.

   a   Increased blood pressure

   b   Decreased level of thirst

   c   Decreased level of agitation

   d   Increased level of restlessness

   e   Decreased pulse rate

   f   Decreased nicotine cravings

   g   Headache improving

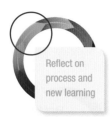

Reflect on
process and
new learning

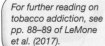

8. REFLECT

Q1   Describe three clinical reasoning errors that influenced the nurses' attitudes towards Shawn and his subsequent management.

Q2   How could this situation have been prevented or managed more effectively?

Q3   What have you learnt from this scenario that you can apply to your future practice?

For further reading on tobacco addiction, see pp. 88–89 of LeMone et al. (2017).

   While reflecting on this scenario, you should also consider how you are feeling and examine your reactions to Shawn. Nursing can be stressful and we often lack the resources to deal with all the stressful experiences we encounter. We are more helpful to others when we are taking care of ourselves physically, emotionally, mentally and spiritually.

Q4   Ask yourself the following questions if you are looking after someone like Shawn.

   a   Are my feelings (positive or negative) about substance abuse so strong that they could influence my reasoning?

   b   Do I have any strong moral beliefs about substance abuse that could affect my reactions to people like Shawn?

   c   Do I have any guilty feelings about my own drinking or smoking? Has anyone ever suggested that I cut down? Have I ever felt annoyed or angry if someone makes comments about my drinking or smoking? Have I ever had a drink first thing in the morning to steady my nerves or to get rid of a hangover?

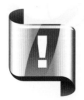

Something to think about . . .

Review the questions below, taken from the CAGE questionnaire (http://pubs.niaaa.nih.gov/publications/ arh28-2/78-79.htm), a screening tool for identifying problems with alcohol intake.

C   *Have you ever felt you should* cut down *on your drinking?*

A   *Have people* annoyed *you by criticising your drinking?*

G   *Have you ever felt bad or* guilty *about your drinking?*

E   Eye opener: *Have you ever had a drink first thing in the morning to steady your nerves or to get rid of a hangover?*

Two positive responses on the CAGE are considered a positive test and indicate further assessment is warranted.

If you have concerns about your own drinking or smoking, take advantage of the programs provided by your workplace or university counselling service. Frequently, people see others in their circle of friends drinking heavily or using substances and see it as the norm. Just because your friends are binge drinking does not make it safe.

SCENARIO 11.2   The story unfolds: More than just substance abuse

CHANGING THE SCENE

1. CONSIDER THE PATIENT SITUATION

It is nearing the end of your shift and you feel concerned that Shawn's 'real' issues may not have been addressed. You also feel a little guilty, as you think your attitude towards Shawn may have been influenced by the comments of other nurses and by your previous experiences with 'challenging' patients. You decide to talk to Shawn and, because you were the nurse who 'sorted out' the nicotine patches for him, he seems to trust you and eventually begins to open up. Here is what he says:

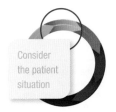

> *Mum and Dad were real battlers and wanted me and my three brothers to do really well. They moved interstate a few years ago. I miss Mum but Dad was a miner and he thought I was a bit of a mummy's boy. He wanted us to do well and it was scary sometimes. My brothers went to uni and I am the loser of the family. Dad made all the decisions and Mum has never worked, and can't even use a computer or get money out of a machine! I was dragged along to see the school counsellor when I was seven with 'school refusal syndrome'. Really Mum just wanted me with her, but it stuffed up my schooling and I left school when I was 16 and just had loser jobs. I didn't fit in there, either. I wanted to be a vet nurse but Dad said that was for 'poofs', so I started drinking to fit in, and always drank heaps before going out so that I wasn't so anxious. That nurse was going on about me having a criminal record, but I got done for trying to protect my so-called mates in a fight at a pub, then they blamed me—the loser, as always. Smokes and beer are my way of coping with my worries really. I have never had a girlfriend. It would've been better if I had a sister, I suppose. I dunno what to say to them!*
>
> *God, I have really stuffed things up now. I have a rotty—Buster—and am really worried that my flatmate won't feed him. Buster will be missing me. He is a brilliant dog, better than any mate. What if I can't get anywhere to live, what will happen to him? He even sleeps on my bed. How am I going to get a job if the cops do me for DUI? Tell you what, though: this is a wakeup call. Mum rang and is going to help and I am never going to get in a mess again—not touching another beer.*

Substance abuse frequently occurs with anxiety disorders. People may use alcohol to help them cope, but this can lead to increased anxiety (Reavley et al., 2013).

2. COLLECT CUES/INFORMATION

(a) Review current information

You have decided that you need more specific information in order to plan Shawn's care. You review the admission documentation, focusing on Shawn's drug and alcohol history. Shawn does not seem to have any symptoms of alcohol withdrawal and he told you that his drinking started when he was trying to fit in with workmates. You start to wonder whether alcohol is the primary problem or if alcohol is actually Shawn's attempt to deal with another problem.

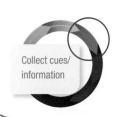

(b) Gather new information

You decide to gather further cues about Shawn's anxiety by using screening questions from the NSW Clinical Guidelines (NSW Health, 2009, pp. 10–11). This is the dialogue with Shawn:

Review the Stages of Change model in LeMone et al. (2017, p. 100).

RN: Have you ever seen a doctor or psychiatrist for emotional problems or problems with your 'nerves', anxieties or worries?

Shawn: *Yes, I have. I saw the school counsellor when I was 10 and a couple of times after that. I have been to my GP a couple of times to try to discuss it, but he gets up me for my drinking.*

RN: Have you ever been given medication for emotional problems or problems with your 'nerves', anxieties or worries?

Shawn: *Not really. A GP once suggested I use an antidepressant, but Dad said I would get addicted to them. I would feel like even more of a loser if I had to take medication for nerves.*

RN: Do you currently have a mental health worker, psychiatrist, psychologist, general practitioner or other health provider?

Shawn: *Nah, just a GP.*

RN: Are you having any difficulties sleeping? Can you tell me about that?

> *Could these symptoms be indicative of depression? Access the following site and take the self-test: <www. blackdoginstitute.org. au/mental-health-wellbeing/depression>.*

Shawn: *Yeah, I lie awake worrying and stuff, and sometimes I get up and have a drink to try to get to sleep. When I wake up, my thoughts just start racing around in my head and I can't get back to sleep.*

RN: Have you experienced any changes in your appetite? Are you eating more or less than is normal for you?

Shawn: *Not really hungry at the moment. I can't be bothered to cook.*

RN: Are you experiencing any changes in your ability to concentrate or complete a task?

Shawn: *Yeah. I hadn't thought about it but I used to like reading and I don't anymore. I keep letting my mates down too. I say I'm going out with them but I get anxious before I even leave the house. I feel sick in my stomach and my head feels light and I get like I am dizzy. When I lived at home, Mum would make excuses for me and ring them and say I was ill. Mum gets anxious too, and she liked to have me at home, I think.*

You know, it has been really difficult here; it is making me really anxious. That night nurse got up me for swearing and all I said was that I felt bloody awful. Things have gone downhill from there.

How common are anxiety disorders? Is feeling anxious sometimes positive?

> *Review the signs and symptoms of anxiety at <www.sane.org/mental-health-and-illness/facts-and-guides/anxiety-disorder?gclid=CLO21 cWT0M8CFZAK0wodR 3kKZQ>.*

Anxiety disorders are the most common type of mental illness, with about one in seven Australians experiencing some type of anxiety disorder every year (Reavley et al., 2013). Anxiety disorders have different symptoms but all cluster around excessive, irrational fear and dread. While everyone feels anxious from time to time, some people experience these feelings so often and/or so strongly that it can affect their everyday lives. It is at this stage that we start to consider that the person may be experiencing an anxiety disorder. It is rather like having an oversensitive burglar alarm on your house which goes off when the next-door neighbour merely turns on a light. Normal anxiety is adaptive—it prevents us taking unnecessary risks and alerts us to danger—but an anxiety disorder can significantly and adversely affect functioning and contribute to other problems such as depression and substance use.

> *View a personal video account of what it is like to live with anxiety and how to overcome it: <www.youtube .com/watch?v=-FyVetL1MEw>.*

Q   Which of the following signs and symptoms are relevant to a diagnosis of anxiety?

   a   Feeling unable to control anxious feelings

   b   Feeling moody or irritable

   c   Having a grandiose sense of self

   d   Changes in eating patterns

   e   Fatigue

f   Insomnia

g   Nausea or abdominal distress

h   Constipation

i   Bradycardia

j   Tachycardia

The relationship between cigarette smoking and anxiety is complex. It is hard for people with anxiety disorders to give up smoking (Piper et al., 2011). People frequently use cigarettes to deal with their anxiety and it may create a temporary calming feeling, but this is short-lived; cigarettes may also play a role in teenagers developing generalised anxiety disorders (GAD) (Johnson et al., 2000). Some of the risk factors associated with anxiety and tobacco use include (a) a stressful childhood, (b) difficulty tolerating negative emotions and (c) impulsiveness. People often self-medicate for anxiety problems like GAD through the use of tobacco, marijuana, alcohol and other substances. The problem with self-medicating is that the relief is usually short-term, the cause of the anxiety is often avoided and there are negative health effects. There is a similar 'bidirectional influence' between alcohol use and anxiety problems. Anxiety can lead people to drink alcohol, and alcohol misuse and withdrawal can increase anxiety.

(c) Recall knowledge

Q1 What can you say to Shawn about his anxiety? Which of following statements are true?

a   Anxiety is a lifelong condition.

b   Anxiety is a common condition that affects more males than females.

c   Adults reporting a high or very high level of psychological distress are more likely to be current daily smokers.

d   Many people treat their mood problems by drinking alcohol and smoking tobacco, and these can bring short-term relief but may cause long-term problems.

e   Shawn will not be able to drink again.

f   Everyone experiences anxiety at times, but if you are having difficulty doing your work, and have problems interacting with family and friends, it is likely that you have an *anxiety disorder*.

g   Anxiety is very treatable.

h   A Mental Status Exam (MSE) cannot be conducted on a client when they are intoxicated.

Q2 What is the difference between anxiety and stress?

Q3 What is the difference between anxiety and an anxiety disorder?

Q4 What is the difference between anxiety and fear?

Q5 Other medical conditions may cause symptoms similar to anxiety. What are they?

3. PROCESS INFORMATION

(a) Interpret

The next step of the clinical reasoning cycle is to interpret the data (cues) that you have collected while applying your knowledge about Shawn. By comparing normal versus abnormal, you will come to a more complete understanding of Shawn's problems.

Q It can be helpful to use a case formulation format to assist you to see what information you have about Shawn and what information may be missing. Fill in the blanks in the following table. Don't worry if something fits into more than one box.

Process
information

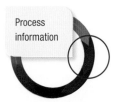

Which stage of change best describes Shawn? <www.mifa.org.au/images/Documents/Wellways/164848%20Substance%20Use.pdf>.

	Predisposing factors	Precipitating factors	Perpetuating factors	Prognostic indicators (including protective)
Biological	Family history of anxiety	Misuse of alcohol		Intelligent
Psychological			Low self-esteem	
Social				

Hint: If any of the boxes are blank, it might be that you need to ask your patient more questions so that you can fill in the missing information.

(b) Discriminate

It is important to now focus on the most relevant information that you have. At this stage, you need to consider the severity of Shawn's anxiety as this will allow you to consider possible treatment options.

Shawn might be diagnosed with GAD if for six months or more, on *more days than not*, he has:

- felt very worried
- found it hard to stop worrying
- found that his anxiety made it difficult for him to carry out everyday activities.

If Shawn answered yes to *all* these questions, we would also ask whether he has also experienced *three or more* of the following:

- felt restless or on edge
- felt tired easily
- had difficulty concentrating
- felt irritable
- had muscle pain (e.g. sore jaw or back)
- had trouble sleeping (e.g. difficulty falling or staying asleep, or restless sleep).

Find out more about anxiety disorders at <www.beyondblue.org .au/the-facts/anxiety/ types-of-anxiety/gad>.

Note: This checklist is not a formal diagnostic tool. It is meant to help identify potential GAD symptoms.

(c) Relate

Q   Based on what you have discovered about Shawn so far, label the following 'true' or 'false':

  a   Shawn's alcohol use has precipitated his problems with anxiety.

  b   Shawn's anxiety has precipitated his problems with alcohol.

  c   Shawn's anxiety has worsened because he was withdrawing from alcohol.

  d   Shawn's anxiety has worsened because he was withdrawing from nicotine.

  e   Shawn's use of alcohol is perpetuating his anxiety.

(d) Infer

Q   From what you know about Shawn's history, identify which of the following inferences are correct. (Select those that apply.)

  a   There is little evidence that Shawn suffered alcohol withdrawal symptoms.

  b   It is likely that Shawn does meet the criteria for a GAD.

  c   Shawn needs to stop drinking before his anxiety can be effectively treated.

d   Shawn's problems with alcohol should be treated at the same time as his anxiety.

e   Shawn's problems with the law precipitated his problems with alcohol.

(e) Predict

Now is the time to consider the consequences of your actions or inaction by predicting potential outcomes for your patient.

Q   If you do not take the appropriate actions at this time, what could happen if Shawn was discharged at this point? (Select the *three* that apply.)

a   Shawn is unlikely to seek treatment for either his alcohol use or his anxiety.

b   Shawn's drinking is likely to get worse.

c   Shawn is likely to end up in the criminal justice system.

d   Shawn will lose his home and his dog.

e   Shawn is at a high risk of post-operative complications.

4. IDENTIFY THE PROBLEM/ISSUE

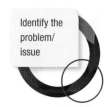

At this stage, you bring together (synthesise) all of the facts you've collected and inferences you've made to make a definitive nursing diagnosis of Shawn's main problems.

Q   Select from the following list the most correct nursing diagnoses for Shawn.

a   Panic attack related to nicotine withdrawal, evidenced by agitation and moodiness

b   Anxiety related to family history, evidenced by insomnia and tachycardia

c   Antisocial personality disorder related to substance misuse, evidenced by aggression and swearing

d   Ineffective coping related to negative role modelling, evidenced by decreased ability to manage stress and financial affairs being in disarray

5. ESTABLISH GOALS

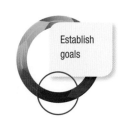

Before implementing any actions to improve Shawn's condition, it is important to clearly specify what you want to happen and when.

Q   From the list below, choose the most important *short-term* goals for Shawn when he leaves the hospital.

a   Referral for psychological treatment in order to understand and change his patterns of behaviours, thoughts and beliefs which trigger anxiety

b   To obtain accommodation for himself and his dog

c   To take prescribed medication to treat anxiety

d   To be abstinent

e   To cut down on his drinking

f   To be admitted to a rehabilitation unit to ensure he is adequately detoxed

g   To cease cigarette smoking

h   To organise family therapy for Shawn and his parents

i   To establish a normal sleep pattern

6. TAKE ACTION

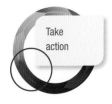

Q   You decide to talk with Shawn about treatment options for his anxiety. Which of the following interventions would be recommended for his anxiety in the first instance? (Select all that apply.)

a   Discussion with GP

b   Referral to a psychiatrist

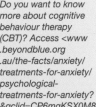

Do you want to know more about cognitive behaviour therapy (CBT)? Access <www.beyondblue.org.au/the-facts/anxiety/treatments-for-anxiety/psychological-treatments-for-anxiety?&gclid=CP6mgKSX0M8CFdAW0wodSEEDLA>.

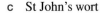

   c   St John's wort

   d   Temazepam to assist with insomnia

   e   Cognitive behaviour therapy (CBT)

   f   Exercise

   g   Relaxation techniques

   h   Meditation, breathing and relaxation techniques

   i   Tricyclic antidepressants

   j   Anxiolytics such as alprazolam, oxazepam or lorazepam

   k   Avoiding illicit drugs

   l   Cutting down on alcohol, sugar and caffeine

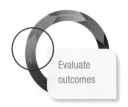

Evaluate outcomes

7. EVALUATE

In complex clinical situations such as the one portrayed in this scenario, it can be difficult to evaluate the effectiveness of your intervention(s) in the short term. This is compounded when there is a short length of stay and you have very little time to build up a therapeutic relationship.

Q   How would you determine whether you have made a positive difference to Shawn's nursing care?

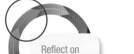

Reflect on process and new learning

8. REFLECT

Reflect on your learning from this scenario and consider the following questions:

Q1   What are three of the most important things that you have learnt from this scenario?

Q2   How does therapeutic communication lead to improved patient outcomes?

Q3   If you come across an 'unpopular patient', what might you change in your approach to their care?

Q4   What actions will you take in clinical practice as a result of your learning from this scenario?

Q5   Next time you hear a handover where the term 'challenging or difficult patient' is used, how could you respond?

Q6   When you are 'challenged' by a patient's behaviour, how do you ensure that you continue to maintain a therapeutic alliance?

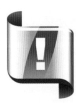

Something to think about ...

You might want to ask yourself the following questions if you are looking after someone like Shawn:

1   Are Shawn's problems too difficult to address with my current knowledge and skills?

2   Am I concerned that I might be acting outside my scope of practice?

3   Am I trying too hard to 'rescue' him?

Time out!

If, while working through this scenario, you have identified that you may be at risk of having a generalised anxiety disorder (GAD) or a substance use disorder, it is important to talk with your doctor and discuss your concerns. It might also be time to evaluate what stresses you are under. Common signs of stress include chronic fatigue, difficulties sleeping, change in appetite, frustration, self-criticism and negativity, inability to 'switch off' from work, over-emotional reactions to stressors and minor physical illnesses (Edward et al., 2011). What are you doing to look after yourself? The following can be useful:

- Have fun outside work.
- Debrief with colleagues/mentor/educator.
- Have regular exercise, get adequate sleep and eat a balanced diet.
- See your mistakes as opportunities to learn.
- Do something enjoyable every day.
- Consider meditation, relaxation, mindfulness or yoga.

Make a resolution that you will look after yourself as well as you look after others!

FURTHER READING

American Psychiatric Association. (2013). *Diagnostic and Statistical Manual of Mental Disorders* (5th edn). Washington: American Psychiatric Association.

Australian Government Department of Health. (2014). *Information for Health Professionals on Assessing Alcohol Consumption in Pregnancy Using AUDIT-C*. Accessed March 2017 at <www.alcohol.gov.au/internet/alcohol/publishing.nsf/Content/wwtk-audit-c>.

Australian Government Department of Health. (2004). *Alcohol and Other Drugs: A Handbook for Health Professionals*. Accessed March 2017 at <www.health.gov.au/internet/main/publishing.nsf/Content/phd-aodgp>.

National Drug and Alcohol Research Centre. (2016). *What Is Alcohol?* Accessed from <https://ndarc.med.unsw.edu.au>.

National Health and Medical Research Council. (2016). *Alcohol Guidelines: Reducing the Health Risks*. Accessed March 2017 at <www.nhmrc.gov.au/health-topics/alcohol-guidelines>.

Stone, T. E. (2010). Insight on mental health nursing. In T. Levett-Jones & S. Bourgeois (Eds), *The Clinical Placement* (2nd edn). Sydney: Elsevier.

Youth beyondblue. (2016). *Alcohol and Drugs*. Accessed March 2017 at <www.youthbeyondblue.com/understand-what's-going-on/alcohol-and-drugs>.

REFERENCES

Althaus, F., Paroz, S., Hugli, O., Ghali, W. A., Daeppen, J.-B., Peytremann-Bridevaux, I. & Bodenmann, P. (2011). Effectiveness of interventions targeting frequent users of emergency departments: A systematic review. *Annals of Emergency Medicine, 58*(1), 41–52.e42.

American Psychiatric Association. (2013). *Diagnostic and Statistical Manual of Mental Disorders* (5th edn). Washington: American Psychiatric Association.

Australian Commission on Safety and Quality in Health Care (ACSQHC). (2016). *National Safety and Quality Health Service Standards Version 2*. Draft, Sydney, Australia.

Australian Drug Foundation. (2011). *Drug Facts*. Accessed October 2016 at <www.druginfo.adf.org.au/>.

Australian Institute of Health and Welfare (AIHW). (2017). *Alcohol and Other Drugs*. Accessed March 2017 at <www.aihw.gov.au/alcohol-and-other-drugs>.

Australian Institute of Health and Welfare (AIHW). (2014). *Australia's Health 2014*. Canberra: AIHW.

Corrigan, P. (2004). How stigma interferes with mental health care. *American Psychologist, 59*(7), 614–25.

Covey, S. (2004). *The 7 Habits of Highly Effective People*. New York: Free Press.

Edward, K., Munro, I., Robins, A. & Welch, A. J. (2011). *Mental Health Nursing: Dimensions of Praxis*. South Melbourne: Oxford University Press.

Goffman, I. (1986). *Stigma. Notes on the Management of Spoiled Identity*. New York: Touchstone.

Hughes, J. R., Higgins, S. T. & Bickel, W. K. (1994). Nicotine withdrawal versus other drug withdrawal syndromes: Similarities and dissimilarities. *Addiction, 89*(11), 1461–70. doi: 10.1111/j.1360-0443.1994.tb03744.x

Johnson, J. G., Cohen, P., Pine, D. S., Klein, D. F., Kasen, S. & Brook, J. S. (2000). Association between cigarette smoking and anxiety disorders during adolescence and early adulthood. *JAMA, 284*, 2348–51.

Johnson, S. L. (2003). *Therapist's Guide to Substance Abuse Intervention*. San Diego: Elsevier.

LeMone, P., Burke, K., Bauldoff, G., Gubrud-Howe, P., Levett-Jones, T., Dwyer, T., ... Raymond, D. (Eds). (2017). *Medical–Surgical Nursing: Critical Thinking in Person-Centred Care* (3rd edn). Melbourne: Pearson.

National Health and Medical Research Council. (2009). *Australian Guidelines to Reduce Health Risks from Drinking Alcohol*. Canberra: Commonwealth of Australia.

NSW Health. (2009). *NSW Clinical Guidelines for the Care of Persons with Comorbid Mental Illness and Substance Use Disorders in Acute Care Settings*. Accessed September 2011 at <www.health.nsw.gov.au/mentalhealth/programs/mh/Pages/comorbidity-report.aspx>.

NSW Health. (2008). *Drug and Alcohol Withdrawal Clinical Practice Guidelines—NSW*. Document No. GL2008_011. Accessed March 2017 at <www1.health.nsw.gov.au/pds/ActivePDSDocuments/GL2008_011.pdf>.

NSW Health. (2003). *Zero Tolerance: Response to Violence in the NSW Health Workplace*. NSW Department of Health.

Nursing and Midwifery Board of Australia (NMBA). (2016). *Registered Nurse Standards for Practice*. Accessed from <www.nursingmidwiferyboard.gov.au/Codes-Guidelines-Statements/Professional-standards.aspx>.

Piper, M. E., Cook, J. W., Schlam, T. R., Jorenby, D. E. & Baker, T. B. (2011). Anxiety diagnoses in smokers seeking cessation treatment: Relations with tobacco dependence, withdrawal, outcome and response to treatment. *Addiction, 106*(2), 418–27.

Prichard, J. & Payne, J. (2005). *Alcohol, Drugs and Crime: A Study of Juveniles in Detention.* Research and Public Policy Series No. 67. Canberra: Australian Institute of Criminology.

Reavley, N. J., Allen, N. B., Jorm, A. F., Morgan, A. J., Ryan, S. & Purcell, R. (2013). *A Guide to What Works for Anxiety* (2nd edn). Melbourne: beyondblue.

Stone, T. E., McMillan, M. & Hazelton, M. (2010). Swearing: Its prevalence in health care settings and impact on nursing practice. *Journal of Psychiatric and Mental Health Nursing, 17*(6), 528–34.

CHAPTER 12

CARING FOR A PERSON WITH A COMPLEX AND CHRONIC HEALTH CONDITION

RACHEL ROSSITER AND TERESA STONE

LEARNING OUTCOMES

Completion of the activities in this chapter will enable you to:

○ explain why an understanding of the impact of chronic and complex health conditions on mental health is essential to competent practice (**recall** and **application**)

○ identify the clinical manifestations of the chronic and complex condition, scleroderma; and co-morbid chronic conditions, Sjögren's syndrome and Raynaud's phenomenon, that will guide the collection and interpretation of cues (**gather**, **review**, **interpret**, **discriminate**, **relate** and **infer**)

○ identify risk factors for patients with chronic conditions such as scleroderma (**match** and **predict**)

○ review clinical information to identify the main nursing diagnoses for a patient with chronic and complex health conditions, for example scleroderma (**synthesise**)

○ describe the priorities of care for a patient with a chronic and complex multisystem autoimmune condition and depression (**goal setting** and **taking action**)

○ identify criteria for determining the effectiveness of nursing actions taken to manage the clinical manifestations of scleroderma and depression (**evaluate**)

○ apply what you have learnt about chronic and complex multisystem autoimmune disease and co-morbid conditions to new situations and with different people (**reflection** and **translation**).

INTRODUCTION

People with chronic and complex autoimmune diseases may also have other co-morbid conditions that manifest in a wide variety of diverse symptoms; and, too often, health professionals have little understanding of the complex interplay between the physical and psychosocial issues encountered. The two scenarios introduced in this chapter will give you the opportunity to explore some of these challenges. While this chapter follows the story of Mrs Elsie Jones who has scleroderma, what you learn will be applicable to the care of people with a variety of chronic diseases across a range of clinical contexts.

For someone with a chronic illness, each day can become a balancing act as they learn to live, and indeed 'take charge of life', with long-term illness (Andersson et al., 2015, p. 3409). For many, the illness may dominate their lives and can become an ongoing source of distress and demoralisation (Newton, Thombs & Groleau, 2012). The importance of nurses providing advocacy and ensuring coordinated care that is tailored to the patient's individual needs cannot be underestimated (Parker, 2013).

Martin and Peterson (2008) suggest that living with a 'chronic illness is a long journey during which care and support needs to be designed to support and optimise a full life' (p. 4). The complexity of chronic illnesses and the impact of living with the day-to-day difficulties place the person at increased risk of mental illnesses such as depression and anxiety. Increasingly, research demonstrates a strong association between chronic physical illnesses and anxiety and depression, as well as the negative impact on outcomes that result from this association (Clarke & Currie, 2009). However, excellent clinical reasoning skills will enable you to systematically address each component of the care required for people with chronic and complex health conditions, and make a real difference to the everyday lives of the people you care for.

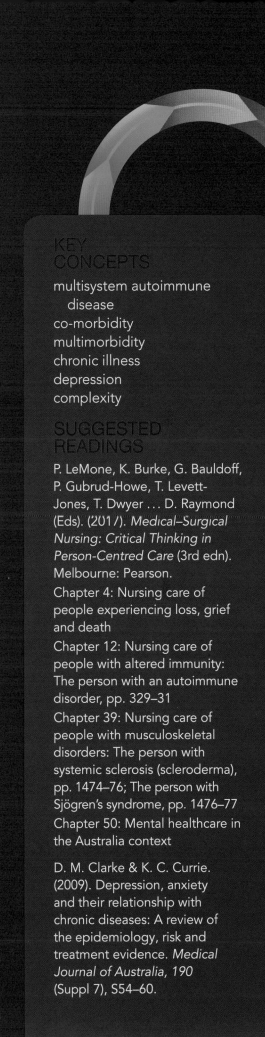

KEY CONCEPTS

multisystem autoimmune
    disease
co-morbidity
multimorbidity
chronic illness
depression
complexity

SUGGESTED READINGS

P. LeMone, K. Burke, G. Bauldoff, P. Gubrud-Howe, T. Levett-Jones, T. Dwyer ... D. Raymond (Eds). (2017). *Medical–Surgical Nursing: Critical Thinking in Person-Centred Care* (3rd edn). Melbourne: Pearson.
Chapter 4: Nursing care of people experiencing loss, grief and death
Chapter 12: Nursing care of people with altered immunity: The person with an autoimmune disorder, pp. 329–31
Chapter 39: Nursing care of people with musculoskeletal disorders: The person with systemic sclerosis (scleroderma), pp. 1474–76; The person with Sjögren's syndrome, pp. 1476–77
Chapter 50: Mental healthcare in the Australia context

D. M. Clarke & K. C. Currie. (2009). Depression, anxiety and their relationship with chronic diseases: A review of the epidemiology, risk and treatment evidence. *Medical Journal of Australia, 190* (Suppl 7), S54–60.

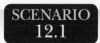

SCENARIO 12.1   Caring for a person with chronic illness

SETTING THE SCENE

Mrs Elsie Jones is a 65-year-old woman with a 30-year history of Raynaud's phenomenon and scleroderma. It took over five years for Elsie to be correctly diagnosed. Although she has struggled at times to cope with the impact of this condition, until recently she has managed to maintain a full and active life, including taking a leading role in a local sporting association and continuing with her life-long hobby of sewing for her daughters and grandchildren.

The prevalence of chronic and complex health conditions

Over 7 million Australians (35 per cent of the population) have a chronic health condition, and the Australian Institute of Health and Welfare (AIHW, 2015) reported that approximately 20 per cent of the population have two or more chronic conditions. As the number of people living with chronic physical conditions has increased, the challenges associated with delivering effective and holistic healthcare have also increased. It is not just the number of illnesses a patient has, or the chronicity of these conditions, that makes for a complex presentation, there are often other issues such as situational complexity, related to factors such as the person's health literacy, social supports and socioeconomic status (Schaink et al., 2012). Health system factors, for example how care is organised and delivered, also contribute to the complexity encountered when caring for people with chronic and complex conditions (Kuipers et al., 2011). For each individual, the burdens associated with chronic physical illness also place them at increased risk of emotional and psychological difficulties such as anxiety and depression, while people living with a mental illness are likewise at increased risk of chronic physical illnesses (Di Benedetto et al., 2014).

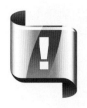

Something to think about …

Chronic: persisting for a long time, either recurring frequently or continuing for the rest of a person's life.

Co-morbidity: two or more diseases experienced at the one time that are connected with each other via pathogenetic mechanisms (Brownie, Scott & Rossiter, 2016).

Multimorbidity: two or more diseases appearing randomly without any connection to each other through pathogenetic mechanisms. It is 'the co-existence of multiple chronic conditions' typically resulting in the person presenting with complex needs and 'significant changes in . . . functional health and quality of life' (Sampalli et al., 2012, p. 762).

The prevalence of multisystem autoimmune diseases and scleroderma (systemic sclerosis)

> Access this site to learn more about autoimmune diseases: <www.allergy.org.au/patients/autoimmunity/autoimmune-diseases>.

> Challenge yourself further and read this article describing the genetics of human autoimmune disease and the progress that has been made in understanding this area of science: <www.sciencedirect.com/science/article/pii/S0896841115300330>.

Once thought to be rare, autoimmune diseases have now been shown to affect 3 to 5 per cent of the world's population (Wang, Wang & Gershwin, 2015, p. 370) and 'are one of the most important health issues in Australia and New Zealand' (Australian Society of Clinical Immunology and Allergy [ASCIA], 2016, p. 1). There are almost 100 distinct autoimmune conditions ranging from those that affect one organ or system to those that affect multiple systems. Multisystem autoimmune diseases (some of which are also described as autoimmune rheumatic diseases) include systemic lupus erythematosus (SLE), anti-phospholipid antibody syndrome, dermatomyositis, scleroderma, polyarteritis nodosa, Wegener's granulomatosis, rheumatoid arthritis, juvenile idiopathic arthritis and Sjögren's syndrome. Diagnosis is often challenging because the symptoms may be ill-defined at the beginning of the illness with frequent overlap between different conditions and some people experiencing more than one of these conditions (Goldblatt & O'Neill, 2013). The main focus of treatment is symptom management, reducing tissue and/or organ damage and maintaining the function of organs affected by the autoimmune disease (ASCIA, 2016, p. 2).

In Australia, there are estimated to be more than 5000 people with scleroderma (Scleroderma Association, 2016). Someone with one autoimmune condition is at increased risk of developing further autoimmune diseases. For example, Sjögren's syndrome, a multisystem autoimmune disease which progressively causes dysfunction of exocrine glands, frequently coexists with scleroderma (Goldblatt & O'Neill, 2013). Up to 50 per cent of those with scleroderma may experience sicca symptoms, which is a frequent cause of morbidity (Swaminathan et al., 2008).

> You may need to brush up on your anatomy here. What is an exocrine gland?

> 'Sicca' refers to dry eyes and dry mouth; it occurs increasingly as people age. Sjögren's syndrome includes dry eyes and dry mouth in conjunction with systemic features. (See LeMone et al., 2017, Chapter 39, for further details.)

The aetiology and pathogenesis of scleroderma

As you read about scleroderma, you will notice that there are a number of different ways in which scleroderma is classified. Scleroderma ('hard skin') is sometimes described as a connective tissue disease or a rheumatic disease, but recently it has been listed as an autoimmune condition. It is classified into categories or subsets and can be either localised (meaning only the skin is involved) or systemic (i.e. internal organ involvement and skin thickening). Scleroderma (systemic sclerosis) is then classified into a number of subsets, including 'diffuse cutaneous systemic sclerosis' and 'limited cutaneous systemic sclerosis' (or CREST syndrome). Three to six times more women than men have scleroderma.

Current 'models of pathogenesis in scleroderma focus on an initiating stimulus in a susceptible individual amplified by vascular, fibrotic and inflammatory processes, resulting in a final common pathway of fibrogenesis and extracellular matrix formation with disruption of tissue architecture and function' (Derrett-Smith & Denton, 2010, p. 129). The ongoing tissue damage 'appears to become sustained and independent of significant ongoing inflammation' (Denton, 2015, p. s59). Although there may not be a family history of scleroderma, it is likely that there will be other family members with autoimmune conditions such as SLE, rheumatoid arthritis or thyroid disease.

Most people who have the limited cutaneous form of systemic sclerosis or scleroderma will have initially developed Raynaud's phenomenon many years prior to the onset of other symptoms.

QUICK QUIZ!

Before progressing to the first stage of the clinical reasoning cycle, test your understanding of the terminologies relevant to this chapter by selecting the correct response for each of the identified terms below.

Q1 'Chronic' means:

   a Short-term

   b Long-lasting, lingering

   c Terminal

   d Very serious

Q2 Autoimmunity is:

   a The failure of recognition of parts of self (self-antigens), resulting in an immune response against one's own cells and tissues

   b An allergic response to a medication

   c A decreased immune response to infectious agents

Q3 Raynaud's phenomenon:

   a Is triggered by excessive heat

   b Occurs only in males

   c Is a disorder of blood circulation affecting the fingers and toes

Q4 Scleroderma/systemic sclerosis is:

   a A skin condition responsive to antibiotics

   b A chronic autoimmune condition affecting connective tissue and microvasculature

   c An inflammatory condition resulting in damage to the myelin sheath

Q5 Sjögren's syndrome is:

 a An autoimmune condition affecting the exocrine glands

 b A form of arthritis caused by a viral infection

 c A tropical infectious disease

1. CONSIDER THE PATIENT SITUATION

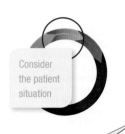

General practitioner appointment

Over the past several months, Elsie has had some worrying symptoms that were believed to be cardiac in origin and she has been reviewed by a cardiologist. Today she is attending the general practice for follow-up with her general practitioner (GP). This is the first time you have met Elsie and you introduce yourself as the practice nurse who will be seeing her prior to her consultation with the GP.

You have recently commenced work as a practice nurse in a busy six-doctor general practice. The practice has a team of practice nurses who are actively involved in ensuring the patients attending have access to comprehensive healthcare. As a practice nurse, your role is to coordinate the care of people with complex chronic health problems, including assessing their health needs and their ability to manage their condition(s), preparing care plans and arranging new referrals as needed. A component of your role is to collect and collate information from the different healthcare professionals who provide care for those with chronic conditions. This is essential for a person with a condition such as scleroderma, which affects multiple body systems, and results in referrals to a number of different medical specialists and different allied health services. Importantly, a vital aspect of effective chronic disease management is to foster the person's capacity for self-management.

Although this scenario is based in a general practice setting, the information will also be relevant to acute care.

Person-centred care

Elsie was born and raised on the Central Coast of NSW. She was the second daughter of three girls who remained close friends throughout their adult lives. Elsie's elder sister died two years ago and her younger sister died 12 months ago. At age 16, Elsie left school to work as an office hand in Sydney. She thoroughly enjoyed her work and rapidly developed skills that led to her being in charge of the office staff where she worked. At age 20, she met Doug, a cabinet-maker, and they married and settled on the Central Coast. They had four daughters—Kate, Jane, Liz and Jill. Elsie stopped work when she had her first daughter and, although she stayed at home with her children, she developed an early interest in sewing and completed a number of courses to become a skilled seamstress. Doug and Elsie enjoyed their family and were financially secure enough so that they later chose to have a fifth child. Tragically, Noel was stillborn on Christmas Day and for the past 30 years Doug has refused to participate in Christmas celebrations. Elsie and Doug have never spoken about their loss. Despite her long-standing sadness, Elsie has maintained close and supportive relationships with her daughters and their children, and has a wide circle of sporting friends that she meets with at least twice a week. Until the onset of cardiac symptoms, she has managed to live well in spite of the limitations imposed by Raynaud's phenomenon and scleroderma.

2. COLLECT CUES/INFORMATION

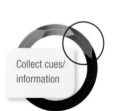

(a) Review current information

Review and think about Elsie's presentation. Although it is spring and the weather is warming up to the extent that you have turned on the air-conditioner in your office, Elsie is wearing thick gloves and a scarf when she arrives. She gingerly takes these off when you ask to take her blood pressure. She has a dressing on her left ring finger stained with serous exudate. There are a number of small, red spots on Elsie's hands and face, including several on her lips. You notice that her hands, which were initially warm and pink, rapidly change colour, with her fingers blanching and the palms becoming dark blue. The skin on her hands and part way up her forearms is tight and shiny, and appears to have limited flexibility.

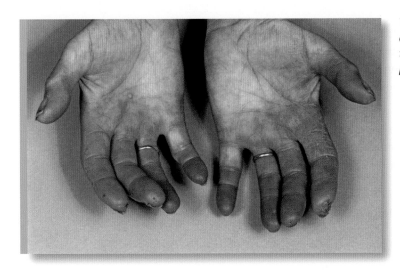

This image depicts an example of the discolouration that occurs in Raynaud's phenomenon

Elsie has a bottle of water with her and you observe that her mouth is so dry that at times she has trouble speaking until she has had a mouthful of water. You also note that her eyes are red and look sore. When you comment, Elsie tells you that they feel as if they have grit in them and she has been trying to stay out of the wind. She also finds that dry weather and air-conditioning make her eyes feel worse. Elsie tells you that over the past few weeks she has noticed that her heartburn has worsened and she experiences acid-reflux straight after eating, if she bends over and even if she sits in a comfortable chair. Elsie has taken to going for a walk after meals to try and minimise the burning sensation and pain associated with heartburn. She has to sleep in a recliner chair in the lounge room, as she wakes up coughing frequently and often feels as if she is choking.

Elsie's clinical notes are somewhat limited. She has a recorded diagnosis of long-standing Raynaud's phenomenon and limited cutaneous scleroderma. She is reviewed annually by an immunologist and was seen by a gastroenterologist several years ago who started her on a proton-pump inhibitor, rabeprazole (Pariet), to treat gastro-oesophageal ulceration. The letter from the cardiologist notes that the cardiac investigations undertaken were negative and that it was likely the chest pain Elsie had experienced was related to gastro-oesophageal disease. There are no nursing notes, because Elsie has not previously seen the practice nurse.

(b) Gather new information

Elsie's vital signs are as follows:

Temperature	36.2°C
Pulse	76
Respiratory rate	18
Blood pressure	L = 135/80, S = 130/75

Q1 As a practice nurse in this situation, what additional cues do you need to collect?

From the list below, identify the five cues that you believe are *most* relevant to your assessment of Elsie at this time.

a Skin condition—integrity and colouration

b Condition of oral mucosa

c Presence of reflux

d Pain score

e Reports of fatigue

f Temperature

g Condition of eyes

h ECG

Q2 What questions would you ask Elsie at this stage?

> *Hint: Think back to the information you have reviewed about Raynaud's phenomenon and scleroderma.*

(c) Recall knowledge

You may have identified some gaps in your understanding about the care of a person with a multisystemic autoimmune condition such as scleroderma. Explore the following websites and then answer the questions that follow. (Note that there may be more than one correct response for each question.)

Scleroderma Australia: <www.sclerodermaaustralia.com.au>
John Hopkins Scleroderma Centre: <www.hopkinsscleroderma.org>
International Scleroderma Network: <www.sclero.org/index.html>

Q1 Limited cutaneous systemic sclerosis, or CREST, includes which of the following?

   a   Antecedent history of Raynaud's phenomenon

   b   Calcinosis

   c   Telangiectasia

   d   Oesophageal involvement

   e   Hypertensive renal crisis

Q2 Severe Raynaud's phenomenon may result in:

   a   Digital ulceration and tissue infarction

   b   Clubbing of the nails

   c   A noticeable tremor

   d   Non-pigmented transverse bands in the nail bed

Q3 Which of the following factors increase the likelihood of digital ulceration?

   a   Activities that constrict blood flow, such as carrying heavy bags

   b   Exposure to cold temperatures resulting in frequent vasospasm

   c   Chronic and persistently high levels of stress

   d   Vaso-constrictors including caffeine and nicotine

   e   All of the above

Q4 Examination of the hands of a person with scleroderma may reveal:

   a   Hyperflexibility of the small joints

   b   Sclerodactyl

   c   Multiple telangiectasia

   d   Normal finger nails

   e   Calcinosis

Q5 Gastro-oesophageal involvement in scleroderma commonly manifests as:

   a   Malaena

   b   Projectile vomiting

   c   Increased appetite

   d   Dysphagia and oesophageal dysmotility

Q6 Which of these systems is not affected by scleroderma?

   a   Integumentary system

   b   Musculoskeletal system

   c   Central nervous system

   d   Gastrointestinal system

Q7 Sicca symptoms place the person at risk of:

  a Sensation of 'grit' in the eyes

  b Corneal ulceration

  c Excessive salivation

  d Difficulty swallowing dry foods

Q8 Scleroderma is thought to be triggered by autoantigens that lead to:

  a Infection and jaundice

  b A self-sustaining autoimmune reaction

  c Local inflammation

  d Fibrosis, tissue damage and organ malfunction

3. PROCESS INFORMATION

(a) Interpret

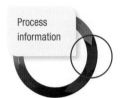

It can be challenging to identify the difference between long-standing signs and symptoms that have been stable for a long period of time and new symptoms that require attention. Be aware that it is common for people with a chronic condition such as scleroderma to blame every new health issue on the disease. This is a situation where you also need to be aware of any tendency to make the clinical reasoning error known as 'diagnostic momentum'. The person can develop other health problems that may or may not be related to the disease. Multisystem autoimmune conditions, by definition, impact on many aspects of a person's wellbeing. It is likely that the person will have more than one issue that requires attention. As health professionals working in a system that continues to focus on a single disease or issue, remember that multimorbidity has been identified in nearly a third of the Australian population (Harrison et al., 2016).

Diagnostic momentum: Once labels are attached to patients, they tend to become stickier and stickier. What started as a possibility gathers increasing momentum until it becomes definite and other possibilities are excluded (Croskerry, 2003).

Your initial assessment revealed that Elsie's basic observations are all within normal limits; however, you notice a number of cues that suggest there may be opportunities to improve Elsie's clinical management.

From your understanding of Raynaud's phenomenon and scleroderma, answer the following questions to identify what Elsie's signs and symptoms could indicate.

Q1 Painful finger with dressing stained with serous exudates may suggest:

  a Digital ulceration

  b Eczema

  c Ulcerating impetigo

  d Herpes simplex

  e Laceration

Q2 Nocturnal coughing and choking may suggest:

  a Sleep apnoea

  b Incompetent cardiac sphincter with gastric acid aspiration

  c Post-nasal drip

  d Dust-mite allergy

Q3 Dry mouth requiring frequent sips of water may suggest:

  a Anxiety

  b Inflammation of the salivary glands with decreased saliva production

  c Dehydration

  d Side effect of medication

Q4 Red and irritated eyes may suggest:

   a   Decreased production of tears

   b   Conjunctivitis

   c   Excessive rubbing of itchy eyes

   d   Irritation from contact lenses

   e   Poor eye hygiene leading to blepharitis

(b) Discriminate

Q   From the list below, select five cues that you believe are *most troubling* to Elsie at this time.

   a   Limited flexibility of joints

   b   Ulcerated finger

   c   Unresolved grief

   d   Rapid change in colour of hands

   e   Nocturnal coughing and choking

   f   Pain

   g   Lack of social support

   h   Red, irritated eyes

   i   Condition of oral mucosa

   j   Difficulty sleeping

   k   Loss of appetite

   l   Fatigue

> Note: It is common for health professionals to underestimate and dismiss the impact of symptoms that are not perceived to be life-threatening.

(c) Relate

Q   Which of the following statements are true?

   a   Elsie is having difficulty sleeping due to anxiety.

   b   Elsie has delayed healing of her digital ulceration because of poor circulation.

   c   Elsie's lachrymal glands are no longer producing sufficient tears to keep her eyes moist and flush out dust particles.

   d   Elsie's telangiectasia is an unexpected sign.

   e   Elsie's nocturnal cough is worsened by her decreased saliva production.

   f   Elsie's irritated and reddened eyes are due to sleep deprivation.

   g   Elsie's insomnia is related to her persistent cough.

   h   Elsie's limited flexibility in her hands is due to swelling from fluid retention.

   i   Elsie's fatigue is worsened because of lack of sleep.

(d) Infer and (e) Match

Q   From what you know about Elsie's history, her chronic health problems and signs and symptoms (as well as your knowledge about Raynaud's phenomenon and scleroderma), identify the correct inferences from the following. (Select the three that apply.)

   a   Elsie is experiencing gastric reflux due to an incompetent cardiac sphincter.

   b   Elsie is allergic to dust mites.

   c   Elsie has digital ulceration due to severe Raynaud's phenomenon.

   d   Elsie has developed an anxiety disorder because she focuses too much on her physical ailments.

  e Elsie has decreased tear and saliva production.

  f Elsie has symptoms that are to be expected in a person who is 65 years old.

(f) Predict

Q If you do not provide Elsie with the appropriate information and education to assist her to manage her symptoms, what may happen? (Select the five that apply.)

  a Elsie's digital ulceration could progress to gangrene.

  b Elsie's ulcer will heal as the weather warms.

  c Elsie's gastric reflux may result in a recurrence of oesophageal ulceration and lead to oesophageal stricture.

  d Elsie may develop a corneal ulceration.

  e Elsie will be at risk of rapid tooth decay.

  f Elsie will require a referral to the Aged Care Assessment Team as she is clearly unable to manage her condition.

  g Elsie's gastric reflux may result in pulmonary aspiration.

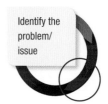

Do you know the difference between Raynaud's disease and Raynaud's phenomenon?

4. IDENTIFY THE PROBLEM/ISSUE

Identify the problem/ issue

Q1 Select from the following list, the three correct nursing diagnoses for Elsie:

  a Gastro-oesophageal reflux related to cardiac sphincter incompetence, evidenced by burning discomfort and pain after eating, and coughing when lying flat

  b Somatisation disorder due to the impact of a long-standing chronic disease, evidenced by a focus on physical sensations in the absence of physiological cause

  c Digital ulceration related to severe Raynaud's phenomenon, evidenced by serous exudate from ulcer on finger

  d Reduced tear and saliva production related to coexisting Sjögren's syndrome, evidenced by gritty sensation in eyes and dry mouth

  e Rheumatoid arthritis worsened by Raynaud's phenomenon, evidenced by painful and swollen joints and blanched fingers

Q2 Identify four factors (at least) that could have led to inadequate management of Elsie's symptoms to date.

5. ESTABLISH GOALS

Before implementing any actions to provide symptomatic relief for Elsie, it is important to clearly specify what you want to happen and when.

Establish goals

Q From the list below, choose three *short-term* goals that are both relevant and achievable for Elsie's management at this time.

  a For effective wound treatment to be commenced to enable Elsie's ulcerated finger to heal

  b For Elsie to understand that focusing on symptoms that cannot be changed is making her miserable

  c For Elsie's gastro-oesophageal reflux to be improved within one week

  d For Elsie's discomfort related to decreased tear and salivary production to be relieved within two days

  e For Elsie to be reviewed by a gastroenterologist within one week

  f For Elsie to understand how to manage her dry mouth and red eyes by the end of your consultation with her

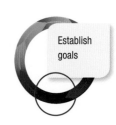

The NMBA's Registered Nurse Standards for Practice (2016) state that RNs must provide comprehensive, safe, quality practice to achieve agreed goals and outcomes that are responsive to the nursing needs of people.

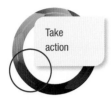

6. TAKE ACTION

You have identified three issues that require attention. Elsie's sleep is severely disturbed by her nocturnal cough and sensation of choking; she has an ulcer on her finger that is painful and inadequately treated; and she has sicca symptoms that are adding to her discomfort. This is the first time you have met Elsie and you are confronted with several issues that each require attention. You decide that you need to ask some more focused questions to help you decide how to proceed.

Gather further information:

- How long has her finger been painful?
- Is the pain worsening?
- Has the ulcer been increasing in size?
- Has she had a fever in the last 24–48 hours?
- What has she been putting on the ulcer?
- How long has she been sleeping in her reclining chair?
- Other than staying upright after meals, is there anything else that helps reduce her gastric reflux?
- Does she use caffeine-containing substances regularly?
- Does she smoke?
- When did she first notice that her mouth was constantly dry?
- How long have her eyes been dry and gritty?

Check what self-care measures Elsie is currently using regularly:

- What does she do to reduce the frequency of Raynaud's episodes?
- Is there anything she has found that helps her digital ulcers to heal more rapidly?
- What treatment is she currently using to manage her gastric reflux?
- Does she belong to a support group such as the Autoimmune Resource and Research Centre?

Review Elsie's medications:

- Is she continuing to take the proton-pump inhibitor that was prescribed?
- Has she ever applied GTN patches (glyceryl trinitrate patches) on the base of her fingers to help the blood vessels to dilate and improve the circulation to the ulcerated area?
- Does she use an artificial tear preparation?
- Does she use a saliva replacement?

Q Number the following list according to the order in which you would undertake the activities.

a Review with Elsie the issues that you have identified as needing attention.

b Prepare Elsie's ulcerated finger for review by the GP and discuss treatment options, including antibiotic, glyceryl trinitrate patches and occlusive dressing.

c Discuss with Elsie and the GP a possible review by a gastroenterologist.

d Refer Elsie to the Autoimmune Resource and Research Centre.

e Ask Elsie to identify which issue she would like addressed first.

f Arrange a follow-up phone call in one week to review the three issues with Elsie.

g Provide Elsie with an information sheet on managing gastro-oesophageal reflux, including how she might access a wedge pillow to reduce gastric reflux when lying down.

h Provide Elsie with a sample of artificial tear preparation.

i Check with Elsie when she last had a dental review.

j Provide Elsie with an information sheet on managing sicca symptoms.

k Review stress management strategies to assist in the healing of the digital ulcer.

Something to think about …

Information sheets for people with autoimmune conditions, scleroderma, lupus, Sjögren's syndrome and Raynaud's phenomenon can be found at the following websites:

Autoimmune Resource and Research Centre: <www.autoimmune.org.au/home/.aspx>

Scleroderma Australia: <www.sclerodermaaustralia.com.au/index.php/publications>

Raynaud's phenomenon: <www.autoimmune.org.au/SiteFiles/autoimmunecomau/raynauds_brochure.pdf>

Sjögren's information: <www.autoimmune.org.au/SiteFiles/autoimmunecomau/sjogrens-brochure.pdf>.

7. EVALUATE

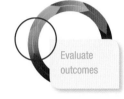
Evaluate outcomes

You arrange to contact Elsie in one week to check whether the medication the GP has prescribed and the recommendations you have given her in regard to managing her symptoms have been beneficial.

Q From the information that Elsie reports when you contact her, rate the following as 'unchanged', 'improving' or 'deteriorating'.

Symptom	
Nocturnal cough and choking	Only awakened twice in the past week
Quality of sleep	Sleeping in bed again
Ulcerated finger	No longer painful, less exudate
Oral dryness	Remains troublesome
Eye irritation	Markedly reduced with regular use of tear replacement
Raynaud's phenomenon	Fewer episodes with warmer weather and use of GTN patches

8. REFLECT

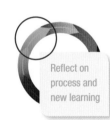
Reflect on process and new learning

Reflect on your learning from this scenario and consider the following questions.

Q1 What are three of the most important things that you have learnt from this scenario?

Q2 What nursing actions might minimise the future impact of Elsie's scleroderma?

Q3 What have you learnt about the importance of effective and person-centred chronic disease management?

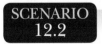
SCENARIO 12.2 The emotional impact of living with a chronic autoimmune condition

CHANGING THE SCENE

The impact of a diagnosis of a chronic illness has been described as a 'life-changing event, signifying the beginning of what will, for most people, be a lifelong process of adapting to significant physical, psychosocial and environmental changes' (Bishop, 2005, p. 219). Increasing numbers of Australians are faced with living with chronic illness and for many the challenges multiply as they attempt to adapt to more than one condition. Nichols and Hunt (2011) suggest that the impact of chronic illnesses also includes recreational, spiritual, sexual and vocational aspects of a person's life.

When considering the spiritual aspect of a person's life, remember that this is not limited to involvement in a particular religious activity. 'For many, spirituality refers to an individual's attempt to find meaning in life, which can involve a sense of involvement with the transcendent outside institutional boundaries' (Williams & Sternthal, 2007, p. S47). A chronic condition that impacts on activities that previously brought meaning and purpose to a person's life can result in grief and a sense of loss. Chronic sorrow or ongoing grief may result from the relentlessness of the impact of chronic illnesses such as scleroderma (Roos & Neimeyer, 2007) and there is an increased risk of psychological conditions such as anxiety and depression (Carrier, 2009, p. 38; Clarke & Currie, 2009; Di Benedetto et al., 2014).

For the person living with a little-known condition such as scleroderma, the difficulties are magnified. Many people experience isolation and fear of the unknown, associated with not having ever heard of the condition with which they have been diagnosed. The fear returns again and again as the person encounters yet another health professional who seems to know little about their condition.

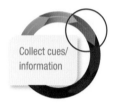

1. CONSIDER THE PATIENT SITUATION

Elsie has lived with scleroderma for many years and she has generally managed by focusing on keeping busy, doing what she could to keep warm and reduce the frequency of her Raynaud's attacks, and just 'soldiering on'. In the past, she has tolerated an occasional digital ulcer in the winter time, relying on the warmer weather to improve her circulation sufficiently for the ulcer to heal.

2. COLLECT CUES/INFORMATION

(a) Review current information

Three-month review of chronic disease management plan

Elsie has returned for the regular three-month review that is an essential component of the chronic disease management program you provide at the GP clinic. You saw Elsie twice following your initial session: to dress her finger and to provide education on the management of her sicca symptoms. At each of these follow-up visits, Elsie was cheerful and pleased with the way in which her symptoms were improving. It is now summertime and you expect that Elsie's Raynaud's phenomenon and scleroderma will be less troublesome, so you plan to take this opportunity to review with Elsie how she is managing her condition. You have reviewed her clinical notes and see that Elsie has seen the GP once on your day off, her digital ulcer has healed and her gastric reflux has responded well to an increase in rabeprazole and careful adherence to the use of the conservative measures the two of you discussed. There is no record of any further chest pain or symptoms suggestive of cardiac problems.

Elsie comes into your office. She sits down and, when you ask her how she is, she looks sad and begins to cry. Elsie starts to apologise for her tears and seems embarrassed that you are seeing the difficulty she is having managing her distress. When Elsie settles a little, you ask if she would like to talk to you about what has upset her. Elsie says, 'I shouldn't be like this. My reflux has settled, my eyes are feeling much better now that I use the artificial tears, and you can see the ulcer on my finger has healed.' After a few moments, Elsie goes on, 'I just can't seem to see the point of going on. I'm so tired of pretending that it's all okay. My daughters get upset if I say anything about how hard it is, and Doug and I are like strangers living in the same house.' Listening closely, you hear that Elsie has been feeling distressed for over a month, is having difficulty sleeping and has lost weight because she has lost her appetite.

(b) Gather new information

Think back to what you know about Elsie's story. While your contact with Elsie thus far has focused on attending to the physical health problems that she experiences, consider what you may have missed.

Q1 Elsie has given you some cues as to what may be troubling her. What questions would you ask her that might help you understand more about her distress?

Q2 Are there other factors in addition to Elsie's chronic autoimmune condition that could be contributing to her sadness?

Q3 What questions will assist you to identify a potential depressive illness?

(c) Recall knowledge

Effective nursing care requires more than a sound understanding of the physical condition affecting the person for whom you are caring.

Q Test your knowledge of the psychosocial dimensions of chronic illness by identifying which of the following are true.

  a Grief is a normal response to significant loss.

  b Signs and symptoms of grief and loss are indistinguishable from depression.

  c The only effective treatment for depression is antidepressant medication.

  d People with depression should be encouraged to snap out of it.

  e The person experiencing depression has both emotional and physical symptoms.

  f Experiencing a chronic illness places a person at greater risk of depression.

  g Depression places a person at risk of self-harm or suicide.

  h Co-morbid anxiety and depression is rare.

  i Chronic sorrow is commonly experienced by people with persistent physical illnesses that limit the person's capacity to undertake normal daily activities.

The following two beyondblue (www.beyondblue.org.au) resources are valuable for people struggling with the impact of grief and chronic illness:

Fact Sheet 23: Chronic physical illness, anxiety and depression.

Fact Sheet 28: Grief and loss.

3. PROCESS INFORMATION

(a) Interpret

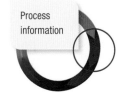

Process information

You have listened closely to Elsie, collected further information and recalled what you know about her life experiences and her journey living with scleroderma. The next step of the clinical reasoning cycle is to interpret the data (cues) that you have collected by careful analysis, all the while applying your knowledge about the impact of chronic illness on the person's wellbeing.

Q1 As you review the information that you have collected, how might you interpret the cues?

Q2 Elsie appears to have previously coped well with her chronic health problems. What has happened recently that might have impacted on her ability to cope?

Q3 Is there anything about Elsie's story and her current distress that raises your level of concern, or do you think what she is telling you is to be expected given her chronic autoimmune condition?

Q4 Are there any indicators of possible co-morbid mental illness?

Q5 Whittemore and Dixon (2008) talk about the tensions between 'living a life and living an illness'. Given Elsie's condition, what might the tensions be for her? What limitations does she have on her day-to-day activities? Is there anything in her story that might lead you to suspect that she is living her illness rather than living her life?

Q6 An acquaintance of Elsie's, who has similar problems, has been a member of the state-wide scleroderma support group for many years, with most of her social activities revolving around raising money for the group. Is this a healthy adjustment to chronic illness or is it 'living an illness'? What are the reasons for your answer?

Q7 Elsie has had minimal contact with the support group over the years, choosing to focus on her family, her hobbies and trying to 'forget about her condition'. Consider whether this decision has perhaps contributed to Elsie's current distress and sense of isolation.

(b) Discriminate and (c) Relate

Q From the list of feelings, thoughts, behaviours and physical symptoms below, select five cues that you believe are *most troubling* to Elsie at this time:

a Guilt

b Irritability

c Feeling miserable

d Indecision

e Sadness and tearfulness

f Saying 'It's all my fault'

g Saying 'Nothing good ever happens to me'

h Saying 'Life is not worth living'

i Talking about suicide

j Relying on alcohol or sedatives

k Withdrawing from family and friends

l Stopping doing things she once enjoyed

m Lack of appetite

> Unfortunately, it is not unusual for health professionals to dismiss cues indicative of psychological conditions on the basis that it is to be expected a person living with a chronic physical condition would be depressed (Roos & Neimeyer, 2007). This is a form of ascertainment bias.

(d) Infer and (e) Match

Q From what you know about Elsie's story, her chronic health problems and current signs and symptoms (as well as your knowledge about mental health issues associated with chronic physical illness and chronic sorrow), identify which of the following inferences are correct. (Select the three that apply.)

a Elsie is developing a psychotic illness due to all the medication she is taking.

b Elsie is experiencing symptoms indicative of clinical depression.

c Elsie appears to be exhibiting symptoms pointing to an emerging dementia.

d Elsie is experiencing chronic sorrow related to the many years of living with scleroderma and exacerbated by recent symptoms initially thought to be cardiac in origin.

e Elsie is experiencing symptoms indicative of manic depression.

f Elsie has a social anxiety disorder that prevents her taking part in previously enjoyed activities.

g Elsie is experiencing distress exacerbated by a loss of meaning and purpose in her life and decreased intimacy, linked to the loss of her son and the impact of this on her relationship with Doug.

(f) Predict

Q If you do not respond to Elsie's distress and assist her to access effective treatment, what might happen? (Select the four that apply.)

a Elsie will feel better in the next few days.

b Elsie's emotional distress will increase the difficulties she experiences in living with scleroderma.

c Elsie will soon realise that she needs to get on with her life.

d Elsie is likely to become increasingly isolated from friends and family.

e Elsie's physical health will deteriorate more rapidly, as she has even less energy to prepare healthy food, exercise or take her medication as prescribed.

   f   Elsie's mood will improve as it gets closer to Christmas.

   g   Elsie's loss of enjoyment of previously enjoyed activities will deepen, with an increasing wish to die placing her at risk of suicide.

4. IDENTIFY THE PROBLEM/ISSUE

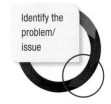

Identify the problem/issue

Q   Select from the following list the *most* correct nursing diagnoses for Elsie.

   a   Exacerbation of limited cutaneous scleroderma

   b   Insomnia secondary to gastro-oesophageal reflux disease

   c   Grief and chronic sorrow related to multiple losses, evidenced by increasing social isolation, sense of hopelessness and sleeplessness

   d   Clinical depression related to grief and chronic sorrow

   e   Medication-related low mood

5. ESTABLISH GOALS

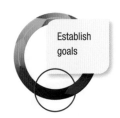

Establish goals

Before implementing any actions to address Elsie's distress, it is important to clearly specify what you want to happen and when.

Q   From the list below, choose the three most important *short-term* goals for Elsie's management at this time.

   a   For Elsie to regain the weight she has lost

   b   For Elsie's embarrassment and shame related to her emotional distress to be alleviated

   c   For Elsie to understand that depression is not a weakness and that effective treatment is available

   d   For Elsie to cheer up

   e   For Elsie to accept referral to a mental health professional for further assessment and treatment of her depression

   f   For Elsie to go back to her previously enjoyed activities when she goes home after today's consultation

6. TAKE ACTION

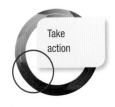

Take action

'Having a physical illness is one of the strongest risk factors for depression' and, conversely, co-morbid depression is linked to 'worse functional outcomes for people with physical diseases' (Clarke & Currie, 2009, pp. S54 and S58). While evidence-based treatments for depression are available, a significant proportion of people experiencing depression are either not diagnosed with the condition or, if diagnosed, fail to receive effective treatment (World Health Organization [WHO] & World Family Doctors [WONCA], 2008). For many people, access to appropriate treatment options has proved difficult. A number of factors, including the stigma related to a diagnosis of mental illness and the cost, have proven to be a strong barrier to people seeking help or indeed following through on a referral for treatment. The Department of Health in Australia has implemented a number of programs designed to improve access to mental health care (Department of Health, 2012).

Why focus on depression? In Australia, depression has been identified as a high prevalence disorder, with significant social, human and economic costs. The public health impact is such that it has been listed as a National Health Priority Area: <www.aihw. gov.au/mental-health-priority-area/>.

As you talk with Elsie, you are increasingly aware that she is feeling very embarrassed about her tears and having opened up to you about her distress. You decide that you need to spend some time allaying her anxiety and making sure that she knows that depression is a treatable illness and not something to be ashamed of.

The NSQHS Standards highlight the importance of shared decision making when developing a comprehensive and individualised plan of care that addresses the significance and complexity of the person's health issues and agreed goals for treatment and care (ACSQHC, 2016).

As Elsie settles, you broach with her the subject of a referral for further assessment and treatment of her possible depression. You have deliberated on the options available before discussing this with Elsie. For several years, the general practice has had two psychologists conducting regular sessions for people needing psychological interventions. Last year, the practice also employed a mental health nurse to work two days a week through the Mental Health Nurse Incentive Program.

Following a quick phone call, you talk to Elsie about meeting the mental health nurse who is in today and available to be introduced to Elsie. She agrees, albeit reluctantly, and you check with her whether there are any issues related to her physical health that you need to attend to before you finish this session.

7. EVALUATE

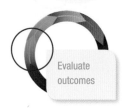

Evaluate outcomes

You have arranged to contact Elsie in two weeks to see how she is feeling following her consultation with the mental health nurse.

Q1 When you make this phone call, what questions will you ask that will help you elicit information to identify whether there has been an improvement in Elsie's mood?

Q2 Long term, how will you evaluate the impact of the referral to the mental health nurse and the subsequent appointments Elsie has with her?

8. REFLECT

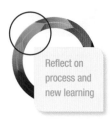

Reflect on process and new learning

Reflect on your learning from this scenario and consider the following questions.

Q1 What are three of the most important things that you have learnt from this scenario?

Q2 When caring for someone with a chronic illness, what nursing actions may minimise the impact of depression on their physical health?

Q3 What have you learnt about the importance of identifying depression secondary to chronic disease?

Q4 What actions will you take in clinical practice as a result of your learning from this scenario?

EPILOGUE

Elsie attended weekly appointments with the mental health nurse for several weeks and then saw her fortnightly for a further three months. During those sessions, Elsie and the nurse talked about the impact that scleroderma had had on Elsie's life. It seemed that the trigger for Elsie's depression had been the investigations for cardiac disease. Until the 'heart scare', Elsie had believed that she could get on with her life in spite of her autoimmune condition, and she had increasingly been troubled by the fear that this 'rotten disease was going to be the end of her'. She had, in fact, packed up her sewing room, resigned from her position on the sports club committee and stopped visiting her grandchildren. Elsie had also spoken about her grief at the loss of Nicholas and the devastating impact that his death had had on her relationship with Doug.

Six months later, just after Christmas, when Elsie attended for her routine chronic illness check, the difference was astounding. Elsie described a 'new lease on life'; not only had she returned to her previously enjoyed activities but for the first time Doug and she had spoken about Nicholas. Doug had attended Christmas with all the family and Elsie was now looking forward to the months and years ahead.

FURTHER READING

Chen, Y.-C. & Li, I.-C. (2009). Effectiveness of interventions using empowerment concept for patients with chronic disease: A systematic review. *JBI Library of Systematic Reviews, 7*(27), 1177–232.

Edward, K.-l. (2013). Chronic illness and wellbeing: Using nursing practice to foster resilience as resistance. *British Journal of Nursing, 22*(13), 741–46.

REFERENCES

Andersson, S., Svanström, R., Ek, K., Rosén, H. & Berglund, M. (2015). 'The challenge to take charge of life with long-term illness': Nurses' experiences of supporting patients' learning with the didactic model. *Journal of Clinical Nursing, 24*(23–24), 3409–16. doi: 10.1111/jocn.12960

Australian Commission on Safety and Quality in Health Care (ACSQHC). (2016). *National Safety and Quality Health Service Standards Version 2*. Draft, Sydney, Australia.

Australian Institute of Health and Welfare (2015). *1 in 5 Australians Affected by Multiple Chronic Diseases*. Available at <www.aihw.gov.au/media-release-detail/?id=60129552034>.

Australian Society of Clinical Immunology and Allergy (ASCIA). (2016). *Autoimmune Diseases. ASCIA Education Resources (AER) Patient Information*. Accessed October 2016 at <www.allergy.org.au/images/pcc/ASCIA_PCC_Autoimmune_diseases_2016.pdf>.

Bishop, M. (2005). Quality of life and psychosocial adaptation to chronic illness and disability: Preliminary analysis of a conceptual and theoretical synthesis. *Rehabilitation Counseling Bulletin, 48*(4), 219–31.

Brownie, S., Scott, R. & Rossiter, R. (2016). Therapeutic communication and relationships in chronic and complex care. *Nursing Standard, 31*(6), 54–56.

Carrier, J. (2009). *Managing Long-Term Conditions and Chronic Illness in Primary Care: A Guide to Good Practice*. Abingdon, Oxon: Routledge.

Clarke, D. M. & Currie, K. C. (2009). Depression, anxiety and their relationship with chronic diseases: A review of the epidemiology, risk and treatment evidence. *Medical Journal of Australia, 190*(Suppl 7), s54–60.

Croskerry, P. (2003). The importance of cognitive errors in diagnosis and strategies to minimize them. *Academic Medicine, 78*(8), 1–6.

Denton, C. P. (2015). Advances in pathogenesis and treatment of systemic sclerosis. *Clinical Medicine, 15*, s58–63.

Department of Health. (2012). Better access to mental health care. Accessed March 2017 at <www.health.gov.au/internet/main/publishing.nsf/content/mental-ba-fact-pat>

Derrett-Smith, E. C. & Denton, C. P. (2010). Progress in the therapy of systemic sclerosis. In C. M. Deighton & M. Doherty (Eds), *Therapeutic Strategies in Rheumatology* (pp. 124–38). Oxford: Clinical Publishing.

Di Benedetto, M., Lindner, H., Aucote, H., Churcher, J., McKenzie, S., Croning, N. & Jenkins, E. (2014). Co-morbid depression and chronic illness related to coping and physical and mental health status. *Psychology, Health & Medicine, 19*(3), 253–62. doi: 10.1080/13548506.2013.803135

Goldblatt, F. & O'Neill, S. G. (2013). Clinical aspects of autoimmune rheumatic diseases. *Lancet, 382*(9894), 797–808.

Harrison, C., Henderson, J., Miller, G. & Britt, H. (2016). The prevalence of complex multimorbidity in Australia. *Australian & New Zealand Journal of Public Health, 40*(3), 239–44. doi: 10.1111/1753-6405.12509

Kuipers, P., Kendall, E., Ehrlich, C., McIntyre, M., Barber, L., Amsters, D., . . . Brownie, S. (2011). *Complexity and Health Care: Health Practitioner Workforce Services, Roles, Skills and Training, to Respond to Patients with Complex Needs*. Brisbane: Clinical Education and Training Queensland.

LeMone, P., Burke, K., Bauldoff, G., Gubrud-Howe, P., Levett-Jones, T., Dwyer, T., . . . Raymond, D. (Eds). (2017). *Medical–Surgical Nursing: Critical Thinking in Person-Centred Care* (3rd edn). Melbourne: Pearson.

Martin, C. & Peterson, C. (2008). Chronic illness and new models of care (Editorial). *Health Issues, 97*, 4.

Newton, E. G., Thombs, B. D. & Groleau, D. (2012). The experience of emotional distress among women with scleroderma. *Qualitative Health Research, 22*(9), 1195–1206. doi: 10.1177/1049732312449207

Nichols, L. M. & Hunt, B. (2011). The significance of spirituality for individuals with chronic illness: Implications for mental health counseling. *Journal of Mental Health Counseling, 33*(1), 51–66.

Nursing and Midwifery Board of Australia (NMBA). (2016). *Registered Nurse Standards for Practice*. Melbourne: NMBA.

Parker, L. (2013). Diagnosis of systemic sclerosis and Raynaud's phenomenon. *Primary Health Care*, *23*(2), 22–24.

Roos, S. & Neimeyer, R. A. (2007). Reauthoring the self: Chronic sorrow and posttraumatic stress following the onset of CID. In E. Martz & H. Livneh (Eds), *Coping with Chronic Illness and Disability: Theoretical, Empirical, and Clinical Aspects* (pp. 89–106). Dordrecht: Springer.

Sampalli, T., Fox, R. A., Dickson, R. & Fox, J. (2012). Proposed model of integrated care to improve health outcomes for individuals with multimorbidities. *Patient Preference & Adherence*, *6*, 757–64. doi: 10.2147/PPA.S35201

Schaink, A. K., Kuluski, K., Lyons, R. F., Fortin, M., Jadad, A. R., Upshur, R., & Wodchis, W. P. (2012). A scoping review and thematic classification of patient complexity: Offering a unifying framework. *Journal of Comorbidity*, *2*(1), 9. doi: 10.15256/joc.2012.2.15

Scleroderma Association. (2016). *Who Suffers from Scleroderma?* Accessed October 2016 at <www.sclerodermaaustralia.com.au/about/about-scleroderma>.

Seldin, M. F. (2015). The genetics of human autoimmune disease: A perspective on progress in the field and future directions. *Journal of Autoimmunity*, *64*, 1–12. doi: 10.1016/j.jaut.2015.08.015

Swaminathan, S., Goldblatt, F., Dugar, M., Gordon, T. P. & Roberts-Thomson, P. J. (2008). Prevalence of sicca symptoms in a South Australian cohort with systemic sclerosis. *Internal Medicine Journal*, *38*(12), 897–903.

Wang, L., Wang, F.-S. & Gershwin, M. E. (2015). Human autoimmune diseases: A comprehensive update. *Journal of Internal Medicine*, *278*(4), 369–95. doi: 10.1111/joim.12395

Whittemore, R. & Dixon, J. (2008). Chronic illness: The process of integration. *Journal of Clinical Nursing, 17*(7b), 177–87.

Williams, D. R. & Sternthal, M. J. (2007). Spirituality, religion and health: Evidence and research directions. *Medical Journal of Australia, 10* (Supplement), s47–50.

World Health Organization (WHO) & World Family Doctors (WONCA). (2008). *Integrating Mental Health into Primary Care: A Global Perspective*. Geneva, Switzerland: WHO.

PHOTO CREDIT

CARING FOR A PERSON EXPERIENCING AN ACUTE PSYCHOTIC EPISODE

ANNA TRELOAR AND PETER ROSS

LEARNING OUTCOMES

Completion of the activities in this chapter will enable you to:

- define the terms 'psychosis' and 'mental state examination' (**gather information, interpret** and **discriminate**)
- explain why an understanding of psychosis is essential to competent nursing practice (**recall** and **apply**)
- outline the clinical manifestations of psychosis that will guide your collection of appropriate cues (**gather information, interpret** and **discriminate**)
- identify possible causes of psychosis (**match** and **predict**)
- review clinical information to identify the main nursing diagnoses for a patient experiencing a psychotic episode (**synthesise**)
- describe the priorities of care for the management of a person experiencing psychosis (**setting goals** and **taking action**)
- identify clinical criteria for determining the effectiveness of nursing actions taken to manage a person experiencing psychosis (**evaluate**)
- consider how inaccurate information may interfere with person-centred care (**reflect**)
- reflect on personal reactions to people experiencing psychosis and identify appropriate management strategies (**reflect**).

INTRODUCTION

The two scenarios in this chapter focus on the care of Jando, a young man with undiagnosed psychosis who has recently been incarcerated. People who enter the prison system are vulnerable groups who often have poor mental and physical health. Although they are entitled to the same standard of healthcare as anybody else in the community, they don't always receive it and significant healthcare problems can be overlooked. In Jando's case, it is particularly difficult to ascertain the true nature of his problem due to situational and contextual factors that influence accurate assessment and diagnosis. Despite the challenges, nurses who work in the prison system are well positioned to provide expert clinical care. For this reason, skills in clinical reasoning are fundamental to the management of the health and wellbeing of people such as Jando.

KEY CONCEPTS

psychosis
mental state examination
co-morbidity
recovery model

SUGGESTED READINGS

P. LeMone, K. Burke, G. Bauldoff, P. Gubrud-Howe, T. Levett-Jones, T. Dwyer . . . D. Raymond (Eds). (2017). *Medical–Surgical Nursing: Critical Thinking in Person-Centred Care* (3rd edn). Melbourne: Pearson. Chapter 50: Mental healthcare in the Australian context

British Psychological Society, Division of Clinical Psychology. (2014). *Understanding Psychosis and Schizophrenia. Why People Sometimes Hear Voices, Believe Things that Others Find Strange, or Appear Out of Touch with Reality, and What Can Help.* Edited by Anne Cook. Canterbury: Christ Church University. Available at <www.bps.org.uk>.

A. Treloar. (2015). Sicoko. *Australian Nursing and Midwifery Journal, 22*(8), 46. Available at <www.anmf.org.au>.

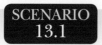
SCENARIO 13.1 Establishing a therapeutic relationship with a person who has a psychotic illness

SETTING THE SCENE

It is Friday night and a new prisoner is escorted into the cell complex of the police station at the coastal resort town of Melaleuca. The prisoner's name is Jando, he is 18 years old and this is his first experience of the adult corrections system. After being assessed by the prison officers who manage the cells, and after having lodgement forms completed, Jando goes into a shared cell. There is a concrete block base for a bed, a plastic covered mattress, a grey blanket and no pillow or sheets. The floor is concrete and there is no window. There is a shower outlet on the wall, a stainless steel toilet with no seat, a water bubbler for drinking water just above the cistern and a television mounted in a metal cage high up on the wall in a corner of the cell. There is nothing else. All personal belongings are kept by the officers and locked up. Jando is scheduled to receive a comprehensive health check on Monday afternoon by the registered nurse who works from 4 pm till 8 pm, Monday to Friday.

The epidemiology of psychosis

> If you are not sure what all these terms mean, access this site: <http://au.reachout.com/tough-times/mental-health-issues/psychotic-disorders>.

The psychotic disorders feature delusions, hallucinations, disorganised thinking and behaviour, and negative symptoms (American Psychiatric Association, 2013). The second national Australian psychosis survey (Survey of High Impact Psychosis) found that in 2010 the estimated treated prevalence of psychotic disorders in a one-month period for people aged 18 to 64 was 3.5 per 1000 population and that the most common disorder was schizophrenia. The onset of illness was under 25 years for 64.8 per cent of people surveyed, and for most the onset was insidious (Morgan et al., 2012).

The aetiology and pathogenesis of psychosis

Many possible causes of psychosis have been put forward over the years, particularly for schizophrenia. It is helpful to consider the aetiology of psychosis as multifactorial, with genetic predisposition, prenatal influences, life events and drug use all implicated. Zubin and Spring (1977) developed the stress-diathesis model, which suggests that everybody has some vulnerability to psychosis—a kind of psychosis threshold—and when this is crossed, psychosis may be triggered. This vulnerability may be increased by a variety of genetic, gestational, infectious and nutritional factors; and those with this vulnerability may have an increased susceptibility, not only to psychosis, but also to other mental illnesses including substance misuse (Ksir & Hart, 2016). Psychological pathways can include early experience of adversity (Beards & Fisher, 2014), and there may also be a range of subtle premorbid developmental deficits and exposure to risks in the time from before birth to early adolescence (Laurens et al., 2015). Schizophrenia may be related to three interacting pathophysiological processes—dysregulation of the dopamine system, disturbed glutamatergic neurotransmission and an increase in the proinflammatory status of the brain (Kahn & Sommer, 2015). Developments in neuroscience and the identification of biomarkers may change the way psychosis is diagnosed in the future (Keshavan et al., 2013).

Person-centred care

Jando has grown up in a quiet coastal village in NSW, with his father, mother and sister. His father moved overseas with his new partner when Jando was in Year 10, saying to Jando before he left, 'You're the man of the house now.' Jando took this responsibility very seriously, along with his commitment to studying (to attain good marks in the HSC) and working with his local Landcare group to protect the dunes. He has two good friends from school and attends a small church regularly with a girl from his street. He hopes to work in environmental science one day.

1. CONSIDER THE PATIENT SITUATION

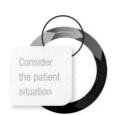

Monday 4 pm

Jonathon is the only registered nurse working at the Melaleuca police cell complex. When he arrives for work, he is told that Jando has spent the whole weekend in the cells, after being taken into custody late on Friday night. Jonathon decides to see Jando first as he is new to the corrections system. The prison officer brings him into the clinic. 'Had to give him a couple of Panadol at lunchtime', says one officer. 'For a headache … that's what he said anyway. Apart from that he hasn't said a thing since he was arrested.' No further information is provided about Jando. There are no medication orders; however, the prison officers keep a box of paracetamol in their office and can supply two tablets if a prisoner complains of pain. This medication is not recorded anywhere.

Tuesday 4 pm

On arrival at work the following day Jonathon finds that, instead of attending court as he was meant to, Jando is on his way back to the cells from the local Emergency Department (ED). 'What happened?', Jonathon asks. 'Not too sure', one of the officers says. 'Seems he fell over on his way into the courthouse and hit his head on the concrete. I didn't see it happen myself. I reckon one of the others could have tripped him up or given him a shove. There was a bit of an argument over food before they all left this morning. We wouldn't have worried about ED except he was talking rubbish after he fell over—kept saying something about a lease.' The prisoners in the main cell complex, usually so ready to volunteer 'helpful information', are strangely silent today.

Prisoners are identified only by their MIN (Master Index Number), not by first or last names. Therefore, part of their experience of being taken into custody is loss of individual identity. How can Jonathon overcome this to provide person-centred care?

2. COLLECT CUES/INFORMATION

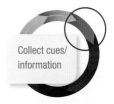

Jonathon wants to check Jando's head wound, so he asks an officer to let him into the cell where he is lying on the bed. Two steri-strips are on the laceration on his forehead 'Nurse, they came after me and punished me', he says sadly. 'I wish to be released but it can never happen.'

Q   Which cognitive bias is this an example of if Jonathon ignores the report from the local ED and doesn't check the head wound because he believes he already knows what the problem is? (*Note*: There is more than one correct answer.)

   a   Anchoring

   b   Ascertainment bias

   c   Confirmation bias

   d   Fundamental attribution error

   e   Psych-out error

   f   Unpacking principle

'Seems so quiet, doesn't he?' says the officer. 'Hard to believe the charges.' 'What did he do?' asks Jonathon. 'Assault—quite a history apparently. Thumped his mum for no reason, then a few weeks later his sister, out of the blue. The reason he's here is because he decked a total stranger in the street. Just went up and punched him.'

The NSQHS Standards emphasise the importance of infection control measures. In prison environments, cleaning standards are less strict than in hospitals, and there is constant prisoner turnover (some having undiagnosed infections), crowded living conditions and a lack of fresh air. Therefore, strict vigilance from Jonathon is required when conducting wound assessments (ACSQHC, 2016).

(a) Review current information

Jonathon has access to limited information about Jando's health status. He is the only RN working in this prison cell complex, so he does not receive a shift handover. The prison officers have no health training and provide few details about Jando's condition. Jonathon's observations of Jando's behaviour, and his ability to establish a therapeutic relationship and gain his trust, are therefore critical to being able to gather the information needed for a comprehensive health assessment.

Before reading the next part of the scenario, consider how Jonathon can best proceed with undertaking a comprehensive health assessment of Jando. How might he ascertain how Jando has behaved over the weekend when he has no access to the records kept by the prison officers and Jando seems reluctant to say much?

The NMBA's Registered Nurse Standards for Practice (2016) state that nurses must work in partnership with patients and use a range of assessment techniques. Jonathon cannot collect all the information he needs if Jando does not trust him.

Q1   How reliable will information provided by the prison officers be?

Q2   What should Jonathon's priorities be when seeking information about Jando?

(b) Gather new information

The standard health assessment form used in the prison health service is divided into four sections: medical and surgical history, alcohol and other drug use (to predict potential for withdrawal), previous psychiatric history and risk assessment (dealing with self-harm and suicidal ideation). Jando answers Jonathon's questions as he works through the health assessment, but volunteers little additional information and most of his replies are monosyllabic. Sometimes when he does offer more information, he seems to stop mid-sentence and lose his train of thought. Jando states that he doesn't have a regular general practitioner (GP) as he prefers to attend the ED at his local hospital for any health problems. He admits to 'some' cannabis use, but can't quantify the amount; he denies using any alcohol or other drugs. When Jonathon asks him how his head feels, Jando smiles and says, 'I have been released.' When Jando is questioned, he doesn't mention any mental health issues or previous psychiatric treatment.

> Poor physical health is common among people who have mental health issues (Martin, 2016). For more information about the health and wellbeing of young people who are incarcerated, access this site: <www.juvenile.justice.nsw.gov.au/Documents/JH_YPICHSRep2009_D10b_00_opening.pdf>.

Q1   Why might Jando be unwilling or unable to answer Jonathon's questions about mental illness? (There is more than one correct answer.)

    a   Jando did not understand what Jonathon was talking about.

    b   Jando has never had any previous psychiatric treatment.

    c   Jando doesn't want the other prisoners to know anything about his health status.

    d   Jando doesn't want the prison officers to think he is a 'spinner'. (This is the prison slang for a person with a mental health problem.)

Jonathon proceeds to check Jando's vital signs and blood glucose level. Review the information provided below:

Temperature	36.3°C
Pulse rate	60
Respiratory rate	18
Blood pressure	110/70
Blood glucose level	6.1 mmol/L
Pain score	0/10 (However, this may not be accurate as Jando seemed unable to concentrate when Jonathon asked him to rate his pain using a numerical rating scale, where 10 is the worst pain ever experienced and 0 represents no pain.)

One of Jonathon's roles is to undertake a risk assessment of all prisoners.

> The NSQHS Standards refer to the provision of comprehensive care and the management of risk. In Jando's situation, this will include consideration of unpredictable behaviours, such as self-harm and suicide, and aggression and violence.

Q2   What types of risk assessment might be relevant in Jando's situation?

Q3   Which of the following statements are true in regards to risk assessments undertaken in a prison context?

    a   Risk assessment is never static and changes depending on the person's mood, level of psychosocial support, situation and circumstances.

    b   Risk assessment is a definitive way to predict whether a person is going to attempt self-harm.

    c   Risk assessment only needs to be undertaken once during the person's time in the healthcare setting.

    d   Risk assessment is unnecessary when the person is in a cell with closed-circuit cameras monitoring behaviour around the clock.

3. PROCESS INFORMATION

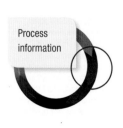

Process information

(a) Interpret

Q1   Which of Jando's vital signs are within normal parameters?

Q2   Jonathon is not focusing solely on the possibility of an undiagnosed mental illness. What other problems does he need to rule out?

Q3 Jando's vital signs suggest that:

a He is a physically fit young man and needs no further observations recorded at this stage.

b He is unlikely to experience any withdrawal state while in custody.

c He is highly anxious.

d He is in acute pain.

Nurses working in the prison system must undertake an assessment of potential substance withdrawal for all inmates and must be familiar with relevant signs and symptoms.

You can find information about withdrawal from legal and illegal drugs at <www.adf.org.au>.

Q4 If Jonathon assumes that Jando's speech and behaviour are due to a withdrawal state simply because many prisoners do have substance misuse problems, this is an example of:

a Anchoring

b Ascertainment bias

c Confirmation bias

d Fundamental attribution error

e Psych-out error

f Unpacking principle

Q5 Signs and symptoms of alcohol withdrawal include:

a Sweating, tremor, nausea, raised blood pressure and anxiety

b Irritability, abdominal pain, anxiety and anorexia

c Mydriasis, piloerection, muscle aches, rhinorrhoea and intestinal cramping

d Extreme tiredness, hunger, mood swings and depression

Q6 Signs and symptoms of withdrawal from cannabis include:

a Sweating, tremor, nausea, raised blood pressure and anxiety

b Irritability, abdominal pain, anxiety and anorexia

c Mydriasis, piloerection, muscle aches, rhinorrhoea and intestinal cramping

d Extreme tiredness, hunger, mood swings and depression

Q7 Signs and symptoms of withdrawal from opioids include:

a Sweating, tremor, nausea, raised blood pressure and anxiety

b Irritability, abdominal pain, anxiety and anorexia

c Mydriasis, piloerection, muscle aches, rhinorrhoea and intestinal cramping

d Extreme tiredness, hunger, mood swings and depression

Q8 Signs and symptoms of withdrawal from methamphetamine include:

a Sweating, tremor, nausea, raised blood pressure and anxiety

b Irritability, abdominal pain, anxiety and anorexia

c Mydriasis, piloerection, muscle aches, rhinorrhoea and intestinal cramping

d Extreme tiredness, hunger, mood swings and depression

(b) Discriminate

Q Which of the following observations might cause Jonathon to be concerned about Jando's health status? (There is more than one correct answer.)

a Jando doesn't talk much.

b Jando is polite to everybody.

c Jando doesn't laugh and joke with the other prisoners in his cell.

d Jando eats the meals provided for him.

e   Jando often goes to the water bubbler and takes a drink of water.

f   Jando spends a lot of time wrapped in the grey blanket issued to him on arrival in the cell, often with his face obscured.

g   Jando passes urine at least twice a day.

h   Jando's facial expression rarely changes and most of the time he looks rather flat.

(c) Relate

At this stage, there seems to be no major concern about Jando's physical health.

Q   Which clusters of information about Jando from the previous section (discriminate) might indicate a possible mental health issue?

(d) Infer

Q   Based on the information you now have about Jando, which of the following inferences are most likely to be 'true'?

a   Jando thinks he is too good for the people he is locked up with, so he doesn't bother chatting or joking with them.

b   Jando is annoyed about being locked up, so he has decided not to co-operate with any interview or assessment process.

c   Jando wants to die, so he is denying himself food and water.

d   Jando is in an environment where he has no privacy and no personal space, so he tries to create it for himself by wrapping himself in his grey blanket.

e   Jando is trying to hide from something.

f   Jando is not sleeping very well, so he looks tired during the day.

g   Jando has an alteration in his affect.

(e) Match

Think back to anybody with a psychiatric diagnosis whom you have known personally or nursed on a clinical placement. Have you seen behaviours that are similar to Jando's before? Was speech or behaviour immediately indicative of a mental health problem?

(f) Predict

Jonathon has limited time available and many other duties to attend to during his four-hour shifts. However, he also knows that he needs to communicate effectively with Jando in every way he can, with frequent interactions and persistence, particularly in this untherapeutic setting (Bowers et al., 2009).

Q   If Jonathon doesn't take the appropriate actions at this time, what could happen to Jando? (There is more than one correct answer.)

a   Jando might go to court and his possible mental health issue not be recognised during the hearing.

b   Jando could be remanded and moved to a large gaol without further health assessment because the receiving nurse at the gaol sees that it has already been completed in the prison cell complex.

c   Jando's mental state might worsen.

d   Jando's mental state might improve.

e   Jando's time on remand is made more difficult because he has an undiagnosed and untreated mental illness.

4. IDENTIFY THE PROBLEM/ISSUE

Q With the limited information Jonathon has been able to collect so far, which of the following are potential nursing diagnoses for Jando?

a Risk of self-harm related to suicidal ideation

b Risk of harm to others related to delusional beliefs

c Ineffective communication related to thought disorder, evidenced by thought blocking, poverty of ideation and possible perseveration

d Impaired therapeutic engagement with RN caused by delusional beliefs, incarceration, fear, social isolation and lack of privacy, evidenced by limited response to questions and reluctance to disclose freely

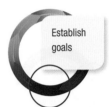

Identify the problem/issue

5. ESTABLISH GOALS

Q What are three important goals for Jando's care at this time?

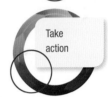

Establish goals

6. TAKE ACTION

Jonathon needs to gain Jando's trust, in spite of the contextual challenges. Without this trust, there is little possibility that Jando will disclose more information about himself. It is particularly difficult for a nurse to gain the trust of a prisoner because of the culture of the correctional setting and because prisoners may assume that the nurse is employed by the corrections system, not by the health service. Jonathon needs to provide physical care, as well as convey an atmosphere of safety and security, a sense of protection and a feeling of companionship (Hawamdeh & Fakhry, 2014). He also wants to be a recovery-focused nurse, even in such a challenging setting, and as such 'holds hope for the client when the client is without hope' (Dalum et al., 2015).

Take action

Q1 Which of the following statements is correct? A therapeutic relationship:

a Is the same as any social relationship

b Is not necessary at this time because Jando is locked up and now being dealt with by the legal system

c Has defined boundaries to protect both nurses and patients

d Is the foundation of mental health nursing practice

e Is based on trust

f Respects a person's rights

g Adheres to confidentiality

h Uses the registered nurse's own personal qualities in such a way as to benefit the patient and promote recovery

i Must always be open to scrutiny.

The NMBA Standards stipulate that RNs must communicate effectively, act as patient advocates and differentiate between personal and professional relationships. Therefore, Jonathon needs to establish a therapeutic relationship and maintain confidentiality, while advocating for Jando's need for mental healthcare.

Q2 Match the correct rationale to its related action in the table below.

Action	Rationale
Observe, engage and continue to assess Jando's mental state	Without a strong therapeutic relationship, assessments and treatment will be more difficult to undertake and it will be hard for Jando to trust Jonathon.

(continues)

(continued)

Undertake regular risk assessments	Jando does not understand that his experiences are caused by a psychotic illness; therefore, he has little insight into his illness and may not accept treatment.
Develop a therapeutic relationship	Although risk assessments cannot ensure safety, they provide early warning of possible risks, allowing staff to take preventive action.
Provide simple education about psychosis	Mental state examination should be done during every shift, as mental state can change rapidly.

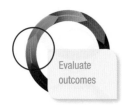

Evaluate outcomes

7. EVALUATE

Jonathon is confident that Jando is safe because he has no means to harm himself; his cell is monitored round the clock on CCTV, and he has shown no sign of harming his fellow prisoners in their shared cell during his time in custody. Jando's vital signs do not suggest any physical illness and, while he doesn't say much, there is nothing so far to suggest an acute confusional state. When Jonathon walks past the cells, Jando looks up and says hello. This suggests to Jonathon that there is some therapeutic engagement, with the beginning of trust and the possibility of further development towards a therapeutic relationship.

Jando sometimes seems unaware of what is happening around him and, when the other prisoners in his cell are chatting among themselves or watching television, he occasionally seems to be whispering to somebody when there is nobody close by him.

Q   What might these observations about Jando indicate?

   a   Jando is responding to internal stimuli.

   b   Jando is lonely, so he is talking to himself.

   c   Jando is reciting a poem to help pass the time as he doesn't enjoy television.

   d   Jando is confused and thinks he is talking to his mother on his mobile which the prison officers removed on his arrival.

   e   Jando has influenza which has caused a sore throat, so he cannot speak loudly without pain.

   f   Jonathon is beginning to establish some rapport with Jando.

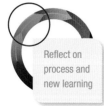

Reflect on process and new learning

8. REFLECT

Jonathon knows that people experiencing their first psychotic episode are likely to feel 'scared, lost and alone' (Lamph, 2010, p. 38) even without being taken into custody. His role is to reach out, establish contact, and offer and start treatment and care (Sebergsen, Norbert & Talseth, 2014).

Reflect on the following questions.

Q1   Why is there a health service in the prison setting?

Q2   What is the best way to provide effective healthcare in the prison setting, and who should be involved?

Q3   If there is no health service in the prison system, what might be the effects on the community as a whole once prisoners are released?

Something to think about …

Your responses to these questions may help you to reflect on, and to understand, equity and access in healthcare (Baum, 2008), and your future role as a registered nurse. Your responses may also reveal certain attitudes or beliefs in relation to your future role which you may not have realised you hold.

SCENARIO 13.2 — Not just an unprovoked aggressive outburst

CHANGING THE SCENE

The following day is Wednesday and when Jonathon gets to work one of Jando's cellmates calls out to you: 'Hey chief! You better take a look at Jando. He's hanging out real bad. He needs something now.' There is a muffled laugh from the other men in Jando's cell. Jonathon is surprised as there have been no objective signs of withdrawal from any drugs or alcohol during Jando's five days in the cells. Jando is brought into the clinic and seems puzzled, almost perplexed. Jonathon asks him if he uses any drug at all on a regular basis. He doesn't reply, so Jonathon repeats the question and, at last, Jando seems able to focus. 'No, not at all', he says. He then repeats this statement, 'No, not at all! No, not at all!' Jonathon concludes that the cellmates are joking, or perhaps trying to secure some diazepam for Jando in the hope that he will divert it to them. Still, just before Jonathon goes off duty, he looks in on Jando once again. He is lying on his bed, facing the wall; his lips are moving, and occasionally he shakes his head and seems to be pushing something away from him.

Although it is after the end of Jonathon's shift, he takes Jando back to the clinic. Jonathon thinks back over what Jando had said about 'being released', which he had assumed referred to being released from custody, and which the officers had misinterpreted as being a mention of 'a lease'. Jonathon wonders about the reason for Jando's unprovoked assaults. He also remembers Jando's look of perplexity when asked about drug use, and how he had been slow to respond to the questions. There was also the mention of using cannabis 'sometimes' at his initial assessment. So Jonathon asks Jando what he was doing when he was lying on his bunk immediately before being brought back to the clinic.

'They came back, nurse', Jando tells him sadly. 'They will not release me.' Jonathon asks who 'they' are and Jando calmly explains that 'they' are the seven devils, who have been with him for a year or more now. Sometimes he looks into people's eyes and he knows that the seven devils are in them too. When he saw them in his mother, he hit her to drive them out and save her from them. It was the same with his sister. And later in the street, he tried to protect a stranger from them too. That was when he was arrested and brought to the cells. Tonight, he says, they have been coming very close to him in the cell which is very frightening, and so he has been praying and trying to push them away. He can hear them whispering to him and telling him he is lost forever now and will never be released from them. He says in a very small voice to Jonathon that he only wants to save his mother and sister from the power of the seven devils, and he no longer expects to survive himself.

Jonathon continues to talk with Jando, and uses the framework of the full mental status examination to gather more information. There is no family history of mental illness, but this episode does coincide with Jando's regular use of cannabis in order to relax from the pressures of Year 12 and the Higher School Certificate. Jando had not liked to say too much about this during his initial assessment on Monday as he feared further charges related to the use of an illegal drug.

1. CONSIDER THE PATIENT SITUATION

Jonathon has been collecting cues since he first met Jando on Monday. His initial concerns have been validated and his preliminary assessment that Jando might have a mental illness has been confirmed. He must now undertake a comprehensive mental health assessment and ensure that Jando is referred to the appropriate services whether he is released from Court on Friday or remanded in custody. He needs to further develop the therapeutic relationship he has established with Jando, and provide some very simple education about what Jando's experiences mean, and what can be done to help him recover.

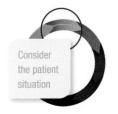

Consider the patient situation

2. COLLECT CUES/INFORMATION

(a) Review current information

Jonathon organises the cues and information he has collected so far in the form of a mental state examination.

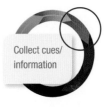

Collect cues/information

What is the difference between the MSE (Mental State Examination) and the MMSE (Mini Mental State Examination)?

Appearance: Slim, fit-looking, young Caucasian male with short blonde hair; clean-shaven, wearing prison green tracksuit, no body odour, no visible lacerations on hands, laceration on right temporal area with two steri-strips, clean and dry, no sign of infection

Behaviour: Initially reserved, apparently shy or fearful, but now engaging better and able to give some account of himself

Speech: Soft voice, somewhat hesitant

Mood: States 4/10 on self-report, using the Self-Report Scale where 0 is 'worst have ever felt' and 10 is 'best have ever felt'

Affect: Blunted

Thought content: Delusional—believes he can see the seven devils in people's eyes; believes they intend to harm his mother and sister as well as a stranger in the street; believes he will never be 'released' from them, does not expect to survive; however, does deny intent to harm himself or any suicidal ideation, as well as denying having a plan or means for suicide; denies any thought of harming any other person

Thought form: Thought blocking, possible perseveration, poverty of ideation

Can you identify some other disorders of thought form?

Perceptual disturbances: Says he can hear the seven devils whispering, feels them coming close to him at times and pushes them away; he also sees them in people's eyes

Insight and judgment: Does not yet understand that his experiences are related to a diagnosable mental illness; however, is amenable to nursing assistance, explanations, education and referrals

Orientation: Knows that he is in Melaleuca Police Station; unsure of day or date; knows month; knows year

Sleep: Usually sleeps well, but has not been able to sleep well since being taken into custody

Insight and judgment are usually recorded together in the MSE. Do you know how judgment should be formally assessed?

Appetite: Says he knows he should try to fast to drive the devils away but adds that sometimes he does get very hungry, so he eats all that is provided

Anhedonia: Not able to comprehend question relating to this; just says he does not deserve to enjoy anything because he has allowed the devils to come too close to his mother and sister when he should have been protecting them

Jonathon also performs a brief alcohol and other drug assessment, and this time Jando opens up to Jonathon because of the rapport that has been established, and because Jonathon explained that health information is not made available to the police so that he will not be charged with illegal drug use. Jando acknowledges that all through Year 12 he used to smoke 'a couple of cones, or sometimes more, each day' to help him cope with the stress of the Higher School Certificate. He denies any other drug use at all, both legal and illegal, since completing the HSC last November, and says he ceased cannabis use when the HSC results came out about six weeks ago. Jonathon is aware that there is a statistical association between cannabis use and the incidence of psychotic disorders (Ksir & Hart, 2016), though it may not play a key part in the development of psychosis in high-risk groups (Phillips et al., 2002).

(b) Gather new information

Jonathon is now confident that he has made an accurate assessment of Jando's mental state, but he also needs to gather some corroborative evidence from others who know Jando well. Jando has no GP, and the summary from his presentation to the local ED after he fell over only notes that he was observed for four hours, all observations were normal and two steri-strips were applied to a laceration on his right temporal area. The prison officers have not observed much that is of relevance to the mental state assessment, and they view Jando as 'a good inmate' because he makes no demands and causes no trouble. Jonathon asks Jando if he may ring Jando's mother to ask how she sees things. Jando agrees and, although he is not allowed to speak to his mother himself, he does sit next to Jonathon while Jonathon makes the call.

Jando's mother is tearful when Jonathon explains who he is and why he is ringing. She has not been able to visit Jando and has only had a single call from him, which is routine for a person newly taken into custody. She tells Jonathon that Jando is always quiet, but 'a lovely boy', very thoughtful and considerate, and very concerned for his 12-year-old sister's safety and wellbeing since their father left and moved overseas with a new partner. Jando is very helpful to his mother and a good student. He enjoys sport, has two good friends and recently became close to a girl from his street whom he met at the church. He has twice visited her at the university where she is enrolled.

Jando himself has elected to take a gap year, and is doing voluntary work with a Landcare group, as the environment and its proper management is very important to him. At school, his teachers did not see him as 'the academic type' but the creative arts department found he had real talent. Jando's mother continues to explain that she hasn't noticed anything very different since he finished the HSC, only that he seems to be even quieter, spends more time in his room listening to music and writing in his journal, and seems to stay up very late—sometimes even all night. Occasionally, she has come into a room and found Jando apparently talking to somebody, but when she asked about this, he mumbled something and left the room. At other times, she has noticed that he seems 'lost for words', as if he has got stuck in the middle of a sentence. In Year 11, Jando used to joke with his sister and play games with her a lot, but she says in the past year he has rarely smiled. When she asked whether he was okay, Jando replied that he was saving the world and was thankful for that opportunity.

Jando's mother knows of no mental health issues on either side of the family and was not aware that Jando had been using cannabis for the past year. The attack on his sister was entirely unexpected and occurred one Saturday afternoon when she was watching a DVD with her mother. Similarly, the attack on his mother was also unexpected and occurred when she asked him if he had had a good day. In both cases, he had shouted loudly, 'NO!', and tried to push his sister and his mother to one side. Neither was injured. Jando's mother was surprised but concluded that he was overtired. She did not discuss these incidents with anybody and never mentioned them to Jando's father on the rare occasions when she did email him. Sounding rather uncertain, she does add that she thinks Jando's paternal uncle may have spent a long period in 'an asylum' during his twenties but that her ex-husband's family were reluctant to discuss the details.

Jonathon now has an account of prodromal symptoms including social withdrawal, decline in functioning, strange behaviours, sleep disturbance and unusual beliefs (Holt, 2013).

Q   How can you be sure you have collected accurate information when the witnesses to the events either have no nursing knowledge or are unreliable historians, and the person whom you are caring for may not be able to give you a full account of what happened?

(c) Recall knowledge

Q1 Which of the following statements are accurate?

a   Cannabis does not cause psychosis but is associated with it.

b   A substance-induced psychotic disorder may resolve with appropriate treatment or may progress to become a chronic condition like schizophrenia.

c   People with psychosis never attempt suicide.

d   Illegal drugs are always involved if a person develops a psychosis.

e   People in a general medical or surgical ward may experience psychosis.

f   There are many causes of psychosis.

g   The most important thing with psychosis is to make the person take their prescribed medication, even if it causes severe side effects.

h   People with psychosis have no hope of recovery.

i   Metabolic monitoring is now part of the mental health nurse's role in caring for a person taking second-generation antipsychotics.

Q2 Co-morbidity refers to a person who has:

a   Both a substance dependence and a mental health problem

b   Both anxiety and depression

c   Both a mental health problem and a legal issue

d   Both schizophrenia and delirium.

Q3 The Recovery Model emphasises which of the following?

a   People who have experienced a psychotic episode will never get better.

b   People who have experienced a psychotic episode will need somebody to tell them what to do for the rest of their lives.

c   People who have experienced a psychotic episode shouldn't be expected to work or study, and usually end up on the Disability Support Pension.

d   People who have experienced a psychotic episode choose their recovery pathway and who will assist them to travel this pathway, so they can achieve the life they want and the outcomes they desire.

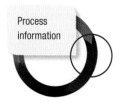

Process information

3. PROCESS INFORMATION

(a) Interpret

Jonathon knows that Jando needs a period of observation and assessment before a final diagnosis can be made. Process the information you currently have about Jando by adding details to the case formulation table below.

	Predisposing factors	Precipitating factors	Perpetuating factors	Prognostic indicators, including protective
Biological	Genetic predisposition?		Not known at this time—continued cannabis misuse could perpetuate	Has ceased cannabis use six weeks ago
Psychological		Stress from HSC and possibly from father's departure	Incarceration, if lengthy	
Social				Stable home Supportive mother Voluntary employment

(b) Discriminate

Jonathon is happy with this formulation but knows that at this stage Jando's prognosis is still uncertain. He considers risk factors for relapse or for the development of a chronic psychotic disorder.

Q   Based on what Jonathon already knows about Jando, which of the following could be significant risk factors for future relapse?

a   Continued cannabis misuse

b   Additional use of other illegal substances such as methamphetamine

c   Family breakdown

d   Insufficient income

e   Lack of community mental health support

f   No regular GP

g   Unstable accommodation

h   Not in work, study or training

i   Not taking medication if prescribed

j   Stigma

k   Lack of psychoeducation

l   Loneliness

(c) Relate and (d) Infer

Q What do you see as most important in contributing to Jando's current mental state?

    a His use of cannabis in the preceding year

    b His unexpected incarceration

    c His head wound

(f) Predict

Q1 What might happen to Jando if he was remanded to a major city gaol and if the receiving RN does not look at his health assessment?

Q2 Based on all the information you now have available, which of the following statements are most accurate predictions for Jando?

    a Jando may have a genetic predisposition to psychosis

    b Jando's cannabis misuse may have contributed to his psychotic episode.

    c Jando's mother is not interested in him and this has caused all his problems.

    d Jando's little sister teased him and this has caused all his problems.

    e Jando's involvement with his church has confused his thinking.

    f Jando will need to have depot injections for the rest of his life to keep him well.

    g Jando will never recover and now can't go to university or get a job.

    h Jando will never marry.

    i Jando should not have children.

4. IDENTIFY THE PROBLEM/ISSUE

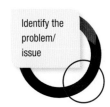

Identify the problem/ issue

Q1 Now that Jonathon has been able to discover much more about Jando, what are the most likely nursing diagnoses?

    a Risk of self-harm related to suicidal ideation

    b Risk of harm to others related to delusional beliefs

    c Problems in effective communication caused by thought disorder, evidenced by thought blocking, poverty of ideation and possible perseveration

    d A problem in establishing a therapeutic relationship with Jonathon, caused by delusional beliefs, incarceration, fear, misunderstanding of reason for his current situation, social isolation and lack of privacy, evidenced by limited response to Jonathon's questions and reluctance to disclose freely

Q2 What do you think might be the most likely final psychiatric diagnoses for Jando?

    a Psychotic episode

    b Substance-induced psychotic disorder

    c Cannabis misuse

    d Cannabis withdrawal

    e Major depressive disorder

    f Generalised anxiety disorder

    g Adjustment disorder

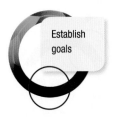

Establish goals

5. ESTABLISH GOALS

Q At this time, what are the most important goals in relation to Jando's nursing diagnoses?

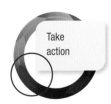

6. TAKE ACTION

Jonathon is obliged to discuss his concerns about Jando's condition with the duty doctor on call at the main gaol in Sydney.

Q1 How would you use ISBAR over the phone to inform the duty doctor (who is hundreds of kilometres away from Jonathon and Jando, and will never meet either of them) of Jando's most urgent needs at this time?

Jonathon receives a faxed medication order from the doctor for an antipsychotic to be commenced tonight. He also needs to educate Jando about the reason for the medication, how it works and possible side effects.

Jando's safety, now and in the future, is Jonathon's main priority. He informs the prison officers of his assessment and flags Jando as a person with a mental illness (without breaching confidentiality).

Jonathon wants to ensure that, when Jando appears in court on Friday, either he is admitted to an inpatient mental health unit or, if he is remanded in custody, on arrival at his gaol of placement he is lodged in an area which is staffed by mental health nurses who can provide a supportive environment for him. Jonathon also needs to explain the need for a mental health admission to both Jando's solicitor and the court liaison nurse.

Q2 Each of the actions above require a specific rationale. In the table below, match the correct rationale to the related action.

> The NSQHS Standards outline the importance of a comprehensive and accurate clinical handover, with communication of critical information and careful documentation of updates or alterations to planned care. This is particularly important in this situation, as the duty doctor must rely solely on what Jonathon tells him in order to prescribe appropriate treatments (ACSQHC, 2016).

Action	Rationale
Describe how Jando presents and summarise assessment data to the duty doctor—including drug and alcohol use, any medical or surgical problems, allergies and any previous psychiatric history.	If the solicitor is not aware of Jando's psychosis, he will be unable to ensure that the magistrate makes the most appropriate decision when Jando appears in court.
Provide information to prison officers to enable them to manage Jando in custody as a person with a mental illness.	Until Jando understands that his experiences are not based in reality, he cannot begin to develop insight into his mental illness or begin his recovery.
Begin psychoeducation with Jando.	Jando requires treatment and this cannot begin effectively without antipsychotic medication.
Notify Jando's solicitor and/or the court liaison nurse of his mental illness.	Because Jando is experiencing a psychotic episode, he needs close observation and appropriate management, and Jonathon cannot provide this round-the-clock care because of the limited hours he works.

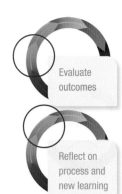

7. EVALUATE

Jonathon's role requires him to provide healthcare that meets the complex physical and psychosocial needs of people who are incarcerated, many of whom have substance abuse and psychiatric problems. How would Jonathon know that his actions in caring for Jando have been effective?

8. REFLECT

Prior to being incarcerated, Jando was becoming mentally ill for over a year while still attending school and spending time with friends and family.

Q1 Why do you think that nobody noticed what was happening to Jando?

Q2 Who could have intervened if they had concerns about Jando's mental health?

Q3 What might those people have done to support Jando?

Q4 What sources of help were available to Jando which he might have accessed himself?

Q5 How could he have found out more about help-seeking, support and recovery?

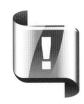

Something to think about ...

Many students are anxious about working with people who have a mental illness. This may be related to many issues: the stigma surrounding mental illness in the community, the sensational press coverage of incidents involving people with a mental illness, a belief that people with a mental illness are always violent, or personal or family experiences. These flawed perceptions can undermine the quality and safety of the care provided to this vulnerable population.

EPILOGUE

Jando accepted the medication which was prescribed for him, but he had trouble understanding that his distressing experiences are symptoms of a mental illness. He also found it difficult to believe that he could recover and his distressing symptoms would pass.

When Jando presented at court, the magistrate considered all the information available to him, including Jando's statement that he regrets shoving the man in the street and that he only intended to protect him from the seven devils. The magistrate directed that he be released from custody and taken to the local mental health inpatient unit, where Jonathon had organised a bed.

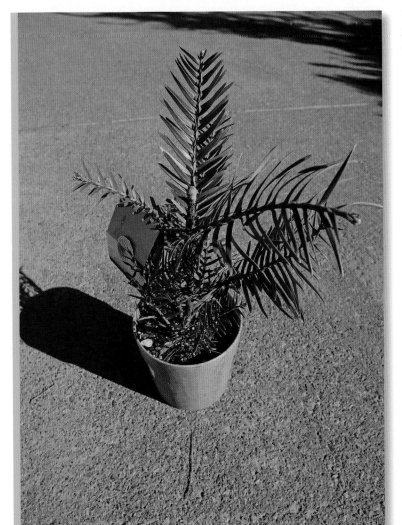

The Wollemi pine, given as a gift to Jando

Jando gained a lot from the ward program, the antipsychotic medication was effective and he experienced no major side effects. He was introduced to his community case manager and found him easy to talk to and confide in. Jando's Landcare group visited him in hospital and said that they were looking forward to his return, as the bitou was getting out of control down at the dunes. Some of his friends visited regularly and expressed their regret for not asking 'RUOK?' when they noticed Jando's unusual behaviour. When his friend from church visited, she brought him a Wollemi pine which he had always wanted.

Jando's mother and sister attended a support group where they were given a lot of information about psychosis, and their church group provided support and reassurance that Jando is well regarded in the church community.

A month later, Jando was discharged home with community support and regular appointments with the community psychiatrist. Jando was referred to a GP to monitor his overall health status. The first thing he did when he got home was to apply for an Environmental Science degree at the university where his friends are studying. Jando recovered and took his place back in the community where he belonged. He was no longer 'confused, scared, depressed, socially isolated, embarrassed and worried about disclosure' (Van Dusseldorp, Goossens & van Achterberg, 2011, p. 2).

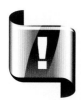

Something to think about …

If you are worried about a friend's mental health, you can:

- *Ask, 'RUOK?'*

- *Suggest you go with your friend to see a GP.*

- *Suggest your friend contacts the local community mental health team.*

- *Advise your friend that, in crisis, the nearest ED will be able to access mental health support.*

- *Tell your friend about websites that are reputable, and can provide information and support. For example, <www.mindhealthconnect.org.au> and <www.mindspot.org.au>.*

- *Make sure your friend has the Lifeline phone number: 131114.*

- *Listen without judging.*

- *Assist with some very simple problem solving.*

- *Let somebody else know if your friend is not amenable to any of your suggestions and you are still very concerned.*

FURTHER READING

Cavanaugh, S. (2014). Recovery-oriented practice. *Canadian Nurse, 110*(6), 28–30. Available at <www.canadian-nurse.com>.

Phillips, N. (2010). *Lost in a Mind Field: Schizophrenia and Other Psychoses*. Concord West: ShrinkRap Press. Available at <www.shrinkrap.com>.

REFERENCES

American Psychiatric Association. (2013). *Diagnostic and Statistical Manual of Mental Disorders* (5th edn). Arlington, VA: American Psychiatric Association.

Australian Commission on Safety and Quality in Health Care (ACSQHC). (2016). *National Safety and Quality Health Service Standards Version 2*. Draft, Sydney, Australia.

Baum, F. (2008). Chapter 18: Creating more equitable societies. In *The New Public Health* (3rd edn, pp. 409–42). South Melbourne, Victoria: Oxford University Press.

Beards, S. & Fisher, H. (2014). The journey to psychosis: An exploration of specific psychological pathways. *Social Psychiatry and Psychiatric Epidemiology, 49*, 1541–44.

Bowers, L., Brennan, G., Winship, G. & Theodoridou, C. (2009). *Communication Skills for Nurses and Others Spending Time with People Who Are Very Mentally Ill*. London, UK: City University of London.

Dalum, H., Pedersen, I., Cunningham, H. & Eplov, L. (2015). From recovery programs to recovery-oriented practice? A qualitative study of mental health professionals' experiences when facilitating a recovery-oriented rehabilitation program. *Archives of Psychiatric Nursing, 29*, 419–25.

Hawamdeh, S. & Fakhry, R. (2014). Therapeutic relationships from the psychiatric nurses' perspectives: An interpretative phenomenological study. *Perspectives in Psychiatric Care, 50*, 178–85.

Holt, L. (2013). Recognising psychosis. *Healthcare Counselling and Psychotherapy Journal, 13*(3), 14–17.

Kahn, R. & Sommer, I. (2015). The neurobiology and treatment of first-episode schizophrenia. *Molecular Psychiatry, 20*, 84–97.

Keshavan, M., Clementz, B., Pearlson, G., Sweeney, J. & Tamminga, C. (2013). Reimagining psychoses: An agnostic approach to diagnosis. *Schizophrenia Research, 146*, 10–16.

Ksir, C. & Hart, C. (2016). Cannabis and psychosis: A critical overview of the relationship. *Current Psychiatry Reports, 18*(12), 1–11.

Lamph, G. (2010). Early psychosis: Raising awareness among non-mental health nurses. *Nursing Standard, 24*(47), 35–40.

Laurens, K., Luming, L., Matheson, S., Carr, V., Raudino, A., Harris, F., & Green, M. (2015). Common or distinct pathways to psychosis? A systematic review of evidence from prospective studies for developmental risk factors and antecedents for the schizophrenia spectrum disorders and affective psychoses. *BMC Psychiatry, 15*(205).

Martin, C. (2016). The value of physical examination in mental health nursing. *Nurse Education in Practice, 17*, 91–96.

Morgan, V., Waterreus, A., Jablensky, A., Mackinnon, A., McGrath, J., Carr, V., … Saw, S. (2012). People living with psychotic illness in 2010: The second Australian national survey of psychosis. *Australian and New Zealand Journal of Psychiatry, 46*(8), 735–52.

Nursing and Midwifery Board of Australia (NMBA). (2016). *Registered Nurse Standards for Practice*. Melbourne: NMBA.

Phillips, L., Curry, C., Yung, A., Yuen, H., Adlard, S. & McGorry, P. (2002). Cannabis use is not associated with the development of psychosis in an 'ultra' high-risk group. *Australian and New Zealand Journal of Psychiatry, 36*, 800–6.

Sebergsen, K., Norberg, A. & Talseth, A. (2014). Being in a process of transition to psychosis, as narrated by adults with psychotic illnesses acutely admitted to hospital. *Journal of Psychiatric and Mental Health Nursing, 21*, 896–905.

Van Dusseldorp, L., Goossens, P. & van Achterberg, T. (2011). Mental health nursing and first episode psychosis. *Issues in Mental Health Nursing, 32*, 2–19.

Zubin, J. & Spring, B. (1977). Vulnerability—A new view of schizophrenia. *Journal of Abnormal Psychology, 86*(2), 103–26.

PHOTO CREDIT

251 Suzanne Long/Alamy Stock Photo

CHAPTER 14

CARING FOR AN OLDER PERSON WITH ALTERED COGNITION

SHARYN HUNTER, FRANCES DUMONT AND JACQUI CULVER

LEARNING OUTCOMES

Completion of the activities in this chapter will enable you to:

○ explain why an understanding of cognitive decline, dementia, delirium, depression (the 4Ds) and mild cognitive impairment are essential to competent practice (**recall** and **application**)

○ identify the clinical manifestations of mild cognitive impairment, dementia, delirium and depression that will guide the collection and interpretation of appropriate cues (**gather, review, interpret, discriminate, relate** and **infer**)

○ identify risk factors for older people experiencing mild cognitive impairment, dementia, delirium and depression (**match** and **predict**)

○ review clinical information to identify the main nursing diagnoses for a person experiencing dementia, delirium and depression (**synthesise**)

○ describe the priorities of care for a person experiencing dementia, delirium and depression (**goal setting** and **taking action**)

○ identify clinical criteria for determining the effectiveness of nursing actions taken to manage dementia, delirium or depression (**evaluate**)

○ transfer what you have learnt about cognitive decline, mild cognitive impairment, dementia, delirium and depression to new clinical situations (**reflect** and **translate**).

INTRODUCTION

This chapter focuses on the care of Mr Dang Tien, an older person who experiences an alteration in cognition. Although nurses often use the term 'confusion' to describe this phenomenon, confusion is an ambiguous term and does not adequately describe the dimensions of this health breakdown condition. When nurses encounter older people with changes in their cognition, it is essential that they have knowledge and understanding of the related pathophysiological and psychosocial issues. A thorough assessment must be conducted as this assists in determining the cause and type of cognitive change presenting. Further, it is important to distinguish between the different types of cognitive changes, as this will determine the appropriate actions required from the healthcare team.

There are four types of altered cognition associated with the older person (Insel & Bager, 2002; Hunter & Miller, 2016). They are: cognitive **D**ecline, **D**ementia, **D**elirium and **D**epression, often referred to as the 4Ds. Each type has specific features and, when the nurse engages in clinical reasoning, the type of altered cognition can be appropriately identified and assessed, the causes determined and the correct interventions implemented. Clinical reasoning skills allow for early recognition and management of the 4Ds, with the aim of preventing complications and further decline. Person-centred care and the development of a therapeutic relationship with the older person are integral to this process.

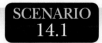

SCENARIO 14.1   Caring for an older person with delirium

THE AETIOLOGY AND PATHOGENESIS OF THE 4Ds

Cognitive decline

During normal ageing, the speed at which individuals acquire information gradually declines, but their ability to recall information remains intact (Insel & Bager, 2002). These changes are referred to as cognitive decline and they are unrelated to disease processes. Mild cognitive impairment (MCI) is a recently identified syndrome that is characterised by cognitive decline which is different from normal ageing, but does not meet the criteria for mild dementia (Patel & Holland, 2012). The key difference between normal ageing and MCI is that the older person with MCI has little or no recognition of memory loss. A cognitive assessment may reveal no significant impairment and there may be no significant changes in instrumental activities of daily living. Currently, it is difficult to differentiate MCI from cognitive decline. Importantly though, MCI can progress to dementia (Patel & Holland, 2012).

Dementia

Dementia refers to a group of diseases, each with a different cause and a unique combination of manifestations. It is a gradual, progressive, irreversible deterioration of cerebral function, which results in disturbance of many higher cortical functions, including memory, thinking and judgment (American Psychiatric Association, 2013). Impairment in cognitive function is commonly accompanied, and occasionally preceded, by deterioration in emotional control, social behaviour or motivation. This deterioration leads to a decreased ability to independently perform activities of daily living (American Psychiatric Association, 2013).

Types and causes of dementia

- **Alzheimer's disease**—causes mostly unknown, but in some cases there is a genetic link
- **Vascular dementia**—chronic decrease in cerebral blood flow, usually related to strokes and hypertension
- **Lewy body disease**—causes mostly unknown but people with Parkinson's disease develop similar symptoms
- **Creutzfeldt-Jakob disease (CJD)**—may be related to a protein called a Prion
- **Fronto-temporal dementia**—causes mostly unknown but there is a genetic link in some cases
- **Korsakoff syndrome**—caused by vitamin B1 deficiency; usually results from alcohol misuse.

Delirium

Delirium is described as an acute, reversible, clinical syndrome of cognitive function, characterised by an acute decline that impairs cognitive and physical function (Inouye, 2006). Delirium occurs as a result of a change in the health status of the older person (Fick, Agostini & Inouye, 2002). It may be the only signal of a developing illness or the exacerbation of a chronic disease. When an older person develops delirium, they will have an acute alteration in attention, and may have changes in perception (visual hallucinations), memory, thinking (delusions usually persecutory), orientation, sleep/wake cycle and (increased/decreased) psychomotor activity (Inouye, 2006). The course of delirium is dynamic and the symptoms may vary and fluctuate (Inouye, 2006).

Delirium can result from the interaction between predisposing factors and precipitating factors, which increases a person's vulnerability and contributes to delirium. Predisposing factors include: advanced age, dementia, depression, functional dependency and a number of medications. Precipitating factors include: surgery, infections, serious illness, pain and physical restraints (Inouye, 2006).

Healthcare professionals frequently under recognise delirium in older people or confuse it with other conditions (Australian Commission on Safety and Quality in Health Care, 2016b). Failure to correctly recognise delirium in its early stages often produces poor outcomes for older people. Episodes of delirium increase the risk of falls, pressure areas, injury, cognitive and functional decline, dehydration, incontinence, malnutrition and mortality (Inouye, 2006).

There are three types of delirium: hyperactive, hypoactive and mixed (Voyer et al., 2008). Hyperactive delirium is characterised by an increased response to stimuli and psychomotor activity, while hypoactive delirium is characterised by a reduced alertness and psychomotor activity, and is commonly known as the 'quiet' delirium. The mixed type has features of both hyperactive and hypoactive delirium.

Depression

Depression in older people is often missed as its signs and symptoms can be attributed to the ageing process, dementia or poor health (Baldwin, 2008). In older people, depression often manifests with vague physical symptoms, memory loss and various behavioural changes. Affective changes also can occur and these include anxiety, irritability, diminished self-esteem and negative feelings about self. The presence of both anxiety and depression has been shown to be associated with increased cognitive impairment (Beaudreau & O'Hara, 2009). Genetics, personality and life experiences are probable causes if the older person has a previous history of depression; however, if the depression is experienced for the first time when older, physical health problems or losses may be the cause.

THE EPIDEMIOLOGY OF THE 4Ds

The epidemiology of the 4Ds varies. It is widely accepted that cognitive decline occurs in all people as they age. However, dementia is not a natural part of ageing, even though most people with dementia are older. After the age of 65, the likelihood of living with dementia doubles every five years. Approximately 1 in 10 people over 65 have dementia and this increases to 3 in 10 people over the age of 85 (Alzheimer's Australia, 2016). Currently, there is no cure for dementia and it is the second leading cause of death in Australia (Alzheimer's Australia, 2016).

Delirium affects up to 18 per cent of older people admitted into Australian hospitals with between 2 and 8 per cent of people developing delirium during hospitalisation (Australian Commission on Safety and Quality in Health Care, 2016b). Data from NSW hospitals shows an increase of 2238 cases from 2007 to 2008, with 11 948 total cases of delirium from 2009 to 2010 (NSW Health, 2011). Although the data is not age-specific, most of these reported cases are older people. Currently, there is no data about the prevalence of delirium among Aboriginal and Torres Strait Islander peoples; however, it is thought to be higher in this population than in other Australians (Australian Commission on Safety and Quality in Health Care, 2016b).

The prevalence of depression in older people is estimated to be between 10 and 15 per cent (National Ageing Research Institute [NARI], 2009).

> Access this link to learn more about cognitive decline in older people from culturally and linguistically diverse (CALD) backgrounds: <http://flinders.edu.au/nursing/mental-health-and-culture/sui/home.cfm>.

SETTING THE SCENE

Mr Dang Tien (Jimmy) is a 75-year-old man with a history of chronic obstructive pulmonary disease (COPD), transient ischemic attacks (TIAs) and hypertension; he also has mild osteoarthritis in his hands and knees.

Mr Dang Tien is currently receiving a visit from the community nurse for medication monitoring, as the dose of his antihypertensive medication was increased last week. The community nurse visits on Monday, Wednesday and Friday and reviews his blood pressure.

> Cultural consideration: What is different about Vietnamese names and how should you address a Vietnamese person?

Medication regimen

atenolol (Tenormin) 100 mg once daily (increased from 50 mg)

fluticasone propionate (Seretide) twice daily

salbutamol (Ventolin) two puffs PRN

Today is Friday and when Kristy, the community nurse, arrives she immediately notices that Mr Tien has a moist cough and he looks exhausted. Kristy asks him how he is feeling and he replies, 'Not too bad.' As they go into the kitchen, Kristy observes that Mr Tien's medicines are in disarray. Usually, he has his medications arranged in an orderly way, just like he used to keep his workplace. He takes a seat and Kristy begins assessing him.

Kristy is able to compare the current observations with those she has previously recorded for Mr Tien, as follows:

Current observations	Normal for Mr Tien
Temperature: 36.9°C	Temperature: 36.4°C
Pulse rate: 100 beats/min	Pulse rate: 85 beats/min
Respiratory rate: 28 breaths/min	Respiratory rate: 22 breaths/min
Blood pressure (sitting): 180/90	Blood pressure (sitting): 130/85
O_2 sats: 89%	O_2 sats: 96%
Bilateral crackles in both lung bases	No crackles in lung bases
Urinalysis: NAD	Urinalysis: NAD

During Kristy's visit, Mr Tien's daughter, Nguyen Qui, arrives. She always comes home to have lunch with her father. She asks her father why he is still in his night clothes as he is always up, showered and dressed when Kristy visits. His breakfast is still on the bench top, too.

Kristy makes the decision to transfer Mr Tien to the local hospital Emergency Department (ED) and he is subsequently admitted with pneumonia. While in the ED, blood and sputum are collected for pathology testing.

Q   Mr Tien has pneumonia but is afebrile. Why is this?

Person-centred care

> The NSQHS Standards state that people receiving care are to be considered partners in planning, design and delivery of care (ACSQHC, 2016a). Being person-centred enables nurses to partner with consumers in a meaningful way.

The goal of person-centred care is to interact with the patient as a person. Collecting personal information, using the person's past life and history in care, respecting the person's choices and focusing on what the person can do, as well as their disabilities, are all part of person-centred care (Edvardsson & Nay, 2010).

Q   What factors might contribute to the risk of older people not being recognised as cognitively competent?

Mr Tien's life story

Mr Dang Tien arrived in Sydney from Vietnam in 1975 with his wife, Dang Doh, and their three children aged 18, 15 and 12. He was 39 years old and his wife was 38. He left Vietnam when the communist regime from North Vietnam moved into Ho Chi Minh City (formerly Saigon). Mr Tien was a respected professional and a Catholic, and he was unable to stay in Vietnam under the communist regime. Mr Tien had good friends in Australia and they were able to assist him and his family to escape from Vietnam. He worked as an engineer prior to his move to Australia, and spoke fluent French as well as Vietnamese. He was able to speak in English but not write it.

When he arrived in Sydney, Mr Tien went to work in a factory as a maintenance engineer, where he was given the nickname 'Jimmy' by his workmates. He worked long hours and saved to buy his own business. In 1990, Mr Tien purchased a dry cleaning shop and his eldest son and daughter joined him in this business. Mrs Tien had always stayed at home and looked after her husband, her children and then the grandchildren when they came along.

Mr Tien retired from the business four years ago because he was unable to physically cope with the work due to his COPD. Since then, his eldest son, Dang Lu, and his son-in-law have run the business. Mr Tien's wife died two years ago from breast cancer and he moved to his daughter's home, where he lives with her, her husband and his two grandsons. His eldest son moved into the family home when his father moved out; it is around the corner from Nguyen Qui's home.

Despite Mr Tien being regarded as a quiet, gentle man, he has always been very sociable, enjoying his days at the shop and the company of his friends and neighbours. He usually speaks Vietnamese at home with the family and English outside the home. Mr Tien plays Chinese chess on Tuesdays and Fridays at the local senior citizens centre.

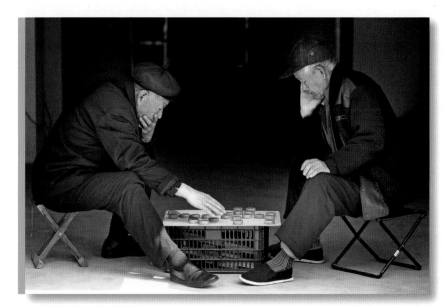

Mr Tien playing Chinese chess with a friend

With some assistance from his daughter and son-in-law, Mr Tien still manages to grow the Asian vegetables that they eat daily. He loves Vietnamese food, which his wife always cooked, but he does eat Western food occasionally. He prefers to eat with chopsticks.

When Mr Tien was diagnosed with COPD, he stopped smoking. He had started when he was a teenager and it became a habit. The progression of the disease has been relatively slow since he stopped smoking and because he is very health conscious.

Mr Tien regularly visits the acupuncturist and the Chinese herbalist for minor ailments. He is not one to complain about his illnesses or the loss of his wife. He feels he is ageing well, as he has a good appetite, is still able to do the things he enjoys, has a good relationship with his children and sleeps about six hours a night, only waking once or twice to go to the toilet. Mr Tien has never been hospitalised.

1. CONSIDER THE PATIENT SITUATION

It is now Friday night in the respiratory unit and while answering a call bell the night duty nurse notices that Mr Tien is out of bed and urinating in the sink near his bed. She says sharply, 'Jimmy, that's not a toilet. That's the sink!' Mr Tien goes back to his bed and the nurse puts the bed rails up. During the night, he is restless and incontinent, and continually pulls off his nasal prongs.

Morning handover report (0700)

Mr Tien behaved inappropriately during the night, using the sink as a toilet. Do not use the sink until it has been cleaned. We are an acute respiratory ward. Why do we get the confused oldies? I put his bed rails up, so he couldn't get out again and he didn't. But I had to keep an eye on him because he didn't sleep much and he was incontinent of urine. He doesn't talk much, just yells in gibberish ... though he could have been speaking Vietnamese, I wouldn't know. He doesn't speak English, although in handover last night they said he did. I think he's demented and will need placement. Just what we need—another bed blocker.

His obs are stable; he is putting out urine in good amounts (all over the bed). I think he needs an IDC. His bowels haven't opened. He was tossing and turning all night. He's still coughing. I spent the whole night putting his nasal prongs back on and keeping him from getting tangled up in his IV. I am exhausted, what a night ...

Cultural consideration: Why is it not appropriate for the night nurse to call Mr Tien 'Jimmy'? Hint: Refer to this web page: <www.diversicare .com.au/wp-content/ uploads/2015/10/ Vietnamese.pdf>.

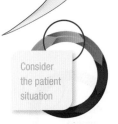

Consider the patient situation

The NSQHS Standards state that clinical handover should be structured to effectively communicate the healthcare requirements of people (ACSQHC, 2016a), for example using the structured communication tool ISBAR to guide clinical handover.

Clinical reasoning errors: The comment about Mr Tien being demented is an example of anchoring and ascertainment bias.

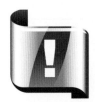

Something to think about ...

Bed rails are considered a form of restraint. According to best practice guidelines, bed rails should only be used: as a last resort; after a thorough assessment of the older person's needs; after other alternatives have been trialed and failed; when appropriate consent is obtained; when it is the only practical, least restrictive and safest strategy available. When bed rails are used, the person being restrained should be closely monitored. Always review your organisation's policies and procedures before considering the use of bed rails.

What questions should Tricia ask the night duty nurse about Mr Tien?

Tricia, a new graduate nurse, is allocated to the care of Mr Tien for the morning shift.

QUICK QUIZ!

Before progressing to the next stage of the clinical reasoning cycle, test your understanding of some of the terms used so far. Select the correct response for each of the following statements:

Q1 COPD is:

   a A disease of the bronchioles

   b An acute disease of the small and large airways

   c A chronic airway disease

Q2 Seretide and Ventolin are used to:

   a Increase airway diameter and reduce inflammation of the bronchioles

   b Reduce swelling and inflammation of the lungs

   c Increase airway diameter and moisture in the bronchioles

Q3 'Bed blocker' is a disparaging term used to describe which of the following?

   a A patient who is always getting out of bed and blocking nurses' movement

   b A bed that is raised on blocks so that patients with respiratory problems can breathe more easily

   c A patient whose hospitalisation extends beyond the standard period of admission, preventing new admissions

Q4 Urinary incontinence is a term typically used to describe:

   a An episode of urination that did not occur in a toilet

   b An inability to control urination

   c A controlled ability to urinate

2. COLLECT CUES/INFORMATION

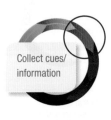

Collect cues/information

(a) Review current information

Now that you have some understanding of Mr Tien's situation, the next stage of the clinical reasoning cycle is to collect relevant cues and information. Tricia has the following information about Mr Tien:

   1 His previous level of functional abilities

   2 Details of current medications and medical history

   3 His usual sleep pattern

   4 His usual bowel and bladder function

   5 Results from his admission urinalysis

Q Can you identify another five important cues that need to be reviewed by Tricia?

(b) Gather new information

At 0800, Tricia goes to Mr Tien's room. The bed rails are still up and Mr Tien's nasal prongs are around his neck. Tricia notices that no water has been drunk from his water jug and his cup is empty on the bedside locker. Mr Tien's breakfast of porridge, tea and toast has not been eaten and he has been incontinent of urine.

Tricia takes Mr Tien's vital signs and completes a respiratory assessment. She also conducts an Abbreviated Mental Test Score (AMTS) and a Confusion Assessment Method (CAM).

The AMTS is a cognitive assessment tool that can be used to quickly assess an older person. It takes five minutes to complete and includes 10 questions. The maximum score is 10 and a score of less than 7 is suggestive of cognitive impairment. The AMTS can identify cognitive impairment but it is not reliable in identifying delirium.

The CAM is a valid 'gold standard' delirium diagnostic tool. It also takes about five minutes to complete.

Tricia finds it difficult to complete these assessments as Mr Tien is only able to tell her his age, address and the year he first arrived in Australia. She can't understand some of Mr Tien's responses, as his English is mixed up with Vietnamese. Some of the questions Mr Tien doesn't attempt to answer; he just stares at Tricia's hands.

Q   Identify two relevant cues that you believe Tricia should collect at this stage to help her understand the care Mr Tien requires:

   a   Level of consciousness and orientation

   b   Urinalysis

   c   Level of psychomotor activity

   d   Bowel pattern

   e   Mr Tien's mood, speech and conversation ability

   f   Skin assessment

   g   Fluid balance status

   h   Falls status

(c) Recall knowledge

Tricia begins to recall what she knows about the causes of altered cognition in older people.

Q1   See how much you know about the 4Ds by completing the following table:

Alteration in cognition	Onset	Level of consciousness	Mood	Self-awareness	Activities of daily living
Dementia		Alert		Unaware of deficits	
Delirium	Acute, hours–days		Fluctuates	Fluctuates	May be intact or impaired
Depression		Drowsy		Aware of cognitive change	
Cognitive decline	Chronic, months–years	Alert	No change		No change

Q2   Which of Mr Tien's medical conditions may alter his cognitive status?

   a   COPD

   b   TIAs

> For more information about AMTS, access <https://www.ncbi.nlm.nih.gov/pmc/articles/PMC2560932/pdf/occpaper00113-0035.pdf>.

> For more information about CAM, access <http://www.viha.ca/NR/rdonlyres/6121360B-B90F-4EF3-88F6-D50CC4825EE7/0/camshortform.pdf>.

> More information about cognition and hosptialised older people can be found at Victorian State Government Department of Health and Human Services (2015). Older people in hospital. Available at <https://www2.health.vic.gov.au/hospitals-and-health-services/patient-care/older-people>.

> Hint: Reading Insel & Bager (2002) or Hunter & Miller (2016) will help you complete the table.

    c Pneumonia

    d All of the above

Q3 How might TIAs contribute to altering Mr Tien's current cognitive status?

    a A TIA can cause cerebral hypoxia and cell death and can lead to the development of delirium.

    b A TIA can cause confusion and can lead to the development of depression.

    c TIAs can cause cerebral ischaemia and cell death and can lead to the development of dementia.

Q4 How might pneumonia contribute to altering Mr Tien's cognitive status?

    a Infections may trigger an episode of delirium in older people.

    b Pneumonia causes hypoxia, which leads to dementia in older people.

    c Pneumonia causes hyperthermia, which triggers an episode of delirium in older people.

    d Pneumonia causes severe fatigue, which predisposes the older person to the development of depression.

Q5 How might COPD contribute to altering Mr Tien's cognitive status?

    a COPD can cause cerebral hypoxia and cell death, which can lead to the development of dementia.

    b COPD can cause confusion and can lead to the development of depression.

    c COPD can cause cerebral hypoxia and can lead to the development of delirium.

> What is the difference between hypoactive and hyperactive delirium?

Q6 Which delirium type or types would Tricia need to recall?

    a Hyperactive

    b Hypoactive

    c Mixed type

    d All of the above

Something to think about …

Healthcare issues can arise when nursing older migrants as they often follow their original culture (Le & Le, 2005). Tricia would need to consider a number of aspects of Vietnamese culture when nursing Mr Tien.

Q7 Review the information you have about Mr Tien and, in the table below, describe how each cultural aspect relates to him.

> If you need help, refer to this web page: <www.diversicare.com.au/wp-content/uploads/2015/10/Vietnamese.pdf>.

Cultural aspect	Mr Tien
Example: Language	Speaks Vietnamese, English and French. Usually speaks Vietnamese with family and English outside the home.
Food and diet	
Attitudes to illness and pain	
Cultural beliefs	
Family (living arrangements)	
Religion	

3. PROCESS INFORMATION

(a) Interpret

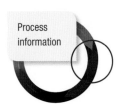

Process information

Q   Which of the following are within normal parameters for Mr Tien?

   a   Temperature: 36.9°C

   b   Pulse rate: 95 beats/min

   c   Respiratory rate: 28 breaths/min

   d   Blood pressure: 175/90

   e SaO_2:   90% (room air)

   f   Lung sounds: Crackles in left lower lung bases

(b) Discriminate

Q1   From the information that you know about Mr Tien and the cues that have been collected by Tricia, which cues are *most relevant* to determine Mr Tien's cognitive status *at this time*?

   a   Vital signs

   b   Level of confusion

   c SaO_2 level

   d   CAM positive result (acute change, easily distracted, rambling and unclear conversation, alert)

   e   AMTS result 3/10

   f   Breathlessness

   g   Urinalysis NAD on admission

   h   Mr Tien's cognition has not been assessed prior to admission

   i   Mr Tien plays chess on Tuesdays and Fridays at the local senior citizens' hall

Hint: A score of less than 6 for the AMTS suggests cognitive impairment but it does not screen for delirium.

Q2   What other information should Tricia consider before making any inferences about Mr Tien?

   a   Mr Tien normally sleeps for six hours and is up to the toilet at least once every night.

   b   His bowels opened yesterday.

   c   No significant abnormalities were noted in urea and electrolytes (U&Es).

   d   Mr Tien usually speaks Vietnamese at home with the family and English outside the home.

   e   Mr Tien lives at home with his daughter.

   f   Mr Tien is a quiet, gentle man.

   g   Mr Tien enjoys living with his daughter and son-in-law.

   h   Mr Tien manages, with assistance from his daughter and son-in-law, to grow the Asian vegetables they eat daily.

   i   Mr Tien has not had any previous hospitalisations.

   j   Mr Tien loves Vietnamese food. He will eat Western food occasionally. He prefers to eat with chopsticks.

Q3   There are many myths about alterations in the cognition of older people. Which of the following statements are true?

   a   All older people will develop dementia.

   b   When people become older, they can expect to feel depressed.

   c   Older people are at increased risk of developing delirium when they experience acute physiological changes.

   d   All older people will lose their short-term memory.

    e   As people age, they cannot learn new information.

    f   Some level of confusion is experienced by all older people.

Q4 Why is it important for Tricia to have knowledge of the myths associated with ageing and cognition?

(c) Relate and (d) Infer

It is important to cluster the cues together and to identify relationships between them (based on the information you have collected so far). From this, you can make inferences about Mr Tien's condition.

Q1 Label the following 'true', 'false' or a 'possibility'.

    a   Mr Tien is incontinent because the bed rails prevent him from getting out of bed to go to the toilet.

    b   Mr Tien is incontinent because he has dementia.

    c   Mr Tien is depressed because he has COPD and is hospitalised.

    d   Mr Tien has language difficulties because he has dementia.

    e   Mr Tien did not eat his breakfast because he does not eat porridge or toast, or drink white tea.

    f   Mr Tien has not been drinking because he is experiencing delirium.

    g   Mr Tien is confused because he is an older person.

    h   Mr Tien is in a delirium because he is older and ill with pneumonia.

    i   Mr Tien has impaired communication because he is experiencing delirium.

Q2 Can an older person be diagnosed with dementia as well as depression or delirium, or with all three?

Q3 Identify three factors that have led to Mr Tien's cognitive alteration.

    a   Advancing age

    b   History of hypertension

    c   Pneumonia

    d   Hospitalisation

    e   Intravenous therapy

    f   Antibiotic therapy

(e) Match

Q Have you ever cared for someone with cognitive alteration? In what way were their presenting signs and symptoms the same as, or different from, Mr Tien's?

(f) Predict

Q If Tricia does not take the appropriate and timely actions regarding his altered cognition, what could happen to Mr Tien? (Select the four correct responses.)

    a   He could have a stroke.

    b   He could be diagnosed with dementia.

    c   He could become hypoxic.

    d   He could become septic.

    e   He could fall.

    f   He could become dehydrated.

    g   He could become suicidal.

    h   He could develop a pressure sore.

> *Important: Whether Mr Tien has dementia, depression and/or delirium will be ultimately determined by the medical officer. The role of the nurse is to work collaboratively with the healthcare team and to report their nursing diagnoses to the team, so they can make an informed and accurate medical diagnosis.*

> *Hint: Think about the causes and risk factors for an older person developing delirium. See Delirium Clinical Care Standard (ACSQHC, 2016b): <www.safetyandquality .gov.au/wp-content/ uploads/2016/07/ Delirium-Clinical-Care- Standard-Web-PDF .pdf>.*

> *NSW Health has adopted the CHOPs (Care of confused hospitalised older persons) program which provides six principles of care for an older person experiencing an alteration in cognition unassociated with normal ageing. For more details, visit <www.aci .health.nsw.gov .au/chops>.*

4. IDENTIFY THE PROBLEM/ISSUE

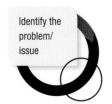

Now is the time for you to bring together (synthesise) all of the information collected and inferences you've made to identify the key nursing diagnoses for Mr Tien.

Q   Select from the following list, the *incorrect* nursing diagnosis for Mr Tien.

a   Functional incontinence related to acute confusional state, evidenced by Mr Tien using the sink to urinate and incontinent of urine in the bed once bed rails raised

b   Impaired communication related to acute confusional state, evidenced by Mr Tien yelling in 'gibberish', not speaking English and ATMS assessment findings

c   Pneumonia evidenced by ATMS 3/10, CAM positive result and communication difficulties

d   Impaired memory related to pneumonia, evidenced by communication difficulties: ATMS and CAM results, and using the sink as a toilet

e   Impaired oxygenation and breathing related to pneumonia, evidenced by respiratory rate 28, SaO_2 90% (room air) and crackles in left lower lung bases

f   Sleep/wake alteration related to acute confusional state, evidenced by night nurse's report

g   Risk of falls related to acute confusional state

h   Risk of skin breakdown related to age, acute confusional state and pneumonia

5. ESTABLISH GOALS

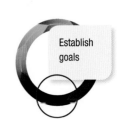

Q   From the list below, choose the most important *short-term* goals (within 24 hours) for Mr Tien's management.

a   For Mr Tien to be orientated and alert

b   For Mr Tien to be able to communicate his needs and wants

c   For Mr Tien to return home

d   For Mr Tien's language skills to return to baseline

e   For Mr Tien to be more interactive with staff

f   For Mr Tien to stop using the sink as a toilet

g   For Mr Tien to be placed in a residential aged-care facility

h   For Mr Tien to eat three-quarters of the food presented at meal times

i   For Mr Tien not to fall

j   For Mr Tien's oral intake to be 1000 mL/24 hrs

k   For Mr Tien's oxygen saturation level to remain above 95% and respiratory rate below 22 breaths/min

6. TAKE ACTION

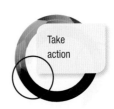

Q1   All of the actions below are appropriate. From this list, identify which of these actions take priority and must be performed *immediately*.

a   Notify Mr Tien's doctor of his condition.

b   Check that the IV cannula is patent.

c   Lower the bed rails on Mr Tien's bed.

d   Regularly orientate Mr Tien to the hospital environment.

e   Ensure Mr Tien is wearing his nasal prongs.

f   Communicate via phone with Mr Tien's daughter.

g   Maintain Mr Tien's fluid balance chart.

h   Engage the interpreter service to assist with communication strategies.

i   Adjust bed to the lowest position.

j   Ask daughter or other family member to sit with Mr Tien.

k   Prompt and assist Mr Tien with drinking and eating.

l   Monitor Mr Tien's vital signs and oxygen saturation level.

m   Move Mr Tien to an area where he can be closely observed.

n   Communicate with family to start discharge planning.

o   Ask Mr Tien's family to bring in his favourite foods for each meal.

Q2   In the table below, match the rationales for care to the corresponding nursing action:

Nursing action	Rationale
Document all nursing observations and actions accurately and contemporaneously	To prevent pressure areas due to reduced mobility
Reassess using the CAM	To ensure clear, accurate and timely communication between all health professionals caring for Mr Tien
Engage interpreter service to assist with the other cognitive assessments	Restlessness and lethargy are indicators of continuing acute confusional state
Prompt and assist Mr Tien with toileting	To identify the progress of the delirium
Prompt and assist Mr Tien with oral fluids	To ensure clear, accurate and timely updates are received by family from all health professionals
Monitor psychomotor activity	To ensure adequate oxygen delivery
Encourage family to stay with Mr Tien	To ensure adequate fluid intake and prevent dehydration
Communicate Mr Tien's progress to his family	To determine Mr Tien's level of cognition
Encourage gentle ambulation and regular position change	To prevent episodes of incontinence
Monitor oxygen saturation levels	To assist with communication, to improve safety and to provide comfort for Mr Tien

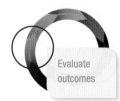

Evaluate outcomes

7. EVALUATE

It is 1430 hrs and the end of Tricia's shift. Mr Tien's current signs and symptoms provide cues that will allow her to make a determination of whether or not her interventions have been effective and his condition is improving.

Q   Rate each of the following signs and symptoms as 'unchanged', 'improving', 'deteriorating' or 'fluctuating'.

Language ability   not speaking

Psychomotor activity   lethargic

Mood   withdrawn

Pulse   90

BP	150/85
Respirations	24
SaO$_2$	94% (via nasal prongs)
Urinary continence	using a urinal with prompting and assistance
Oral intake	eating and drinking food brought in by daughter and with her assistance

8. REFLECT

Reflect on your learning from this scenario.

Q1 What have you learnt that you can apply to your future nursing practice?

Q2 What actions might the night duty nurse have taken to better manage Mr Tien?

Q3 If you suspect that an older person has an alteration in cognition, what three actions would you take and why would you undertake them?

Q4 Imagine you overheard one of the nurses calling Mr Tien 'Sweetheart'. What would your reaction be and why?

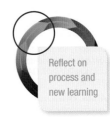

Reflect on process and new learning

If unsure, read Gardner et al. (2001), 'Don't call me sweetie!' Patients differ from nurses in their perceptions of caring.

SCENARIO 14.2 Caring for an older person with dementia

CHANGING THE SCENE

Mr Tien's condition improves and after five days he is discharged and returned home with his daughter, Mrs Nguyen Qui. He has made a good recovery from his pneumonia and delirium but has not returned to his normal level of cognitive or physical functioning. Mr Tien and his family are told by the nurse and medical officer at the hospital that it may take several weeks before he will start to feel strong and clear-headed again.

1. CONSIDER THE PATIENT SITUATION

Three weeks following discharge, Kristy, the community nurse, is visiting Mr Tien. His daughter, Mrs Qui, answers the door and immediately says: 'I'm worried. Dad isn't getting any better and he is more forgetful. Some days he forgets to eat breakfast, doesn't shower or shave, and keeps putting on the same clothes. When I get home, I try to get him to change or bathe but he gets upset and tells me to leave him alone. He tells me I'm not a good daughter, that a good daughter would not question her father. I can't leave him alone all day like this. And he hasn't been going to his chess days since his return from hospital. I am so worried about him.'

Kristy then visits Mr Tien in the next room. He smiles when she enters and nods his head in greeting. Kristy asks him how he is feeling and he replies, 'I'm okay, but my daughter keeps telling me what to do.'

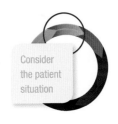

Consider the patient situation

2. COLLECT CUES/INFORMATION

(a) Review current information

Q What information should Kristy review that is most relevant to Mr Tien at this stage?

   a Current cognitive abilities

   b Details of current medications

   c History of vascular risk factors

   d History of sleep pattern

   e History of bowel and bladder function

   f Mr Tien's past life in Vietnam

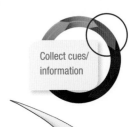

Collect cues/ information

Hint: Think back to all that you know about Mr Tien and his situation.

See the following for more information on these instruments:

GCS, <www.strokecenter .org/wp-content/ uploads/2011/08/ glasgow_coma.pdf>

MMSE, <www.ihpa.gov .au/sites/g/files/net636/f/ publications/smmse- tool-v2.pdf>

DASS21, <https://maic .qld.gov.au/wp-content/ uploads/2016/07/DASS- 21.pdf>

ATMS, <www.ncbi.nlm .nih.gov/pmc/articles/ PMC2560932/pdf/ occpaper00113-0035 .pdf>

CAM, <www.viha.ca/ NR/rdonlyres/6121360B- B90F-4EF3-88F6- D50CC4825EE7/0/ camshortform.pdf>.

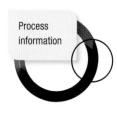

Process information

g Medical history

h Hydration/nutritional status

i Current level of functional abilities

j The fact that Mr Tien has not been to his chess sessions since discharge

(b) Gather new information

Q1 What new information should Kristy gather that would assist her in understanding Mr Tien's current condition more fully?

Q2 Which assessment instruments could Kristy consider using to help her come to a deeper understanding of Mr Tien's current level of cognition?

    a Glasgow Coma Scale (GCS)

    b Mini Mental Status Examination(MMSE)

    c Depression, Anxiety, Stress Scales (DASS21)

    d Abbreviated Mental Test Score (ATMS)

    e Confusion Assessment Method Instrument (CAM)

3. PROCESS INFORMATION

(a) Interpret

Q Which of the following assessment findings (recorded by Kristy at 1200 hours) would provide her with information about what is happening to Mr Tien?

    a Temperature: 36.4°C

    b Pulse rate: 87 beats/min

    c Respiratory rate: 22 breaths/min

    d Blood pressure: 170/85

    e SaO_2: 96% (room air)

    f Respiratory: lungs clear

    g CAM: negative result

    h ATMS: 5/10

    i DASS21: negative for depressive symptoms but mild anxiety and stress levels

    j Food and fluid intake: adequate with prompting from daughter

    k Urinalysis: NAD

    l Bowels: opened today

    m Mood: irritable

Hint: A score of 5 for the ATMS suggests cognitive impairment.

(b) Discriminate

Q From the cues and information you now have, you need to narrow down the information to what is most important. From the list below, select the cues that you believe are *most relevant* to Mr Tien's cognitive status *at this time*.

    a Vital signs

    b Level of confusion

    c SaO_2

    d CAM negative result

    e ATMS 5/10

    f Urinalysis

g   DASS21 results

h   Mood

(c) Relate and (d) Infer

Q   Cluster the cues together and identify relationships between them. Label the following 'true', 'false' or a 'possibility'.

a   Mr Tien has cognitive decline associated with ageing.

b   Mr Tien is confused because he is hypoxic.

c   Mr Tien is confused because he is an older person.

d   Mr Tien is depressed because he has not been able to return to his normal activities.

e   Mr Tien's cognition has deteriorated because he may have experienced a cerebral vascular event.

f   Mr Tien remains in a delirium because he is older and was ill with pneumonia.

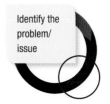

Kristy has also noted that Mr Tien's blood pressure is elevated and she will need to report this to Mr Tien's GP.

(e) Predict

Q   If Kristy does not take the appropriate actions regarding Mr Tien's altered cognition at this time, what could happen to Mr Tien? (Select the correct response.)

a   Mr Tien could have a stroke.

b   Mr Tien could develop depression.

c   Mr Tien could fall.

d   Mr Tien could become suicidal.

e   Mr Tien could develop delirium again.

f   Mr Tien's cognitive impairment may be missed.

4. IDENTIFY THE PROBLEM/ISSUE

Identify the problem/ issue

Q   Select from the following list, the correct nursing diagnoses for Mr Tien.

a   Impaired communication with daughter related to an alteration in cognition, evidenced by Mr Tien's saying, 'I'm okay, but my daughter keeps telling me what to do', and that Mrs Qui is 'not a good daughter'

b   Mood disorder related to an alteration in cognition, evidenced by the DASS21 results and Mr Tien not going to his regular chess days

c   Personal hygiene deficit related to an alteration in cognition, evidenced by Mr Tien's not bathing and shaving, and putting on the same clothes each day

d   Acute confusional state related to an alteration in cognition, evidenced by Mrs Qui stating that Mr Tien is more forgetful

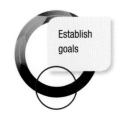

The NMBA's Registered Nurse Standards for Practice (2016) indicate that RNs must be able to comprehensively assess patients and develop a plan of care based on their assessment findings.

e   Cognitive impairment related to a currently unknown pathophysiology, evidenced by Mrs Qui's statement that Mr Tien is more forgetful; CAM negative; T, PR, RR and SaO_2 normal for Mr Tien; ATMS 5/10; DASS21 results; urinalysis–NAD

f   Altered nutrition/hydration intake related to an alteration in cognition, evidenced by Mr Tien forgetting to eat breakfast and needing prompting from his daughter to eat

5. ESTABLISH GOALS

Establish goals

Q   From the list below, choose the four most important *short-term* goals for Mr Tien's management at this time.

a   For Mr Tien to be orientated and alert

b   For Mr Tien to be assessed by his GP

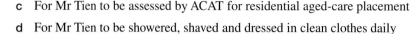

c   For Mr Tien to be assessed by ACAT for residential aged-care placement

d   For Mr Tien to be showered, shaved and dressed in clean clothes daily

e   For Mr Tien's cognition to be assessed by a geriatrician

f   For Mr Tien to receive services from an ACAT

g   For Mr Tien not to state that his daughter is a bad daughter

h   For Mr Tien to have an understanding of his cognitive change

i   For Mr Tien to eat his meals and drink at least 1600 mL/day

An assessment by ACAT (Aged Care Assessment Team) is required before placement into a residential aged-care facility can occur.

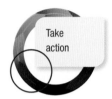

Take action

6. TAKE ACTION

Q   Select the nursing actions that must be performed before Kristy concludes her visit with Mr Tien and label these actions with a 1; label the actions that Kristy will perform once she returns to the office as a 2; and label the incorrect actions with a 3.

a   Ring Mr Tien's eldest son.

b   Discuss the results of the assessments with Mrs Qui.

c   Explain to Mr Tien that he is not to speak to his daughter in a negative way.

d   Suggest some strategies for Mrs Qui to help with Mr Tien's personal hygiene.

e   Plan for readmission to hospital.

f   Make a referral to an ACAT.

g   Arrange for Mr Tien to receive Meals on Wheels.

h   Suggest some communication strategies to help Mrs Qui receive positive responses from Mr Tien.

i   Discuss the need to organise Mr Tien's admission to a residential aged-care facility in the near future.

j   Suggest some strategies that Mrs Qui can use to ensure Mr Tien is eating and drinking adequately.

k   Notify Mr Tien's GP of his condition.

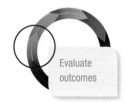

Evaluate outcomes

7. EVALUATE

It is now one week later and Kristy is visiting Mr Tien and his daughter. Mr Tien's signs and symptoms provide you with data to make a determination about whether the above interventions have been effective, and if Mr Tien's condition is improving.

Q   Rate each of the following signs and symptoms as 'unchanged', 'improving' or 'deteriorating'.

ATMS	5/10
CAM	negative result
Mood	calm
Pulse	87
Blood pressure	140/75
Respirations	20
SaO$_2$	96%
DASS 21	no depressive, anxiety or stress symptoms
Personal hygiene	Mr Tien's son, grandsons or son-in-law assist Mr Tien with his showering, shaving and dressing daily.

| Communication | Mrs Qui has not been called a bad daughter since Kristy explained what was happening and Mrs Qui has not been bathing him. |
| Nutrition/hydration | Mrs Qui reports that Mr Tien is eating and drinking as he would usually do. |

8. REFLECT

Reflect on your learning from this scenario.

Q1 What are three of the most important things that you have learnt from this scenario?

Q2 What three actions will you take in clinical practice as a result of your learning from this scenario?

Q3 What have you learnt about cultural awareness from this scenario that you can apply to your practice?

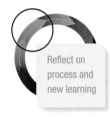

Reflect on process and new learning

EPILOGUE

Following further assessment by Mr Tien's GP, he was diagnosed with vascular dementia. The doctor suggested that Mr Tien probably suffered a vascular event triggered by his hypertension during or after hospitalisation. Mr Tien continues to live with his daughter and his family is very supportive. They prefer to care for him at home, with help from community services. Mr Tien is enjoying spending more time with his son and grandsons. He does not attend his chess sessions anymore, but some of his close friends come over for lunch once a month. Mr Tien still works in his garden.

FURTHER READING

Australian Commission on Safety and Quality in Health Care (ACSQHC). (2016). *Delirium Clinical Care Standard.* Sydney: ACSQHC. Accessed December 2016 at <www.safetyandquality.gov.au/wp-content/uploads/2016/07/Delirium-Clinical-Care-Standard-Web-PDF.pdf>.

Calley, C. T. G., Womack, K., Moore, P., Hart, J. & Kraut, M. (2010). Subjective report of word-finding and memory deficits in normal aging and dementia. *Cognitive Behavioural Neurology, 23*(3), 158–91.

Smith, K., Flicker, L., Shadforth, G., Carroll, E., Ralph, E., Atkinson, D, … LoGiudice, D. (2011). Original research, 'Gotta be sit down and worked out together': Views of Aboriginal caregivers and service providers on ways to improve dementia care for Aboriginal Australians. *Rural and Remote Health: The International Electronic Journal of Rural and Remote Health Research, Education, Practice and Policy, 11*(1650), 1–14.

REFERENCES

Alzheimer's Australia. (2016). *Key Facts and Statistics 2016.* Accessed December 2016 at <www.fightdementia.org.au/about-dementia/statistics>.

American Psychiatric Association. (2013). Diagnostic and Statistical Manual of Mental Disorders: Fifth Edition. *American Journal of Psychiatry.* Accessed March 2017 at <http://doi.org/10.1176/appi.books.9780890425596.744053>.

Australian Commission on Safety and Quality in Health Care (ACSQHC). (2016a). *National Safety and Quality Health Service Standards Version 2.* Draft, Sydney, Australia.

Australian Commission on Safety and Quality in Health Care. (2016b). *Delirium Clinical Care Standard.* Sydney: ACSQHC.

Baldwin, R. (2008). Mood disorders: Depressive disorders. In R. Jacoby, C. Oppenheimer, T. Dening & A. Thomas (Eds), *Oxford Textbook of Old Age Psychiatry* (pp. 529–56). Oxford: Oxford University Press.

Beaudreau, S. A. & O'Hara, R. (2009). The association of anxiety and depressive symptoms with cognitive performance in community-dwelling older adults. *Psychology and Aging.* 24, 507–12.

Edvardsson, D. & Nay, R. (2010). Acute care and older people: Challenges and ways forward. *Australian Journal of Advanced Nursing, 27*(2), 63–68.

Fick, D. M., Agostini, J. V. & Inouye, S. K. (2002). Delirium superimposed on dementia: A systematic review. *Journal of the American Geriatrics Society, 50*(10), 1723–32.

Gardner, A., Goodsell, J., Duggen, T., Murtha, B., Peck, C. & Williams, J. (2001). 'Don't call me sweetie!' Patients differ from nurses in their perceptions of caring, *Collegian, 8*(3), 32–38.

Hunter, S. & Miller, C. (2016). *Miller's Nursing for Wellness in Older Adults.* Sydney: Lippincott Williams & Wilkins Pty Ltd (Chapters 11–15).

Inouye, S. K. (2006). Delirium in older persons. *New England Journal of Medicine, 354*(11), 1157–65.

Insel, K. & Bager, T. (2002). Deciphering the 4Ds: Cognitive decline, delirium, depression and dementia: A review. *Journal of Advanced Nursing, 38*(4), 360–68.

Le, Q. & Le, T. (2005). *Cultural Attitudes of Vietnamese Migrants on Health Issues.* Tasmania: University of Tasmania. Available at <www.aare.edu.au/05pap/le05645.pdf>.

National Ageing Research Institute (NARI). (2009). *Depression in Older Age: A Scoping Study—Final Report.* Accessed December 2016 at <www.beyondblue.org.au/docs/default-source/research-project-files/bw0143---nari-2009-full-report---minus-appendices.pdf?sfvrsn=4>.

NSW Health. (2011). *Admitted Patient Data Collection.* Sydney: NSW Health.

Nursing and Midwifery Board of Australia (NMBA). (2016). *Registered Nurse Standards for Practice.* Accessed December 2016 at <www.nursingmidwiferyboard.gov.au/Codes-Guidelines-Statements/Professional-standards.aspx>.

Patel, B. B. & Holland, N. W. (2012). Mild cognitive impairment: Hope for stability, plan for progression. *Cleveland Clinic Journal of Medicine, 79*(12), 857–64.

Voyer, P., Richard, S., Douce, L., Danjou, C. & Carmichael, P. -H. (2008). Detection of delirium by nurses among long-term care residents with dementia. *BMC Nursing, 7*(4), 1–14.

PHOTO CREDIT

CHAPTER 15

CARING FOR A PERSON WITH A DISABILITY

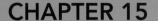

STEPHEN GUINEA, JESSICA McKIRKLE AND CHRISTINE IMMS

LEARNING OUTCOMES

Completion of the activities in this chapter will enable you to:

○ describe techniques for effective therapeutic nurse/patient communication in the context of young adults with a disability (**recall** and **application**)

○ explain and describe common physiological, developmental and psychosocial manifestations of cerebral palsy, particular to a young adult, that will guide the collection of cues (**gather**, **review**, **interpret**, **discriminate**, **relate** and **infer**)

○ review information to identify the main nursing diagnoses for a person with a disability and their family (**synthesise**)

○ describe the priorities of care for a young adult with a disability, taking into account legislation, and the role of the registered nurse in advocacy for patient autonomy (**goal setting** and **taking action**)

○ identify criteria for evaluating the effectiveness of nursing actions taken to enhance person-centred care (**evaluate**)

○ consider potential challenges to planning and implementing person-centred care for a person with a disability (**reflection** and **translation**)

○ reflect on your ability to practise person-centred care that promotes advocacy for the young adult with a disability (**reflection** and **translation**).

INTRODUCTION

The two scenarios introduced in this chapter focus on the care of a young adult with a physical disability. You will meet Amelia, a 22-year-old woman who has cerebral palsy, and explore her story of transition to an autonomous young adult. Cerebral palsy is the most common physical disability in children in Australia (Australian Cerebral Palsy Register Group [ACPRG], 2013). It is caused by 'non-progressive disturbances in the fetal or infant brain' (Rosenbaum et al., 2007, p. 1) and is a complex, permanent condition that primarily affects an individual's movement and posture. People who have cerebral palsy often have additional conditions such as vision or hearing loss, epilepsy, communication difficulties, intellectual impairment or behavioural problems.

For teens and young adults with a chronic illness or disability, this period of their life is often characterised as one of transition; transition from paediatric to adult care, and from dependence to autonomy, interdependence or independence (Rosenbaum & Rosenbloom, 2012). Structured social age markers, which historically have been used to define the timing of a child transitioning to adolescence and young adulthood, may be less relevant for those with a disability as these transitions may occur at later ages. Defining the timing and duration of transitions may be more effectively based on a series of decisions made by the individual and their family (Furlong, 2009).

Person-centred care of a young adult requires an in-depth and holistic approach, respecting them as individuals, as well as members of families and wider communities. Knowledge of the person's physical, psychosocial and cultural history and preferences is essential to person-centred nursing care. Nurses require insight into the young adult's needs as an *autonomous person*, rather than as someone for whom a series of tasks needs to be completed (Hewitt-Taylor, 2008). Well-developed clinical reasoning skills can assist nurses to understand and consider different perspectives such as those portrayed in this chapter, resulting in empathic, considered and appropriate nursing care.

KEY CONCEPTS

disability
cerebral palsy
person-centred care
healthcare transition
interprofessional
    healthcare team
discharge planning

SUGGESTED READINGS

Agency for Clinical Innovation. (2014). *Key Principles for Transition of Young People from Paediatric to Adult Health Care.* Accessed March 2017 at <www.aci.health. nsw.gov.au/__data/assets/ pdf_file/0011/251696/Key_ Principles_for_Transition.pdf>.

A. Merritt & M. Boogaerts. (2014). Psychosocial care. In E. Chang & A. Johnson (Eds), *Chronic Illness & Disability: Principles for Nursing Practice* (2nd edn). Chatswood, Australia: Churchill Livingstone.

D. Tasker & T. De Bortoli. (2014). Communicating with people who have communication impairment. In T. Levett-Jones (Ed.), *Critical Conversations for Patient Safety: An Essential Guide for Health Professionals.* Frenchs Forest, Australia: Pearson.

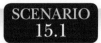

SCENARIO 15.1   Discovering the person behind the disability

SETTING THE SCENE

Amelia Traynor is a 22-year-old woman who was admitted to hospital three days ago for treatment of aspiration pneumonia and the insertion of a percutaneous endoscopic gastrostomy (PEG) tube. Amelia has a diagnosis of cerebral palsy. She underwent the surgical insertion of the PEG tube yesterday morning. You have been allocated the care of Amelia during the morning shift. The time is 1130 hrs and you are preparing to assist Amelia with her shower.

The epidemiology of cerebral palsy

Cerebral palsy is the most common physical disability in children, affecting 1 in 500 births in Australia (ACPRG, 2013) and approximately 17 million people worldwide. The number of people with cerebral palsy in Australia is expected to increase due to continued population growth and the low mortality rate associated with cerebral palsy (Rosenbaum & Rosenbloom, 2012).

For most people, the causes of cerebral palsy remain unknown. However, four groups that are at statistically greater risk of cerebral palsy are: males (approximately 55%), premature babies, babies of low birth weight and children from a multiple birth (ACPRG, 2013). The financial cost of caring for a person with cerebral palsy in Australia has been estimated at over $43 000 per person per year, of which approximately 37 per cent is borne by the person or their family (Access Economics, 2008). It must be acknowledged that there may be significant psychosocial, emotional and physical costs to individuals and their families associated with living with cerebral palsy.

The aetiology and pathogenesis of cerebral palsy

Cerebral palsy is a term that refers to a group of permanent disorders of development, movement and posture. It is caused by non-progressive disturbances to the developing brain during pregnancy or soon after birth. Cerebral palsy is a complex disability, where the manifestations are dependent on the areas of the brain affected. It can affect body movement, muscle control, muscle coordination, muscle tone, reflex, posture and balance (Rosenbaum & Rosenbloom, 2012). In addition to motor disorders, people living with cerebral palsy often experience disturbances of sensation, perception, cognition, communication and behaviour (Rosenbaum et al., 2007).

Cerebral palsy is classified according to the part of the body affected and is defined as bilateral or unilateral. Bilateral cerebral palsy affects both sides of the body. It may be further classified as diplegic where both legs are affected with the arms affected to a lesser extent, or quadraplegic where all four limbs, as well as the muscles of the trunk, face and mouth, are affected. Unilateral (or hemiplegic) cerebral palsy affects the left or right side of the body only.

Cerebral palsy is also classified according to the way it affects people's movements, with each related to the damaged part of the brain. These are presented in Table 15.1.

Functional presentations associated with cerebral palsy

Along with understanding what part of the body is affected and the type of motor disorder, there are four important functional classification systems used with people with cerebral palsy that provide a clear description of their abilities and paint a picture of the severity of the condition. In each of these classification systems, the individual's usual ability is described. The Gross Motor Function Classification System—Expanded and Revised (GMFCS-ER) provides a way of classifying the individual's ability to make self-initiated movements related to sitting and walking. The GMFCS is a five-level system as presented below (adapted from Palisano et al., 2008):

- **Level I**—Walks without restrictions; limitations in more advanced gross motor skills
- **Level II**—Walks without assistive devices; limitations walking outdoors and in the community

- **Level III**—Walks with assistive mobility devices; limitations walking outdoors and in the community
- **Level IV**—Self-mobility with limitations; individuals are transported or use power mobility outdoors and in the community
- **Level V**—Self-mobility is severely limited even with the use of assistive devices

Table 15.1 *Motor disorders associated with cerebral palsy*

Movement disorder	Prevalence (of all people living with cerebral palsy)	Aetiology	Manifestations
Spastic	70–80%	Damage to the motor cortex	Muscle tone is increased, so movements feel stiff or limbs resist movement. • Stiff, rigid muscles due to hypertonia • Stiff, jerky or absent limb movement • Difficulty controlling individual muscles or muscle groups required, e.g. when handling objects or speaking
Dyskinetic (dyskinesia)	6% (in isolation)	Damage to the basal ganglia	Involuntary patterns of movement of groups of muscles or body parts. Dyskinesia manifests in different ways depending on the locus of damage to the basal ganglia. • Dystonia: slow twisting or repetitive movements, or abnormal posture of a limb (or digit, mouth or eyes) or the body, that may be triggered when the person attempts to move, or by excitement, startle, stress or other events • Athetosis: slow, continuous writhing movements that are present at rest and worsened by attempts to move. Muscle tone fluctuates between hypotonia (floppy muscle tone) and hyperkinesia (extremely variable muscle tone) • Chorea: involuntary movements that are brief, abrupt, irregular and unpredictable. Chorea can affect speech and swallowing as well as limb movement, and is often worsened when attempting to move, or with anxiety or stress.
Ataxic (ataxia)	6%	Damage to the cerebellum	Ataxia is an incoordination of muscle control when a person attempts to perform voluntary muscle movements involving the arms and legs. Movements are not smooth and may appear tremulous, jerky, imprecise, unbalanced or uncoordinated.
Mixed	Common	Multiple areas of damage	Depending on the areas of brain damage, mixed motor type will involve a combination of movement disorders. Most commonly those with spasticity will also have dystonia.

Sources: Adapted from Cerebral Palsy Alliance. (2016). *Types of Cerebral Palsy.* Retrieved from <www.cerebralpalsy.org.au/what-is-cerebral-palsy/types-of-cerebral-palsy>; Crosbie, J., Alhusaini, A. A. A., Dean, C. M. & Shepherd, R. B. (2012). Plantarflexor muscle and spatiotemporal gait characteristics of children with hemiplegic cerebral palsy: An observational study. *Developmental Neurorehabilitation, 15*(2), 114–18.

The Manual Ability Classification System (MACS) is designed to describe the individual's ability to handle objects in important daily activities, such as eating, dressing or at school/work. The five levels of the MACS are presented below (adapted from Eliasson et al., 2006):

- **Level I**—Handles objects easily and successfully
- **Level II**—Handles most objects but with somewhat reduced quality and/or speed of achievement
- **Level III**—Handles objects with difficulty; needs help to prepare and/or modify activities
- **Level IV**—Handles a limited selection of easily managed objects in adapted situations
- **Level V**—Does not handle objects and has severely limited ability to perform even simple actions

The Communication Function Classification System (CFCS) describes the individual's communication ability. The five levels of the CFCS are listed below (adapted from Hidecker et al., 2011):

- **Level I**—Sends (can talk or use device) and receives (understands) with familiar and unfamiliar communication partners effectively and efficiently
- **Level II**—Sends and/or receives with unfamiliar and/or familiar communication partners but may be slower
- **Level III**—Sends and receives with familiar communication partners effectively but not with unfamiliar communication partners
- **Level IV**—Inconsistently sends and receives communication even with familiar communication partners
- **Level V**—Seldom effective sender and receiver even with familiar communication partners

The Eating and Drinking Ability Classification System (EDACS) is relatively newly developed and assists in understanding the ability individuals have with managing eating and drinking. The five levels of the EDACS are presented below (adapted from Sellers et al., 2014):

- **Level I**—Eats and drinks safely and efficiently
- **Level II**—Eats and drinks safely but with some limitation to efficiency
- **Level III**—Eats and drinks with some limitations to safety; there may be limitations to efficiency
- **Level IV**—Eats and drinks with significant limitations to safety
- **Level V**—Unable to eat or drink safely; tube feeding may be considered to provide nutrition

> The NSQHS Standards specify that health professionals must provide coordinated healthcare that is 'aligned with the patient's expressed goals of care and healthcare needs, considers the impact of the patient's health issues on their life and wellbeing, and is clinically appropriate' (ACSQHC, 2016, p. 36).

Knowing the motor type, the distribution of the disorder and an individual's classification provides a wealth of important information about someone with cerebral palsy. A person may have limited ability to walk (GMFCS Level III), good communication (CFCS Level I), adequate ability to handle objects (MACS Level II) and significant difficulties managing food and drink (EDACS Level IV). In addition, 49 per cent of individuals may have intellectual impairment (Novak et al., 2012), which may also impact on their daily functioning. As can be appreciated, no two people with cerebral palsy are the same and cannot be treated as such. Whilst the damage to the brain does not deteriorate over time, the effects of cerebral palsy on the body may result in increasing impairment. Therefore, an individualised care plan is required to meet the needs of people with this disability and those of their family.

Person-centred care

> What is an APGAR test? What assessment information does it provide?

Amelia Traynor was born at 33 weeks gestation via Caesarean section, secondary to pre-eclampsia, to Kathryn and Jim Traynor. Initial APGAR score at birth was 7 with no movement of limbs and 'floppy' muscle tone.

> Due to the complex nature of cerebral palsy, confirming a diagnosis can take some time. When it is severe, a diagnosis may be made soon after birth, but for the majority of children, diagnosis may take up to two years and require a neuro-developmental assessment, MRI, cranial ultrasound or CT scans.

This score remained unchanged at 5 and 10 minutes post-birth. Over the coming months, Amelia failed to meet developmental milestones and subsequently underwent a number of tests, observations and evaluations.

Amelia's diagnosis of spastic quadriplegic cerebral palsy was made when she was 12 months old. Her condition has resulted in the following functional impairments:

- Amelia converses with people effectively; however, she has slow and slurred speech. People who don't know Amelia take about 15 minutes to get used to how she speaks—they can then usually understand what she says (CFCS Level II).

- Amelia requires a fully supported wheelchair to help her with sitting balance, and someone to push the chair (GMFCS Level V).
- Amelia has difficulty handling objects. She needs someone to set up activities and support her to do them (MACS Level III).
- Amelia does not have an intellectual impairment.

Amelia lives with her parents in a single-story house in a metropolitan area. As a child, Amelia's mother Kathryn stopped work to provide full-time care. Both Kathryn and Jim are central to Amelia's care and have, with considerable effort, managed to juggle the demands of work and family life through a strict routine. Typically, Jim has been responsible for Amelia's physical transfers—they have a hoist in the family home to assist with this—whilst Kathryn has managed her daughter's hygiene, nutritional and health requirements. Both parents assist with socialisation, including transporting Amelia to activities. Amelia is rarely alone, accompanied by either her parents or siblings most of the time. Both parents are active in the cerebral palsy community, engaging in fundraising and community awareness programs; and Jim and Kathryn have ensured Amelia has been a central figure in these activities.

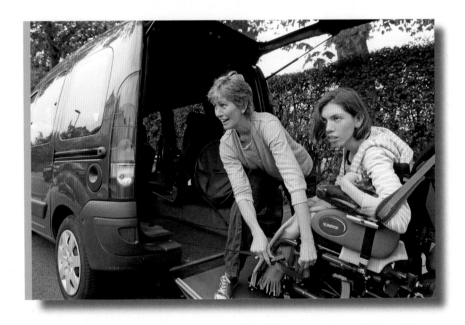

Amelia is the eldest of three children and her two siblings are Sebastian, 18 years, and Naomi, 15 years of age. The relationship between Amelia and Naomi is very close. In contrast, Sebastian, at times, speaks to his friends of resenting his older sister as he feels he has missed out on some of the opportunities and 'normal' life that his friends have had.

At the age of 19, Amelia completed secondary school. For Amelia, secondary school was characterised by her differences. While she was, on occasion, teased about her disability, a greater challenge to her self-concept was the ways in which accommodations were made for her disability; accommodations that she did not always want. Whilst Amelia knew that people meant well, she often felt that, when people went out of their way to make her feel included, it highlighted the fact she was different. As Amelia reached her late teens, these same feelings extended towards her parents as well. Consequently, over the past two years, Amelia has been yearning for greater autonomy and more independence from her mother and father.

For children and teenagers living with disability, the transition to becoming an autonomous adult may be delayed, with parents continuing to assume a significant role in decision making on behalf of their child. Amelia feels she is ready and capable of making her own decisions in relation to who provides her care, who she socialises with and when. Recently, Amelia has been chatting to friends

The Agency for Clinical Innovation and Trapeze (2014) provides useful information about planning for transition: <www.aci.health.nsw. gov.au/__data/assets/ pdf_file/0011/251696/ Key_Principles_for_ Transition.pdf>.

The Cerebral Palsy Alliance has a useful website: <www. cerebralpalsy.org.au>.

online about further studies. One friend in particular introduced her to a not-for-profit organisation called the Cerebral Palsy Alliance.

Amelia has explored programs offered by this organisation and has wondered if she might be able to receive assistance that would help her obtain future employment, and enable her to move out of home and into supported accommodation. Amelia tried to discuss this with her parents and, while her father appeared to consider the idea, her mother would not engage in any discussion. Amelia had to put such ambitions on hold due to the recent deterioration in her health.

While Amelia has always had some difficulty with eating and drinking (EDACS Level III), she has been able to maintain her ability to do so. Over the past six months, Kathryn noticed Amelia attempting to clear her throat and 'gurgling' much more frequently than usual when drinking. Following a series of assessments by her paediatrician and a speech pathologist, Amelia was gradually progressed to Grade 5 thickened fluids to minimise the risk of choking and aspiration, and to provide adequate nutritional intake. However, Amelia's dysphagia worsened and resulted in aspiration pneumonia, requiring hospitalisation.

On admission to hospital, Amelia was febrile with a temperature of 39.2°C, was tachycardic, dehydrated and lethargic. A formal assessment by a speech pathologist and radiographer, comprising video fluoroscopy, found a delayed onset of laryngeal closure and aspiration into both lungs. These assessment findings concluded that Amelia was unable to clear fluids and protect her airway due to her impaired swallow and weak cough. It was recommended that Amelia undergo a surgical insertion of a PEG for enteral nutrition and remain nil-by-mouth from this time.

1. CONSIDER THE PATIENT SITUATION

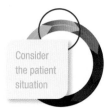

Consider the patient situation

It has been a busy morning in the surgical ward; however, you are feeling like you are doing a good job today as you have provided care according to Amelia's nursing-care plan. This has included: attending to Amelia's toileting needs; obtaining vital signs; administering her morning medications and enteral nutrition; assessing the PEG insertion site; and attending to pressure area care. You have just returned from your morning break and have collected the shower chair, towels, a clean hospital gown and the lifter to assist with transferring Amelia from bed to the shower chair.

You approach Amelia to inform her that you will be showering her shortly and that you are waiting for a second nurse to assist with the transfer. Amelia becomes agitated and states forcibly 'I have been stuck in this bed all morning. I never stay in bed this late. I feel sweaty and uncomfortable and I just want to get up, showered and in my chair.' You are unsettled by this outburst as it was handed over that Amelia is a pleasant and compliant patient. However, the awkwardness of responding to this outburst is avoided as the nurse arrives to assist with the transfer.

Once in the shower, you are relieved that Amelia appears more settled. You have almost finished the shower when Amelia asks 'Can you hand me the shower head? I like the feeling of water on my face. I can do things you know.' Whilst you're drying Amelia, she begins to open up. Here is what she says:

> What I really like is when people ask me for my opinion. I like to get up early in the morning, have a shower before breakfast and get in my chair. I don't like being in bed all day. I don't like these hospital gowns. I am not sick and would like my own clothes. Just because I have CP, people think that everything, every decision needs to be made for me. I am not a kid. I know I can do things for myself, and make decisions for myself, but even mum and dad don't see this. I love mum and dad but I feel like they control every part of my life. This PEG tube is a good example. I was not really given any choice; I had to get the tube. I hate it! I was hoping to move out of home, to have some carers my own age, to be showered and dressed by someone my own age. I want to be around people my own age rather than being dependent on my parents. I know people who have CP and they can do this. I know I can do this too, but the tube is going to make it even harder.

2. COLLECT CUES/INFORMATION

(a) Review current information

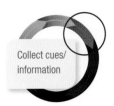

Collect cues/information

Following the shower, you reflect on the very personal information that Amelia has just shared. You realise that Amelia has a desire for autonomy—a desire that is not being met in this hospital admission, or within the family unit. You also feel unsure about what to do in this situation. You decide to start by reviewing what you know in terms of related subjective and objective data (see Table 15.2).

Table 15.2 *Subjective and objective information about Amelia*

Subjective	Objective
Amelia states her desire to: • be asked her opinion in planning her care • be showered before breakfast • select her clothes for the day • make decisions independent of her parents • move out of home and into supported accommodation • be showered and dressed by someone her own age • not be dependent on her parents.	**Medical/surgical history:** • Elective admission to an adult surgical unit for treatment of aspiration pneumonia and insertion of PEG tube • Diagnosed with spastic quadriplegic cerebral palsy at 12 months of age • Deterioration of swallow reflex and weak cough **Vital signs at 1000 hrs:** • Temperature: 37.4°C • Pulse rate: 82 (strong and regular) • Respiratory rate: 22 • Blood pressure (at rest): 134/78 mmHg • O_2 saturations: 96% (room air) • Numeric pain scale: 4/10 **Lung auscultation:** • Late inspiratory fine crackles in bases of both lungs **Integumentary:** • Skin dry and intact **Wounds:** • PEG insertion site—clean with slight serous fluid

Q Which objective assessment findings suggest Amelia's aspiration pneumonia is improving? Why?

(b) Gather new information

Nurses are familiar with conducting health history assessments. However, engaging in conversations that focus on developmental and psychosocial issues relating to disability can be challenging. Such conversations can be particularly challenging when assessing physical, emotional and social dimensions of adolescents and young adults.

> *The RCH Melbourne provides guidance for engaging with and assessing an adolescent, including communication style, how to convey confidentiality and requirements for consent: <www.rch.org.au/clinicalguide/guideline_index/Engaging_with_and_assessing_the_adolescent_patient>.*

Q1 You suspect that Amelia's health history on admission has omitted some important information needed to provide person-centred care. How would you initiate a conversation with Amelia in order to conduct a more holistic assessment?

  a 'Amelia, I want to discuss further what you were saying in the shower. You are visibly upset, so let's talk about this now and see if we can come up with a solution together.'

  b 'Let's have an open and honest conversation about what is going on in your life. Let's invite your mum as she can give some great insight into the issues you are facing.'

  c 'Amelia, thank you for opening up to me in the shower and sharing some concerns you have. I was wondering if we could talk about this some more, so we can come up with an appropriate solution together. Is now a good time?'

d   'Amelia, from what you are saying, there appears to be some urgency to this situation. I can see you're upset, but if you talk to me now I can get a routine in place to meet your needs.'

Q2   Using the following table, identify questions for each category of the HEADSSS assessment (The Royal Children's Hospital Melbourne, 2016) that would contribute to the planning of person-centred care by providing useful insights to Amelia's values, beliefs and desires.

The HEADSSS (Home; Education & Employment, Eating; Activities; Drugs & Alcohol; Sexuality; Suicide, Depression & Self-Harm; Safety from Injury & Violence) assessment tool can guide the process of psychosocial screening: <www.rch.org.au/ clinicalguide/guideline_ index/Engaging_with_ and_assessing_the_ adolescent_patient>.

Focus	Psychosocial assessment
Home	
Education and employment	
Eating	
Activities	
Drugs and alcohol	
Sexuality	
Suicide, depression and self-harm	
Safety from injury and violence	

(c) Recall knowledge

You begin to recall what you know about the role of the nurse in promoting person-centred care.

Q1   A person-centred approach to nursing care emphasises:

a   The nurses' knowledge and experience

b   The point of view of the individual as a partner in their own care

c   The nurse as the provider of care

d   An unequal power relationship between nurse and individual

Q2   An essential part of a therapeutic relationship is collaborative decision making. Collaborative decision making involves:

a   Nurse and individual agreeing on a goal

b   Negotiating the approach to achieving the goal that is most acceptable to nurse and individual

c   Combining the nurse's knowledge and experience with the individual's knowledge, perspectives and desires

d   All of the above

Q3   One of the most effective approaches to the management of disability is self-management. Self-management is when:

a   The person takes responsibility for the management of their own condition

b   There is shared responsibility between the nurse and the person in the management of their care

c   The person is independent in the management of their own care

d   The person hands the responsibility for the management of their own condition over to another

Q4   Nurses contribute to person-centred care by empowering the person so that they can manage their own care. Empowerment may involve:

a   Defining what the nurse will or will not do

b   Defining what the person will or will not do

   c   Family members speaking on behalf of the person

   d   The nurse understanding and empathising with the person's point of view, as well as negotiating and resolving conflicting expectations relating to healthcare

Q5 A critical role of the nurse is that of an advocate for the individual. Which of Amelia's statements indicate the need for patient advocacy?

   a   I feel like they (mum and dad) control every part of my life.

   b   What I really like is when people ask me for my opinion.

   c   I was not really given any choice; I had to get the (PEG) tube.

   d   I was hoping to move out of home.

   e   I like to get up early in the morning; I don't like being in bed all day.

   f   I was hoping to have some carers my own age.

   g   I was hoping to be showered and dressed by someone my own age.

   h   I am not sick and would like my own clothes.

3. PROCESS INFORMATION

(a) Interpret

The next step in the clinical reasoning cycle is to interpret the data you have collected about Amelia. Interpretation of information can be more difficult when working with data that is subjective rather than objective. In such situations, our sometimes unconscious biases may inadvertently influence the way in which data is interpreted, due to one's previous life experiences or prior expectations. This is called *ascertainment bias*, with examples including stereotyping, ageism, stigmatism and gender bias. Understanding and considering different perspectives allows nurses to plan and implement empathetic, considered and appropriate person-centred care. To better understand ascertainment bias in relation to Amelia, consider the following questions:

Q1 What are your previous life experiences and prior expectations that could influence your interpretation of the information about this situation?

Q2 The situation involves differing values, beliefs and priorities. We are aware of Amelia's values, beliefs and priorities, but those of Amelia's family are not as well known. How might they affect the situation?

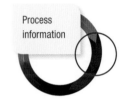

The NMBA's Registered Nurse Standards for Practice (2016) state that RNs must respect each person's dignity, culture, values, beliefs and rights. This means that, as nurses, we need to be aware of the ways our biases may influence our nursing practice.

(b) Discriminate

Amelia's scenario is complex. The subjective nature of the situation, the essential role of the family in Amelia's life and the complexity of this situation require the discrimination between what is achievable in the short term and what will take longer to achieve.

Q From the list below, select four cues that you believe are most troubling to Amelia at this time.

   a   Not being asked her preference for activities of daily living

   b   Her desire to move from home to supported accommodation

   c   Parents' involvement in the planning and implementation of Amelia's care

   d   Pain score of 4/10

   e   Temperature: 37.4°C

   f   The insertion of the PEG tube

   g   Bilateral fine crackles in the bases of both lungs

(c) Relate and (d) Infer

It is important to cluster the cues together and to identify relationships between them (based on the information you have collected so far). From these cues, you can make inferences about Amelia's situation.

Q   Label the following 'true' or 'false':

a   Due to her cerebral palsy, Amelia cannot legally provide informed consent.

b   The insertion of the PEG tube signifies for Amelia a deterioration in her condition.

c   Amelia's agitation can be attributed to a temperature of 37.4°C, abnormal lung sounds and pain score of 4/10.

d   Amelia's transition from adolescence to adulthood has been delayed due to her disability-related needs.

e   Amelia's desire for independence from her parents is not realistic due to her disability and insufficient community services.

f   Amelia requires the PEG tube as she cannot feed herself.

g   Amelia's medical diagnosis of spastic cerebral palsy will result in an inability to conceive and a limited life span.

(e) Match

If this is the first time you have encountered this kind of situation, you will probably experience feelings of uncertainty towards engaging in conversations that involve negotiating the different perspectives and desires of the person and their family.

Q   Think about people you have encountered in your everyday life who may have the same disability as Amelia. How do they appear to function independently?

(f) Predict

Now is the time to consider the consequences of your action or inaction by predicting potential outcomes for Amelia and her family.

Q   Amelia is due to be discharged tomorrow. If there is no change initiated during this admission, what might be the consequences? Using the following table, indicate whether each of the following is 'Highly Likely', 'Possible' or 'Unlikely' by placing an 'X' in the respective box.

	Highly likely	Possible	Unlikely
a Amelia's mother and father will continue to manage all aspects of Amelia's life.			
b Amelia will enrol herself into an online learning program.			
c Amelia will be empowered in self-management of her activities of daily living.			
d Amelia's psychosocial issues will not be resolved.			
e A partnership between Amelia and her mother will occur in the form of negotiating how and when nutrition will be provided.			
f Amelia will be at risk of depression or self-harm due to not 'being heard'.			

4. IDENTIFY THE PROBLEM/ISSUE

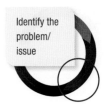

At this stage, you bring together (synthesise) all of the facts you have collected and inferences you have made to make a definitive nursing diagnosis for Amelia.

Q   Select from the following list *one* nursing diagnosis that best reflects Amelia's current situation.

   a   Ineffective health management related to aspiration, as evidenced by a medical diagnosis of aspiration pneumonia

   b   Potential for disturbed personal identity of parents related to change of roles, as evidenced by Amelia's increasing independence

   c   Infection related to PEG tube insertion site, as evidenced by temperature of 37.4°C

   d   Impeded transition to autonomous adulthood related to disability and family dynamics, as evidenced by Amelia's desire for increased independence

5. ESTABLISH GOALS

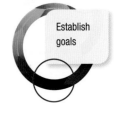

Q   From the list below, choose the three *most important* short-term (up to one week) goals for Amelia's management at this time.

   a   For Amelia to be an active participant in education relating to the care of her PEG tube and enteral nutrition

   b   Discharge Amelia to supported accommodation for people living with disability

   c   To communicate Amelia's preferences in relation to her activities of daily living by documenting these in her nursing care plan

   d   For Amelia to demonstrate autonomy in decision making and lifestyle choices, including social relationships

   e   To arrange a family meeting with Amelia and her family prior to discharge, to facilitate the beginning of discussions about Amelia's desire for increased autonomy and independence

   f   For Amelia's parents to provide Amelia greater autonomy and independence

   g   For Amelia to reach the milestones that signify progression from adolescence to adulthood

6. TAKE ACTION

> SOAP (subjective, objective, assessment and planning) is a problem-oriented technique, designed to allow nurses to describe the patient's condition and progress, and identify a plan designed to resolve the problem (Courtney-Pratt, 2015, pp. 288–89).

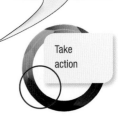

You have identified three important short-term goals to be implemented prior to Amelia's discharge tomorrow. To promote person-centred care, you communicate your assessment findings from this morning and the three goals by documenting them in the (a) nursing care plan, (b) progress notes and (c) handover to the afternoon shift. You complete the notes using the SOAP format.

Q   Using the following table, complete a progress notes entry, according to the SOAP acronym, for communicating your assessment findings and plan for Amelia.

S	
O	
A	
P	

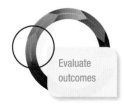

7. EVALUATE

Q It is now the end of your shift. Which of the following strategies would indicate to you that you have made a positive difference to Amelia's nursing care?

a Amelia reports that her preferences for activities of daily living are being considered by the nursing staff.

b Amelia's parents are insisting that they attend to Amelia's hygiene needs as they understand her preferences.

c Nursing staff actively engage Amelia in education regarding care of the PEG tube and enteral nutrition.

d A family meeting will be planned prior to discharge.

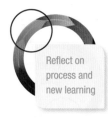

8. REFLECT

In the last stage of the clinical reasoning cycle, it is important to consider what you have learnt and how your learning will inform and shape your future practice.

Q1 What are the three most important things that you have learnt about caring for a young adult with a disability?

Q2 In what ways does therapeutic communication contribute to person-centred care for a person living with a disability who is transitioning from adolescence to young adulthood, and their family?

Q3 What do you see as the greatest challenges to nurses providing person-centred care when caring for someone with a disability?

Q4 What actions will you take in your future practice as a result of your learning from this scenario?

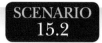

SCENARIO 15.2   Amelia's discharge

CHANGING THE SCENE

It is the morning of Amelia's discharge and you receive the handover report from the night shift:

In Bed 8 is Amelia Traynor, a 22-year-old female who was admitted four days ago for treatment of aspiration pneumonia and insertion of a PEG. Amelia slept really well overnight. She is afebrile for the first time this admission and her other vital signs are stable. PEG site is clean and dry. Her peripheral IV cannula has been removed and she continues on antibiotics via the PEG. No complaints of pain overnight. Amelia is being discharged home today, most likely this afternoon as it will take a while to get her organised. I am pretty sure her mum will be in soon if she is not already.

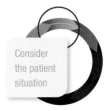

1. CONSIDER THE PATIENT SITUATION

At the completion of handover, you review Amelia's discharge paperwork. You notice that there are no entries in Amelia's progress notes that respond to the issues you communicated yesterday and you are concerned that there has been no follow-up about a family meeting, as recommended in your nursing notes and your handover.

Today, on entering Amelia's room, you see that she has been showered, is dressed in her own clothes and is already in her chair. Amelia appears pleased to see you. Whilst you are assisting Amelia with her enteral nutrition, the following conversation unfolds:

You: *The things you were talking about yesterday, you know, about wanting greater autonomy, do you still feel that way today?*

Amelia: *Yes.*

You: *Has anyone come to talk to you about a family meeting so that some of these issues can be discussed?*

Amelia: *No, I haven't spoken to anyone but you since yesterday. I'm supposed to be going home today, so I guess that means nothing will happen.*

You: *I'm not sure, but leave it with me and I'll see what we can do.*

2. COLLECT CUES/INFORMATION

(a) Review current information

You acknowledge that your concern for Amelia is based on your interpretation of what Amelia has told you. You recognise a need to gather the perspectives of Amelia's family and members of the interprofessional healthcare team for the planning of effective person-centred care.

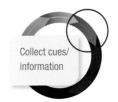

Collect cues/ information

(b) Gather new information

You decide that you need more information in order to follow up on your recommendations from yesterday. You re-read Amelia's progress notes and discharge documentation, searching for any referrals to the interprofessional team. You realise that your entry in Amelia's progress notes yesterday did not propose a plan for organising a family meeting, and you did not identify who would arrange and coordinate the meeting. You start to think about what it is that you want to achieve, and how to go about doing this.

Q1 What is a family meeting? How might it contribute to increasing Amelia's desire for autonomy?

Q2 What are the two *most relevant* reasons a family meeting should occur in Amelia's situation?

  a Family meetings are one way in which Amelia and her family can be involved in the process of planning for person-centred care, whilst being supported by nurses and members of the interprofessional healthcare team.

  b Family meetings are utilised only when family situations are complex or problematic.

  c Family meetings can be a proactive way of managing and planning person-centred care within inpatient, community and extended care contexts.

  d Family meetings provide an opportunity for family involvement in the planning of care, as it is the family who understand the person's needs best.

(c) Recall knowledge

Members of the interprofessional healthcare team involved in the planning and implementation of care will differ depending on the needs of the person, and in Amelia's case, the family. You consider the healthcare professionals who would positively contribute to a family meeting for Amelia.

See Gonda and Hales (2015) for a summary of the roles of health providers in Australia.

Q Using the following table, match the healthcare professional with their role description.

Health professional		Description
1	Registered nurse	**a** Assists people with impaired function to gain the skills to adapt and perform activities of daily living, or modifies the environment to enable this
2	Case manager	**b** Diagnoses and treats dental health problems

Health professional		Description
3 Dentist	c	A range of professionals (e.g. lab technicians/ radiographers) who use specialised tests and objective data to inform the diagnosis and treatment of health problems
4 Dietitian	d	Prepares and dispenses pharmaceuticals in the hospital and community setting
5 Pharmacist	e	Assists clients with musculoskeletal, cardiovascular or respiratory problems. Services are provided in inpatient or community settings
6 Occupational therapist	f	Counsels individuals and their support persons regarding finances, accommodation services and community supports. A significant role is connecting individuals and their families to government services
7 Health technician	g	Has specialised knowledge regarding diets required to maintain health and treat disease
8 Physiotherapist	h	Responsible for health promotion and health prevention, as well as the medical diagnosis and the medical therapy required for a person with a disease or injury
9 Medical officer	i	Diagnoses and treats foot conditions
10 Social worker	j	Assesses a patient's health status, identifies health problems and develops and coordinates care
11 Patient care attendant/assistant in nursing	k	Ensures that patients receive fiscally sound, appropriate care in the best setting. This role may be fulfilled by any member of the healthcare team, but usually one who is most involved in the person's care
12 Podiatrist	l	Health staff who assume delegated aspects of basic care
13 Speech pathologist	m	Has specialised knowledge in the study, diagnosis and treatment of communication and swallowing disorders

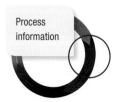

Process information

3. PROCESS INFORMATION

(a) Interpret and (b) Discriminate

The next step of the clinical reasoning cycle is to interpret the information that you have collected and, while applying your knowledge about Amelia, narrow down this information to what is most important.

Q1 Based on the information collected, which do you believe are the most relevant health professionals to be present at the family meeting?

a Case manager

b Dentist

c Dietitian

d Health technician

e Medical officer

    f   Occupational therapist

    g   Patient care attendant

    h   Pharmacist

    i   Physiotherapist

    j   Podiatrist

    k   Registered nurse

    l   Social worker

    m   Speech pathologist

Q2   Who would you suggest performs the role of case manager?

(c) Relate and (d) Infer

Q   Drawing on your knowledge from the previous stages of the clinical reasoning cycle, which of the following are realistic contributions from each participant in the family meeting?

    a   The *speech pathologist* will provide information about the aetiology of Amelia's aspiration and the pathophysiology of her impaired swallow. The speech pathologist will provide exercises to enable Amelia to safely manage oral secretions. The speech pathologist may also assist Amelia to identify 'safe' foods for social eating or eating pleasure.

    b   The *social worker* will provide information about government services, not-for-profit support groups, options for supported accommodation and strategies for facilitating Amelia's transition, increasing autonomy and independence. Importantly, the social worker will facilitate the transfer of Amelia's case to a case manager in the community.

    c   The *registered nurse* will provide documented evidence related to Amelia's trajectory of care during the hospitalisation, and advocate for the person by reporting Amelia's stated desire for autonomy in her healthcare decisions and greater independence.

    d   *Amelia* will have the opportunity to voice her perspectives, values and desires to her parents, in an environment that is supported by the interprofessional healthcare team.

    e   The *medical officer* will inform the meeting about Amelia's medical needs from this admission and options for medical support in the community.

    f   *Kathryn, Jim, Sebastian* and *Naomi* will be provided with an opportunity to voice their perspectives, values and desires in an environment that is supported by the interprofessional healthcare team.

    g   The *occupational therapist* will provide advice and support related to adaptive strategies for promoting autonomy and interdependence, either at home or in supported accommodation. This can include accessing health packages and the NDIS, and consideration of vocational preparation planning. They may also assist with designing an adaptive approach if Amelia wishes to contribute to the practical aspects of managing the administration of enteral nutrition and PEG care.

    h   The *case manager* will co-ordinate the meeting and ensure everyone's voice is heard. Importantly, the case manager will facilitate a process of negotiation in order to establish a plan of action that is agreed upon by all participants of the family meeting.

    i   The *dietitian* will provide advice about meeting nutritional requirements, frequency and timing of enteral feeds, and issues relating to infection control. This will include education and a plan for meeting daily nutritional needs, as well as follow-up requirements post discharge.

(e) Match

Q   Have you ever participated in a family meeting (also known as a case conference)? If so, who was present and what did they contribute?

(f) Predict

Now is the time to consider the possible consequences for the planning process by predicting the probable outcomes of the family meeting.

Q   Which of the following possible outcomes of the family meeting is the most probable?

    a The concerns of each participant will be heard and resolved during the family meeting.

    b The concerns of each participant will be heard and a plan comprising short-term goals will be developed.

    c The concerns of each participant will be heard and a plan comprising short- and long-term goals will be developed.

    d The concerns of each participant will be heard and a plan comprising long-term goals will be developed.

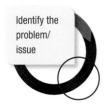
Identify the problem/issue

4. IDENTIFY THE PROBLEM/ISSUE

At this stage of the clinical reasoning cycle, you bring together (synthesise) all of the facts you have collected, and all of the inferences you have made to make definitive nursing diagnoses for Amelia and her family.

Q   From the following list, identify two nursing diagnoses that best reflect the situation confronting Amelia and her family.

    a Altered family processes, and change to family roles and structure related to increased autonomy and independence, as evidenced by changes to long-standing roles and uncertainty.

    b Knowledge deficit (of parents) related to disability services, as evidenced by parents fulfilling role as primary carer.

    c Risk of self-concept disturbance (of parents) related to altered role performance and self-esteem disturbance, as evidenced by implementation of strategies to promote Amelia's autonomy.

    d Decisional conflict related to multiple or divergent sources of information, as evidenced by verbalised uncertainty about choices or decisions.

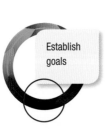
Establish goals

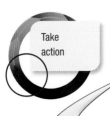
Take action

5. ESTABLISH GOALS AND 6. TAKE ACTION

As has been seen in this chapter, young adults such as Amelia who are living with a disability encounter a number of unique challenges that can impede, hinder and delay achieving the milestones of adulthood. The primary goal of person-centred care is to support the person's rights to self-determination and autonomy, by providing them with sufficient information to participate in decision-making processes and maintain a feeling of being in control.

In relation to planning care that is person-centred, the management goals should be SMART:

- **S**pecific
- **M**easurable
- **A**chievable
- **R**ealistic
- **T**imely

Stanley (2015, p. 346) provides insight into the impact of illness on the individual and their family.

It is important to begin the process of planning care by asking Amelia and her family to identify three goals: one short-term (achievable in two to three weeks), one medium-term (achievable within two months), and one long-term (achievable within six months). For people who are transitioning from adolescence to young adulthood, the goals need to be specific and realistic and, most importantly, things that both Amelia and her family want to achieve.

Q The plan represented in the following table provides examples of possible goals for Amelia and her family. Add to the table one more short-, medium- and long-term goal for Amelia.

> *For further information about quality care plans for community care, go to Chapter 3 of The Goal Directed Care Planning Toolkit: <http://kpassoc.com.au/wp-content/uploads/2014/07/Goal-Directed-Care-Planning-Toolkit-Web-version.pdf>.*

Goal	Actions	Person(s) responsible	Time frame	Review date	Outcomes
Short term					
1. Amelia will increase her autonomy in decision making for her own care.	Ask Amelia what decisions she would like to make about her care.	Amelia Kathryn and Jim Healthcare team	2–3 weeks		
2. Amelia will begin to be involved in the management of PEG and enteral nutrition.	Provide Amelia with opportunities to participate in the day-to-day care of her PEG and enteral nutrition.	Amelia Kathryn Community nurse Dietitian	2–3 weeks		
3.					
Medium term					
1. Amelia will receive community support to assist with ADLs and socialisation.	Involve Amelia in the process of selecting carers.	Case manager Social worker Community support services	2–3 months		
2. Amelia will develop an identity as an autonomous young adult.	Provide Amelia with opportunities to socialise independently of her family.	Parents Amelia Case manager Friends	2–3 months		
3.					
Long term					
1. Amelia will enrol in an online course of her choosing.	Provide Amelia with assistance to research courses and enrol.	Amelia Person of Amelia's choosing	6 months		
2. Amelia will begin the transition to supported accommodation.	Provide Amelia with assistance to research supported accommodation options.	Amelia Case manager/ social worker	6 months		
3.					

Source: Adapted from Pascale, K. (2013). *The Goal Directed Care Planning Toolkit: Practical Strategies to Support Effective Goal Setting and Care Planning with HACC Clients.* Melbourne, Victoria: Eastern Metropolitan Region (EMR) HACC Alliance, Outer Eastern Health and Community Services Alliance.

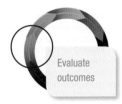

7. EVALUATE

In complex situations such as the one portrayed in this chapter, it can be difficult for members of the interprofessional healthcare team to predict the effectiveness of the planned actions to be put into place. It is therefore important to think about how the actions may be evaluated at the time of establishing goals.

Q1   Based on the statements in the following table, evaluate the effectiveness of the planned actions after a period of three months, based upon the following statements. Label each as 'effective' or 'ineffective'.

Amelia is . . .	Rating
. . . guiding carers or her siblings on how to administer her enteral nutrition and clean the equipment after use.	a
. . . planning her ADLs around a schedule that she has determined, in collaboration with her parents and community support services.	b
. . . feeling guilt about her parents refusal to acknowledge her desire to move to supported accommodation.	c
. . . meeting new friends through new social groups and activities.	d
. . . uncertain about her role in contributing to Sebastian's decision to move out of home.	e
. . . engaging in conversation with her family about the new challenges she is encountering through her increasing independence.	f
. . . researching online accounting courses through VET and university providers.	g

Q2   In this chapter, we have explored issues of delayed transition from adolescence to adulthood for people living with disability. Why do you believe the parents of a child with a disability may contribute to the delayed transition of their child?

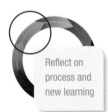

8. REFLECT

In the last stage of the clinical reasoning cycle, it is important to consider what you have learnt and how your learning will inform your future practice.

Reflect on your learning from this scenario and consider the following questions.

Q1   What are the three most important things that you have learnt from this scenario?

Q2   If you were caring for a person living with a disability, what might you change in your approach to person-centred care?

Q3   What might you do if you come across a person (patient) or their family where there appears to be a conflict in perspectives, values or desires?

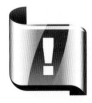

Something to think about . . .

For people who do not live (or have not lived) with disability, understanding the impact of disability on everyday life is difficult to appreciate. In 2009, the Australian Government Department of Social Services published a consultation paper titled SHUT OUT: The experience of people with disabilities and their families in Australia *(Commonwealth of Australia, 2009), available at <www.dss.gov.au/sites/default/files/documents/05_2012/nds_report.pdf>.*

This paper provides stark insight into the worlds of people living with disability. Pay particular attention to the story of 'D' (Chapter 2.7: 'Isolated and alone'—the social experience of disability, 53).

EPILOGUE

Amelia continues to live with her family. She feels she has a better 'relationship' with her PEG tube and, while she cannot administer the enteral nutrition herself, she knows she can time her 'feeds' to the mealtimes of her family or friends, and can direct people to administer the enteral nutrition. Amelia has also developed the confidence to tell people her preferences for positioning the PEG tube and setting up her feeding equipment in a way that is inconspicuous.

Strategies developed through regular community-care meetings, coordinated by her community case manager, have enabled Amelia to select and manage her personal carers (of her own age), manage her finances and begin navigation of the social services available to her. For the first time in her life, Amelia has been going out at night with friends, independent of her parents. Amelia still plans to move to supported accommodation in the future, but she understands that this transition will take time.

FURTHER READING

Gonda, J. & Hales, M. (2015). Health care delivery systems. In A. Berman, S. J. Snyder, B. Kozier, G. L. Erb, T. Levett-Jones, T. Dwyer, … D. Stanley (Eds), *Kozier and Erb's Fundamentals of Nursing* (3rd Australian edn). Melbourne, Australia: Pearson.

Stanley, D. (2015). Health, wellness and illness. In A. Berman, S. J. Snyder, B. Kozier, G. L. Erb, T. Levett-Jones, T. Dwyer, … D. Stanley (Eds), *Kozier and Erb's Fundamentals of Nursing* (3rd Australian edn). Melbourne, Australia: Pearson.

REFERENCES

Access Economics. (2008). *The Economic Impact of Cerebral Palsy in Australia in 2007*. Access Economics Pty Ltd, for Cerebral Palsy Australia.

Agency for Clinical Innovation and Trapeze. (2014). *Key Principles for Transition of Young People from Paediatric to Adult Health Care*. Accessed March 2017 at <www.aci.health.nsw.gov.au/__data/assets/pdf_file/0011/251696/Key_Principles_for_Transition.pdf>.

Australian Cerebral Palsy Register Group. (2013). *Australian Cerebral Palsy Register: Report 2013*. Accessed March 2017 at <wwwthoracic.org.au/documents/papers/aprghomeventilationguideline.pdf>.

Australian Commission on Safety and Quality in Health Care (ACSQHC). (2016). *National Safety and Quality Health Service Standards Version 2*. Draft, Sydney, Australia.

Commonwealth of Australia. (2009). *SHUT OUT: The Experiences of People with Disabilities and Their Families in Australia*. Australian Government Department of Social Services. Accessed March 2017 at <www.dss.gov.au/sites/default/files/documents/05_2012/nds_report.pdf>.

Courtney-Pratt, H. (2015). Documenting and reporting. In A. Berman, S. J. Snyder, B. Kozier, G. L. Erb, T. Levett-Jones, T. Dwyer, … D. Stanley (Eds), *Kozier and Erb's Fundamentals of Nursing* (3rd Australian edn). Melbourne, Australia: Pearson.

Eliasson, A. C., Krumlinde-Sundholm, L., Rosblad, B., Beckung, E., Arner, M., Ohrvall, A. & Rosenbaum, P. (2006). The Manual Ability Classification System (MACS) for children with cerebral palsy: Scale development and evidence of validity and reliability. *Developmental Medicine & Child Neurology*, *48*(7), 549–54.

Furlong, A. (2009). Introduction. In *Handbook of Youth and Young Adulthood: New Perspectives and Agendas*. Milton Park, New York: Routledge.

Hewitt-Taylor, J. (2008). *Providing Support at Home for Children and Young People Who Have Complex Health Needs*. West Sussex, UK: John Wiley & Sons Ltd.

Hidecker, M. J. C., Paneth, N., Rosenbaum, P. L., Kent, R. D., Lillie, J., Eulenberg, J. B., … Taylor, K. (2011). Developing and validating the Communication Function Classification System for individuals with cerebral palsy. *Developmental Medicine & Child Neurology*, *55*(8), 704–10.

Novak, I., Hines, M., Goldsmith, S. & Barclay, R. (2012). Clinical prognostic messages from a systematic review on cerebral palsy. *Pediatrics*, *130*(5), e1285–312.

Nursing and Midwifery Board of Australia (NMBA). (2016). *Registered Nurse Standards for Practice*. Retrieved from <www.nursingmidwiferyboard.gov.au/Codes-Guidelines-Statements/Professional-standards.aspx>.

Palisano, R. J., Rosenbaum, P. L., Bartlett, D. & Livingston, M. H. (2008). Content validity of the expanded and revised gross motor function classification system. *Developmental Medicine & Child Neurology*, *50*(10), 744–50.

Rosenbaum, P., Paneth, N., Leviton, A., Goldstein, M. & Bax, M. (2007). A report: The definition and classification of cerebral palsy, April 2006. *Developmental Medicine & Child Neurology*, *49*(Suppl 49), 8–14.

Rosenbaum, P. L. & Rosenbloom, L. (2012). *Cerebral Palsy: From Diagnosis to Adult Life*. London, UK: Mac Keith Press.

Sellers, D., Mandy, A., Pennington, L., Hankins, M. & Morris, C. (2014). Development and reliability of a system to classify the eating and drinking ability of people with cerebral palsy. *Developmental Medicine & Child Neurology*, *56*(3), 245–51.

The Royal Children's Hospital Melbourne. (2016). *Clinical Practice Guidelines: Engaging with and Assessing the Adolescent Patient*. Accessed March 2017 at <www.rch.org.au/clinicalguide/guideline_index/Engaging_with_and_assessing_the_adolescent_patient>.

PHOTO CREDIT

CHAPTER 16

CARING FOR A PERSON REQUIRING PALLIATIVE CARE

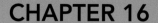

PAMELA VAN DER RIET AND VICTORIA PITT

LEARNING OUTCOMES

Completion of the activities in this chapter will enable you to:

○ explain why an understanding of palliative care and complementary therapies is important for competent practice (**recall** and **application**)

○ identify the clinical manifestations of constipation, terminal dehydration and terminal restlessness that will guide the collection and interpretation of cues (**gather, review, interpret, discriminate, relate** and **infer**)

○ review clinical information to identify the main nursing diagnoses for a person requiring palliative and end-of-life care (**synthesise**)

○ describe the priorities of care for a person requiring palliative and end-of-life care, taking into account their physical, psychological, social and spiritual needs (**goal setting** and **taking action**)

○ discuss the role and responsibilities of the palliative care team (**taking action**)

○ identify factors that impact on the quality of end-of-life care

○ identify clinical criteria for determining the effectiveness of nursing actions taken to manage pain, constipation, terminal restlessness and terminal dehydration (**evaluate**)

○ apply what you have learnt about palliative care to new situations (**reflection** and **translation**).

INTRODUCTION

This chapter focuses on the care of a 37-year-old woman with metastatic breast cancer. You will be introduced to Sally Abraham and follow her journey through palliative care.

The World Health Organization (WHO, 2011) defines palliative care as an approach that improves the quality of life of people who face life-threatening illness, and their families, by providing pain and symptom relief, and spiritual and psychosocial support, from diagnosis to the end of life and bereavement. Palliative care enables people facing death to be as free as possible from unnecessary suffering, to maintain their dignity and independence throughout the experience, to be cared for in an environment of their choice, to have their grief needs recognised and responded to, and to be assured that their family's needs are being met (Palliative Care Australia, 2011).

Caring for a person undergoing palliative care not only requires effective clinical reasoning skills but also requires the nurse to practise in a way that is holistic, person-centred and respectful. Holistic healthcare emphasises the importance of the individual as a whole being within a social, cultural, spiritual and environmental context, rather than a person with isolated malfunction of a particular system or organ (Walton & Sullivan, 2004; Mason, 2014; Kittelson, Eli & Pennypacker, 2015). Dying with dignity involves physical comfort, autonomy, meaningfulness, usefulness, preparedness and interpersonal connection, and is a critical principle of palliative care (Proulx & Jacelon, 2004; Oechsle et al., 2014).

Dying is influenced by the patient's beliefs, values, history, emotions and culture (van der Riet et al., 2009). Although this can be challenging for novice nurses, the clinical reasoning cycle provides a coherent framework for working confidently through the complexities inherent in palliative care.

This chapter also discusses the use of complementary therapies in the context of palliative care. Complementary therapies have been referred to as 'those healing practices, technologies, perspectives and products (within a given country and time) that are not an established component of conventional medicine' (Adams, 2007, p. xix). The use of complementary therapies is founded on a belief in holism and the nurturing of the mind, body and spirit as inseparable elements of health. Complementary therapies create opportunities for nurses to provide a more holistic and innovative approach to patient care (Smith, 2009; van der Riet, 2011). However, nurses need to be familiar with specific practices so that they can assist patients to make informed decisions about the use of these therapies, thus preventing adverse outcomes.

KEY CONCEPTS

palliative care
complementary therapies
holistic care
terminal dehydration
terminal restlessness
dying with dignity

SUGGESTED READINGS

P. LeMone, K. Burke, G. Bauldoff, P. Gubrud-Howe, T. Levett-Jones, T. Dwyer ... D. Raymond (Eds). (2017). *Medical–Surgical Nursing: Critical Thinking in Person-Centred Care* (3rd edn). Melbourne: Pearson.

Chapter 5: Nursing care of clients experiencing loss, grief and death

SCENARIO 16.1   The palliative care journey begins

SETTING THE SCENE

Sally Abraham is a 37-year-old single mother who was recently referred to the palliative care outreach team with metastatic breast cancer. When asked about her experiences by the palliative care nurse, Sally recounted her story as follows:

I was 25 when I was diagnosed … I found a lump in my breast and I went to my GP. My daughter was 2 years old and I thought it was probably a blocked milk duct. The GP wasn't worried. I had a mammogram but it didn't show anything. So I had an ultrasound because the GP could feel the lump. The ultrasound found that there were three lumps in my breast.

So I went into hospital to have a biopsy done and found out it was breast cancer. I had a partial mastectomy and two months of radiotherapy. Everything was clear for two and a half years, but then two lumps came up in the initial site and one under my arm. So I had a full mastectomy, followed by six months of chemotherapy. Six weeks later, another lump came up in the scar. This went on for about six years … it seemed never ending.

Around this time the oncologist told me I couldn't have any more radiotherapy, that I had already had my limit. He said I could have one more round of chemotherapy but he didn't like my chances and that I probably had around six months to live. I walked out of there really angry with him. I was told to just go home and wait basically …

I cried all the way home from the hospital. When I pulled up in the driveway, I was thinking, 'How do I tell my daughter Olivia that I am not going to live long enough to raise her? She's only 11 years old and I'm a single mum.' I couldn't work out a way to do it. So I called my family and said, 'This is what the doctor said. I am going to do everything I can to fight it, but I'm not going to have another round of chemo.'

At first, I cried and cried for weeks, thinking, 'Oh … I am dying … This is really going to happen. I am really going to die.' But then I went to a herbalist, and there on the bookstand in the health food shop was a book with this guy with one leg on the cover and the words, 'You can conquer cancer'. So I bought the book, and took it home and read it. It's by Ian Gawler, and that's when I started looking at complementary therapies, because the medical profession couldn't offer me anything at all.

Two years later and I have used a lot of complementary therapies; and I've visited a herbalist and psychotherapist. I began to actually say, 'OK, well, we are all going to die anyway. We are all born terminal.' So I planned my funeral, I wrote my will and did all of that. I told Olivia that I loved her every day and started playing meditation tapes all the time; so she was meditating too, whether she liked it or not [joking tone]. She had all these positive affirmation tapes. We only live in a little caravan but she's one of the calmest children I know.

But I have lost my family. They became angry with my decision and said, 'What are you doing, not having the chemo? You're drinking all these carrot juices and seeing this guru fella [psychotherapist]. We see you sitting with your legs crossed and it's just so strange. You've got unrealistic expectations and you're giving your daughter false hopes too.'

I love my family but I needed to be positive and I couldn't deal with their negativity. I don't understand why they are like this. So I had to make a terrible decision: I just don't go there anymore. So I don't have any support from family, and I don't have any real friends; people don't know what to say, how to act or what to do. So Olivia and I are on our own. Her dad is not in the picture and I worry what will happen to her if … when … I die.

To find out more about the investigations used to identify breast cancer, see <https://canceraustralia.gov.au/publications-and-resources/position-statements/early-detection-breast-cancer>.

The stages of grief vary between individuals. Can you trace the stages of Sally's grief as she narrates her story, referencing Elisabeth Kübler-Ross' stages of grief: denial, anger, bargaining, depression and acceptance? (Elisabeth Kübler-Ross Foundation, 2012): <www.ekrfoundation.org/five-stages-of-grief>.

Mindfulness meditation has many benefits, including reduced stress (Yazdanimehr et al., 2016; Bower et al., 2015), enhanced personal wellbeing (Sears et al., 2011), reduced cortisol levels and improved immune response (Ernst, Pittler & Wider 2006).

The epidemiology of breast cancer

In Australia, breast cancer is the cancer with the highest incidence for women (Australian Institute of Health and Welfare [AIHW], 2010). It can occur at any age, but it is more common in women over the age of 60. Men can also develop breast cancer, although this is quite rare. Although the pathogenesis of breast cancer is not known, in about 5 per cent of women there is a genetic link involving two breast cancer genes, known as BRCA1 and BRCA2 (Cancer Institute NSW, 2008). There have been many risk factors identified in the literature, which include getting older, geographic location (country of origin), socioeconomic status, reproductive events, exogenous hormones, lifestyle risk factors (alcohol, diet, obesity and physical activity), familial history of breast cancer, mammographic density and history of benign breast disease (Dumitrescu & Cotarla, 2005).

Access Australia's Health (AIHW, 2010) to find out more about the incidence, mortality, death rate and survival rate for breast cancer.

Complementary therapies

Australia has the highest utilisation of complementary therapies in the developed world (Reid et al., 2016) with one in four people using complementary therapies and over $2 billion being spent on complementary therapies annually (Adams, 2006). In the period 1995 to 2005, the number of people visiting a complementary health professional in Australia increased by 51 per cent (Australian Bureau of Statistics, 2008). There is a growing body of evidence indicating that complementary therapies make a significant and cost-effective contribution to the health of the community, especially in relation to cancer management and palliative care (Mansky & Wallerstedy, 2006). With the increased interest in complementary therapies, there is a need to ensure that these practices are safe, cause no harm and are used to enhance wellbeing (McCabe, 2005; van der Riet, Francis & Levett-Jones, 2011).

Access the Cancer Council NSW website to learn more about the use of complementary therapies in cancer.

Many complementary therapies include a combination of pharmacological and non-pharmacological components, such as the oils used in aromatherapy, herbal therapies or 'medicines' prepared by Chinese traditional healers. It is common for people to believe that, because complementary medicines are 'natural' products, they must be good for you. However, like all medicines there are potential risks associated with some complementary medicines (van der Riet, Francis & Levett-Jones, 2011; Sheppard-Hanger & Hanger, 2015). For example, while there is evidence to support the effect of St John's wort in depression and kava for use in the treatment of anxiety disorders (Larzelere, Campbell & Robertson, 2010), there are safety warnings against these products being taken in conjunction with prescribed antidepressants or anti-anxiolytics. Another common example of a self-prescribed and self-administered complementary medicine is echinacea, a remedy for the common cold, which has over 20 known side effects, including asthma attacks, aching muscles and stomach upsets (National Prescribing Service, 2010).

For more information about specific complementary therapies, see <www.mskcc.org/cancer-care/interactive-medicine/about-herbs-botanicals-other-products>.

The use of complementary therapies in palliative care is common in oncology patients (Tovey, Chatwin & Broom, 2007; Lui et al., 2016). Many of these therapies, in particular massage (Kotsirilos, Vitetta & Sali, 2011; Henneghan & Harrison, 2015), music therapy (Gallagher, Lagman & Walsh, 2006), meditation (McDonald, Burjan & Martin, 2006), and aromatherapy (Kotsirilos, Vitetta & Sali, 2011), do contribute to a reduction in anxiety and improved quality of life for this group of patients. However, safety should always be an important consideration. For example, people who have had chemotherapy may have a reduction in their platelets and a vigorous massage could cause bleeding. This is not to say that massage should not be used; however, nurses should use this modality with care and carefully assess the patient's condition first.

Who are the members of the palliative care team? What are their roles? See <www.caresearch.com.au/caresearch/ProfessionalGroups/tabid/55/Default.aspx>.

Models of palliative care

1. The palliative approach (primary model of care)

This model involves a palliative approach where cure is not an option. Symptom-management-focused care is usually implemented within residential care facilities for the older person, where the goal is to improve the resident's level of comfort by providing holistic and person-centred care. General care is provided by the usual professional carers of the resident and family. The level of palliative care required is regarded as low to moderate.

2. Specialised palliative care provision (tertiary)

In this model, the patients and their symptoms require extra attention. Symptoms may involve pain, breathlessness, nausea and/or vomiting. In this model, care is provided for patients and their families with moderate to high palliative care needs. Referral to the interprofessional palliative care team is required. The goal is one of assessment and management of complex symptoms.

3. End-of-life care (terminal care)

This usually involves the final days or weeks of life. Here the focus is very much on physical, emotional and spiritual comfort, and support for the family (Palliative Care Curriculum for Undergraduates [PCC4U], 2011).

> *The NSQHS Standards highlight the importance of coordinated delivery as an integral part of caring for an individual at the end of life (ACSQHC, 2016). Coordinated delivery of care involves collaboration, partnership and communication between all team members, with compassionate care the central tenet.*

1. CONSIDER THE PATIENT SITUATION

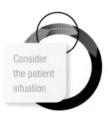

Consider the patient situation

Morning handover for the outreach palliative care team

Sally Abraham is a 37-year-old woman recently referred to the Outreach Community Palliative Care Service with a primary diagnosis of breast cancer and bone secondaries. Her initial visit was last week. She called last night with increasing generalised pain, nausea and vomiting. She is on MS Contin 120 mg BD and morphine (Ordine) elixir 40 mg PRN for breakthrough pain. Sally said she is also using complementary therapies; I'm not sure which ones. She is not keen to be admitted to the hospice for symptom management and wants to stay at home as long as she can. But she lives in a caravan with her 14-year-old daughter and has limited family support. Sally's mum and dad live locally but they are estranged.

2. COLLECT CUES/INFORMATION

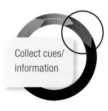

Collect cues/ information

(a) Review current information

You are one of the nurses from the palliative care service. When you visit Sally, she tells you that her pain is worse and that she hasn't been getting around much. Olivia tells you that her mum has been nauseated; she made her ginger tea but she hasn't been able to eat anything solid for a few days.

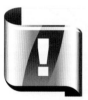
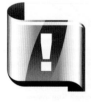

Something to think about ...

People requiring palliative care may experience a range of symptoms depending on the underlying pathology of the disease, co-morbidities and other psychological, social and environmental factors. Preventing, minimising and treating these symptoms is an important part of the nurse's role. Some of the most common physical symptoms include fatigue, pain, dyspnoea, anorexia and constipation. Each of these alone or in combination causes suffering. The onset or exacerbation of symptoms can signal disease progression and this can cause additional emotional distress, anxiety and depression. A person's symptoms don't always follow a predictable pattern; they are experienced differently by each person and have multiple contributing factors and effects (PCC4U, 2011).

(b) Gather new information

> *Review the comprehensive Symptom Assessment Scale (SAS) at this link: <http://ahsri.uow.edu.au/pcoc/sas/index.html>.*

Effective and accurate clinical assessment skills are imperative for the nurse working in palliative care. The comprehensive Symptom Assessment Scale (SAS) (Palliative Care Outcomes Collaboration, 2011) is one of the recommended assessment tools of the Australian Palliative Care Outcomes Collaboration.

A comprehensive symptom assessment typically includes:

- An evaluation of contributing factors

- Characteristics of the symptoms (such as intensity, location, quality, temporal nature, frequency and associated pattern of disability)

- The meaning of the symptom(s) to the person (including beliefs about the symptom(s) and the effect on the person's physical, psychological and social wellbeing)

- Behavioural responses to the symptom(s) (such as the actions that the person is taking to manage or cope) (PCC4U, 2011).

Q   You begin your physical assessment of Sally. Rank the following assessments according to level of importance based on your response to the handover report.

   a   Vital signs

   b   Mobility assessment

   c   Falls assessment

   d   Pain assessment

   e   Abdominal distention and bowel (elimination) assessments

   f   Assessment of nausea/vomiting

   g   Medication history

   h   Assessment of fatigue

   i   Assessment of breathlessness/dyspnoea

   j   Family/carer/social supports

There are seven main principles of pain management in palliative care:

1. Listen to the patient; involve the family.

2. Determine the cause of the pain and treat.

3. Anticipate pain and anticipate side effects of drugs.

4. Start using the least invasive route and follow the WHO analgesic ladder.

5. Give medication regularly 'by the clock' and give PRN doses; use a combination of drugs.

6. Give the right drug and dose to treat the type of pain without unpleasant side effects.

7. Conduct regular reassessment of pain.

> *Review the World Health Organization's pain ladder at <www.who.int/cancer/palliative/painladder/en/>.*

You review Sally's medication regime and note that she has been taking MS Contin 120 mg BD and morphine (Ordine) elixir 40 mg for breakthrough pain. She has had three breakthroughs in the last 24 hours. She tells you that this is 'just not holding her pain though'.

(c) Recall knowledge

How confident are you about your knowledge of palliative care nursing?

QUICK QUIZ!

Q1   Individuals with which life-limiting illnesses may access palliative care services?

   a   Breast cancer

   b   Motor neuron disease

   c   Leukemia

   d   Melanoma

   e   Chronic obstructive pulmonary disease

   f   All of the above

Q2   Your own values and beliefs about death and dying may impact on your interactions with a dying person, which is why self-awareness is such an important strategy for the palliative care nurse. True or false?

Q3   Fill in the missing word. _____ is the most common strong opioid used to treat cancer-related pain.

Q4 Fill in the missing word. _____ are found within opioids (morphine, oxycodone and hydromorphone) and have the potential to accumulate in patients, with renal impairment causing tremors and delirium.

Q5 For MS Contin, which of the following statements are true and which are false?

    a   MS Contin is an opioid drug.

    b   MS Contin is a non-opioid drug.

    c   MS Contin is used for breakthrough pain.

    d   MS Contin is a slow-release drug.

    e   MS Contin can be crushed for easier administration.

    f   MS Contin should never be cut or crushed.

Q6 Which of the following is the reason that pethidine is rarely used for pain relief in palliative care?

    a   It has a strong odour.

    b   There is the potential for accumulation of toxic metabolite.

    c   It is a drug of addiction.

    d   It is too long acting.

Q7 What are the potential side effects of opioids? (Select the five correct answers.)

    a   Tachycardia

    b   Nausea

    c   Polydipsia

    d   Drowsiness

    e   Hypertension

    f   Constipation

    g   Confusion

    h   Hallucinations

    i   Vivid dreams

    j   Anxiety

Sally uses a number of complementary therapies, including:

- Bovine cartilage powder (oral)
- Ginger tea
- Juices (carrot, beetroot and celery) three times a day
- Slippery elm powder, bovine powder and lavender oil made into a paste for skin irritation on her chest wall
- Echinacea

Although you are not expected to have an extensive knowledge of all complementary therapies, it is important that you have a general understanding of their use.

Something to think about …

People seek complementary therapies for a number of reasons, for example to maintain control, to provide hope and to retain an active part in one's treatment process. To gain an understanding of information you might provide to a person seeking advice about complementary therapies, access the Cancer Council's site:

    <www.cancercouncil.com.au/1302/get_informed/treating_cancer/cancer_treatment/understanding_ complementary_therapies_how_treated/?pp=1303>.

Q8 Sally thinks about visiting another complementary therapy provider and asks you what questions she should ask. What would be the appropriate reply?

   a What side effects could there be?

   b What is the evidence for the success of the therapy?

   c They are only after your money, so I wouldn't waste your time.

   d How much will the therapy cost?

   e a, b and d.

Q9 The action of bovine cartilage powder is to:

   a Reduce inflammation and pain in the joints and lower back

   b Assist in the prevention of cold and influenza

   c Cure breast cancer

   d Treat nausea and vomiting

Q10 The action of echinacea is to:

   a Reduce inflammation and pain in the joints and lower back

   b Boost the immune system and help the body fight infections such as the common cold

   c Promote gastric emptying

   d Manage pain

> *When caring for an individual with a life-limiting illness, you also need to care for the caregivers. Consider the experience of Sally's family and how the stages of grief are evident in their experiences.*

A major concern for Sally is her current lack of social support. She tells you that her family became very dismissive when she wanted to talk about her use of complementary therapies and told her she was just giving herself and her daughter false hope. Sally also tells you that she has not talked to her GP about her complementary therapy use as she is sure he does not believe in their effectiveness.

Understanding why a person uses complementary therapies can assist health professionals to gain a more comprehensive understanding of their patient's needs. There are various reasons why people with cancer use complementary therapies, but research (O'Callaghan, 2011) has demonstrated that these therapies are primarily used to improve quality of life by reducing the physical and emotional side effects of the disease. O'Callaghan's review of the literature noted that individuals rarely sought complementary therapies as a cure, and that negotiating control of their lives and health was a more important reason for use.

> *See O'Callaghan (2011) for further information regarding 'Patients' perception of complementary and alternative medicine': <www.cancerforum.org.au/Issues/2011/March/Forum/Patients_perceptions_complementary_alternative.htm>.*

Many patients may be reluctant to discuss their use of complementary therapies with health professionals because of a perception that it will not be supported. It is important that health professionals initiate these conversations to demonstrate their support for open communication regarding complementary therapies.

3. PROCESS INFORMATION

(a) Interpret

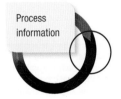

Process information

Q1 Within palliative care, you may find that a full set of vital signs are attended on an irregular basis. In a home visit situation, taking a full set of vial signs is rare. Select the vital signs that would be the most important for Sally.

   a Temperature, pulse, blood pressure

   b Pain assessment, bowel assessment, respiration rate

   c Oxygen saturation, respiration, temperature

   d Bowel assessment, blood pressure, temperature

Q2 To assist with understanding Sally's condition, a full set of vital signs are provided below, along with those assessments that are a priority in palliative care. Which of these is considered to be within normal parameters for Sally?

a   Temperature: 37.3°C

b   Pulse rate: 120

c   Respiratory rate: 30

d   Blood pressure: 140/95

e   Oxygen saturation level: 95%

f   Abdominal sounds: high-pitched tinkling sounds

g   Skin condition: dry skin

h   Oral mucosa condition: dry with tongue furrowed

i   Abdominal distension: evident on visual inspection

Q3 Sally tells you she feels bloated; she has pain near her rectum and has been passing small amounts of liquid diarrhoea that she can't always control. She also feels nauseated and has vomited small amounts. For a person with metastatic breast cancer, these symptoms are:

a   Unpleasant but expected

b   Typical of bone pain

c   A potential side effect of medications

d   Confirmation of cancer spread

e   A potential side effect of complementary therapies

(b) Discriminate

Q From the list below, select cues that you believe are *most relevant* to Sally's situation at this time.

a   Respiratory rate

b   Pulse

c   Skin irritation

d   Oxygen saturation

e   Nausea and vomiting

f   Lack of appetite

g   Urine output

h   Pain

i   Frequency of bowel movements

> See the following CareSearch site to gain a further understanding of constipation: <www.caresearch.com.au/caresearch/tabid/744/Default.aspx>.

It is important at this stage of the clinical reasoning cycle to recognise *any gaps* in the cues you have collected. From the information you have collected, you begin to think that Sally may be constipated. She cannot remember the last time she had her bowels opened, although she does admit she is never regular. You palpate Sally's abdomen, which reveals an easily palpable colon with a soft and mobile faecal mass. Digital examination of the rectum reveals hard stools.

(c) Relate

> Clinical reasoning errors: Sally's diagnosis of metastatic breast cancer and her referral to palliative care may limit cue collection. Anchoring could lead you to focus on the pain related to metastatic breast cancer and overlook assessment of the potential side effects of medications.

Q It is important to cluster the cues together and to identify relationships between them (based on the information you have collected so far). Which of the following statements are true?

a   Sally could be in pain because she has metastatic breast cancer.

b   Sally could be in pain as a result of her skin irritation.

c Sally could have nausea and vomiting as a side effect of the MS Contin and oral morphine that she is taking.

d Sally could be hypertensive because she is anxious about dying and leaving her daughter.

e Sally could have nausea and vomiting because she is constipated.

f Sally could be hypertensive as a result of her pain.

g Sally could be tachycardic as a result of her vomiting and pain.

h Sally is probably febrile because she is developing a chest infection.

i Sally is probably constipated as a side effect of the MS Contin and oral morphine that she is taking.

(d) Infer

Q It is time to think about the cues that you have collected and clustered about Sally's condition, and to make inferences based on your interpretation of those cues. From what you know about Sally's history, signs and symptoms, as well as your knowledge about palliative care, identify which of the following inferences are correct. (Select the one correct answer.)

a Sally is septic.

b Sally is constipated.

c Sally is in shock.

d Sally has metastatic spread.

e Sally is suffering from anorexia nervosa.

> *Hint: Think about the side effects of morphine.*

(e) Predict

Q1 Predict what might happen if Sally's pain, nausea and vomiting are not corrected. (Select the four that apply.)

a Sally could go into shock from an electrolyte imbalance.

b Sally's condition will gradually deteriorate over the next few days.

c Sally could go into acute renal failure (acute tubular necrosis).

d Sally could develop pulmonary oedema.

e Sally could die.

f Sally could become hypoxic.

> *Despite the prevalence of constipation in palliative care patients, it is often underdiagnosed and undertreated (Droney et al., 2008; Andrew & Morgan, 2013).*

Q2 Predict what might happen if Sally's constipation is not treated. (Select the four that apply.)

a Sally could become hypotensive.

b Sally could develop a bowel obstruction.

c Sally could have a seizure.

d Sally could become hypoxic.

e Sally could develop toxic megacolon.

f Sally could become confused.

g Sally could become agitated.

4. IDENTIFY THE PROBLEM/ISSUE

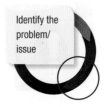

Identify the problem/ issue

Q Sally is currently experiencing a number of problems. From the following list, select the most appropriate nursing diagnosis at this stage.

a Acute pain related to metastatic spread of cancer, evidenced by high pain score

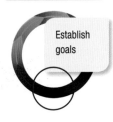

The NMBA's Registered Nurse Standards for Practice (2016) state that RNs must provide comprehensive, safe, quality practice to achieve agreed goals that are responsive to the individual needs of people. This is particularly important in end-of-life care decisions.

b Constipation related to opiod use, reduced oral intake and limited mobility, evidenced by pain, nausea and vomiting

c Metastatic spread of cancer related to abdominal distension, evidenced by high-pitched tinkling sounds

d Sally is experiencing 'typical' cancer pain

5. ESTABLISH GOALS

Establish goals

Q1 From the list below, choose the two most important *short-term* goals for Sally at this time.

a For Sally to be free of pain, nausea and vomiting

b For Sally to resume a normal diet

c For Sally's faecal impaction to be cleared

d For Sally to be admitted to a hospice

You are aware that Sally's accommodation could be contributing to her constipation, as she explains that walking to the public toilets is becoming more and more difficult. You are also concerned about how she will manage as her condition deteriorates and there is a lack of social support for her and her daughter.

Q2 Once Sally's immediate physical needs are addressed, it is important for you to do which of the following? (Select the two correct answers.)

a Contact Sally's parents.

b Organise alternative accommodation for Sally and Olivia.

c Plan where Olivia will go when Sally's condition deteriorates.

d Spend time talking with Sally so that you understand her wishes and needs for herself and Olivia.

e Contact anyone that Sally wants to speak to.

f Refer Sally to the social worker for help with possible accommodation.

6. TAKE ACTION

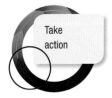

Take action

Q At this stage of the clinical reasoning cycle, you need to decide on the most important course of action. Number the following nursing actions in order of priority:

a Negotiate an action plan in case of further episodes of constipation.

b Administer two glycerine suppositories to soften hard rectal stools.

c Ensure the glycerine suppositories are against the wall of the bowel.

d Administer an enema to clear the faecal impaction.

e Educate Sally about the importance of adequate fluids, mobility and use of aperients.

f Contact Sally's doctor to discuss her condition, and for an order for an enema as well as oral aperients or laxatives.

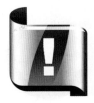

Something to think about ...

Although rectal enemas are sometimes necessary for treating faecal impaction, they should not be part of the regular treatment of every cancer patient with constipation. They are undignified and inconvenient, and may have a considerable negative effect on quality of life.

7. EVALUATE

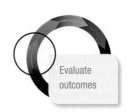

It is now two hours since Sally was given a rectal examination and two microlax enemas.

Q1   Rate each of the following signs and symptoms as 'unchanged', 'improving' or 'deteriorating'.

Cognitive status	patient restless and anxious
Pulse	90
Bowels	good result but sticky stools
Oral mucosa	mouth is dry and tongue furrowed
Oral intake	tolerating sips of water
BP	110/70
Colour	pale
Pain	on scale of 10, Sally reports 2
Nausea	slight nausea
Vomiting	nil

Q2   You now need to synthesise these parameters to decide whether Sally's status has improved overall. Which of the following statements is most correct?

a   Sally's pain, nausea and vomiting have improved significantly.

b   Sally's pain, nausea and vomiting have not improved and you need to contact the doctor again.

c   Sally's pain, nausea and vomiting have improved significantly but still require careful monitoring and will require oral aperients.

d   Sally's status has not improved but you will monitor her condition carefully for the next four hours.

8. REFLECT

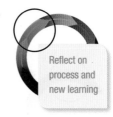

Reflect on your learning from this scenario and consider the following questions.

Q1   What actions will you take in clinical practice as a result of your learning from this scenario?

Q2   Why is therapeutic communication and holistic care important when caring for someone requiring palliative care?

Q3   Why is interprofessional communication imperative to the care of the person needing palliative care?

Q4   Standard 1 of Palliative Care Australia's *Standards for Providing Quality Palliative Care for All Australians* (2005) states that 'care, decision-making and care planning are each based on a respect for the uniqueness of the patient, their caregiver/s and family'. What strategies will you use in your clinical practice to meet this standard when caring for people requiring palliative care?

Q5   What advice would you give if a patient or a friend asked you about the use of complementary therapies for the treatment of cancer or the management of symptoms?

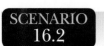

The palliative care journey comes to an end

CHANGING THE SCENE

Since referral to palliative care, Sally has continued working with the Outreach Palliative Care Team, including nurses, doctors, allied health, pastoral care, social work and complementary therapists. With their help, she has been able to reconnect with her family who are now more accepting and supportive. Sally shares her story with the palliative care nurse:

The housing commission organised this house for me, and my family now support my use of complementary therapies. So now when I get stressed Mum says, 'Come and I'll put a

Support groups can be another valuable resource for patients and carers. For more information, access <www.caresearch.com.au/caresearch/ClinicalPractice/PsychologicalSocialSpiritual/SocialSupport/tabid/643/Default.aspx>.

For introductory information on metastatic spread of breast cancer, see Dumitrescu & Cotarla (2005).

Respite care is offered to carers of individuals with life-limiting illness. What is respite care? What are the benefits for the carer and the client? Access <www.caresearch.com.au/caresearch/tabid/1113/Default.aspx>.

What does the literature say about medical hydration for dying patients? If unsure, access these articles: van der Riet, Brooks & Ashby (2006) and Higgins et al. (2014).

meditation tape on for you'; and Dad says, 'You're running out of vitamin C. I'll go up the road and get you some.'

I've also been connected to the support group through palliative care and it's been great. When you're at home and you're doing everything that you can, your family is as supportive as they can be and so are your friends—but it's the same old stuff … they just don't know what it is like. And you go along to a support group and you are not a minority anymore; you're part of the majority. Everybody in the room is going through a similar journey; so you don't feel isolated and lonely.

Although the referral to palliative care has had a positive effect on Sally's psychosocial health, her breast cancer has continued to progress …

I remember when the cancer first spread to my bones … my ribs were hurting a bit. I had a bone scan straightaway … the radiotherapist had written down on the report, there could be signs of metastatic disease. Then everything was going along fine but I started to get aches and pains all over; it was hard to lift my leg up to get dressed, get in and out of bed, just basic things … I thought I had just been bashing myself a bit too much. I didn't think too much about it but I had an appointment a week and a half later with the oncologist. So I thought, I will leave it till then … I went and had another bone scan done and it was everywhere … all through my hips, in the top of my femur in one of my legs, in about eight vertebrae in my spine and six ribs. It has gone into my shoulder, and I think … it's getting worse; I can feel more pains and aches; it has gone into my neck as well, um … and I am kind of in shock that this is it …

It has been six months since Sally was first referred to palliative care, and in the last month she has noted a decline in her mobility and her independence, and an increase in her pain. Sally and her daughter moved in with her parents as she required more care and support. However, over the last week her parents have found it increasingly difficult to manage her pain, discomfort and restlessness, and Sally has agreed to be admitted to the hospice.

1. CONSIDER THE PATIENT SITUATION

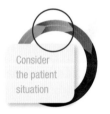

Consider the patient situation

Morning handover at hospice

Sally Abraham is a 37-year-old woman with metastatic breast cancer; secondary sites include multiple bone metastases. The outreach team commenced analgesia via a syringe driver the day prior to her admission, but Sally's pain was not covered and she became increasingly restless. Her family stated that she has been eating only a spoonful of food a couple of times a day and having occasional sips of water. Sally was limited to her bed because of pain and weakness; previously she was walking short distances around the house. Sally was admitted to the hospice yesterday with increasing pain and decreasing consciousness. She has been moved to a single room.

Since admission, she has commenced on morphine/midazolam infusion and, although she is sleeping most of the time, she is easily roused. Her mother approached me before I came into handover asking if we are going to commence intravenous fluids, because Sally is no longer taking anything orally.

Her parents (Nancy and Brendan) and Sally's daughter, Olivia, are staying in the room, and although they are all aware that Sally is dying, her parents are becoming distressed with Sally's agitation and the fact that she is not drinking and eating.

QUICK QUIZ!

Review the medications being delivered via the syringe driver.

Q1 A syringe driver in palliative care delivers a continuous infusion of medication over a 24-hour period, thus providing continuous dosing and avoiding the 'peak and trough' effect of four-hourly dosing. True or false?

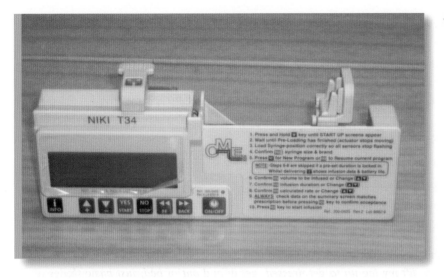

Syringe driver

> Access Palliative Care Guidelines Plus for information on syringe drivers and compatible medications: <http://book.pallcare.info/index.php?tid=96&searchstring=syringe%20drivers>.

Q2 A syringe driver is helpful for:

  a Post-operative pain

  b Intractable vomiting

  c Providing hydration and nutrition

  d When a patient is too weak to swallow

  e b and d

Q3 Circle the *true* statements concerning midazolam.

  a It is a benzodiazepine drug.

  b It is a non-benzodiazepine drug.

  c It is used for terminal restlessness due to its sedating and muscle-relaxing effect.

  d It is used for pain relief.

Q4 Fill in the missing word. For palliative care patients, _____ delivery of medication is preferable to intravenous administration.

Q5 Fill in the missing word. Increased agitation, twitching, restlessness and groaning are a form of _____, which may be present in the terminal phase of illness.

> Note: Multiple terms are used to describe terminal restlessness, including 'terminal agitation', 'delirium' and 'confusion'. See <www.pallcareact.org.au/images/pdfs/ConfusionAndRestlessness.pdf>.

2. COLLECT CUES/INFORMATION

(a) Review current information

Sally's condition has deteriorated and her family are aware that she is close to death. Bereavement support of carers often commences prior to a patient's death. Therapeutic communication skills make a significant impact on the experience of carers in the terminal phase of their loved one's life.

Q What current information might you consider prior to entering Sally's room?

  a Age of Sally

  b Relationships of bereaved to Sally

  c Gender of bereaved

  d Your own self-care strategies when dealing with grief reactions

  e Age of the bereaved

  f All of the above

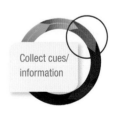

Collect cues/information

Access CareSearch for communication strategies when talking with children: <www.caresearch.com.au/caresearch/ForPatientsandFamilies/LivingWithIllness/WhyIsCommunicationImportant/TalkingWithChildren/tabid/1139/Default.aspx>.

(b) Gather new information

The terminal phase of an illness describes the final days of a person's life. The focus during this stage is to provide symptom management for the patient to ensure that suffering is minimised, but supporting the carers or family is also a focus.

It is important to explain to the family the signs that will indicate Sally is in the terminal phase of her illness.

Q1 Indications that Sally is dying may include:

   a Thirst, fatigue and increased pain

   b Mainly asleep, bedbound and little oral intake

   c No bowel movements and increased pain

   d Increased confusion

Hint: Being aware of signs of imminent death are essential for palliative care nurses so that they can fully support the carers or family.

Q2 Sally's parents and daughter have expressed a need to be with Sally when she dies; however, they are extremely tired. What actions could you recommend for them based on your knowledge of the terminal phase?

   a Encourage them to go home and shower and have some rest.

   b Encourage them to walk in the garden outside the room for 15 minutes while you sit with Sally.

   c Encourage them to go to the cafeteria for a break.

Ascertainment bias

The transition and assessment during this phase can be difficult. The clinical reasoning error of ascertainment bias may occur when a nurse bases his or her judgment of terminal phase on assumptions rather than on a full assessment of the client and the carer or family's needs.

(c) Recall knowledge

The provision of physical, psychological and spiritual care for patients during the terminal phase is essential.

Spirituality

For the palliative care patient, spirituality is often likened to a search for inner meaning, and complementary therapies can sometimes assist them in this process, particularly meditation as it provides a space for contemplation. Many of these therapies, as previously stated, reduce anxiety and this then opens up the space for self-reflection.

Spirituality is an important component of professional nursing (Smyth & Allen, 2011); however, it is also an elusive term with no clear definition (Baldacchino, 2008; Stephensen & Berry, 2015) that can mean different things to different people. Amoah (2011) points out that spirituality helps the dying person make sense of their life and that it is an integral component of palliative care. Smyth and Allen's research into nurses' experiences in assessing dying patients found that 'spirituality forms a significant component of the wellbeing of patients and as such is integral to delivering nursing care in any setting' (2011, p. 342). Importantly, this study reported that nurses implement 'spiritual care through listening, observing and communicating' (p. 341). For Wright, spirituality is 'what gives people balance when finding meaning in the existential challenges of life' (2005).

How would you communicate with Sally to ensure that you deliver spiritual care that acknowledges her individual needs and wishes?

Hint: A spiritual assessment tool may assist you. Access <http://book.pallcare.info/index.php?tid=170&dg=9>.

Q1 When exploring spirituality, which aspects do you need to consider?

   a The patient's perspectives

   b The views of the interdisciplinary team

   c The patient's own thoughts or concepts of spirituality

> d Your own perceptions of spirituality and how they might impact on discussions with the patient
>
> e All of the above

Now that Sally is dying, your nursing priorities include:

- Promotion of comfort and relief of suffering
- Careful assessment and management of symptoms
- Pain assessment and management
- Consideration of existential issues: spiritual issues, affirmation of life, meaning, unfinished business, reconciliation, culturally appropriate care
- The needs of family and carers: anticipatory grief, emotional support.

Advanced care planning is a strategy that can assist individuals with life-limiting illness to ensure that their wishes are respected when they are no longer able to verbalise them. Sally's parents and daughter have a clear understanding of Sally's wishes in relation to the terminal phase of her illness.

Q2 Advanced care planning is best discussed with the patient in the later stages of their illness.

   True or false?

3. PROCESS INFORMATION

(a) Interpret

Sally's mother has approached you as she is upset that intravenous fluids have not been commenced. You have been doing regular mouth care for Sally and are aware that she is not complaining of thirst or hunger.

QUICK QUIZ!

Q1 Artificial or medical hydration should be considered in the palliative approach where dehydration results from potentially correctable causes. Identify which of the following are correctable.

   a Over-treatment of diuretics and sedation

   b Recurrent vomiting

   c Diarrhoea

   d Hypercalcaemia

   e All of the above

Q2 Medical provision of hydration (intravenous fluids) can make a difference to a dying patient's thirst. True or false?

Q3 Dehydration in dying patients does not produce discomfort for the patient. True or false?

Q4 Intravenous fluids in the dying patient can cause burdensome and distressing symptoms. True or false?

Q5 In terminal dehydration, patients experience an alteration in their serum sodium levels. True or false?

Q6 Terminal dehydration stimulates the production of endorphins. True or false?

Q7 A decrease in endorphins can cause some degree of analgesia. True or false?

Q8 Anorexia in the dying person results in ketoacidosis and this removes a feeling of hunger, resulting in analgesia. True or false?

Q9 Medical provision of hydration (IV fluids) can produce distressing and life-threatening symptoms for patients with end-stage illness and multi-organ failure. True or false?

Q10 Medical provision of hydration (IV fluids) can produce distressing symptoms because the physiological and metabolic processes of the body are no longer efficient. True or false?

Process information

(b) Discriminate

Q   From the cues and information you now have, you need to narrow down the information to what is most important. From the list below, select four cues that you believe are *most relevant* to Sally's situation at this time.

    a   Blood pressure

    b   Dyspnoea

    c   Sally's agitation

    d   Oxygen saturation

    e   Condition of oral mucosa

    f   Level of consciousness

    g   Sally is not eating or drinking

    h   Urine output

    i   Pain

    j   Family distress

(c) Relate

Q   It is important to cluster the cues together and to identify relationships between them (based on the information you have collected so far). Which of the following are true statements?

    a   Sally is restless because she has terminal restlessness.

    b   Sally is restless because she may be frightened of dying.

    c   Sally's family are worried about her not eating and drinking.

    d   Sally's family feel helpless that Sally is not eating.

    e   Sally's family feel that she is suffering because she is not eating and drinking.

(d) Infer

Access CareSearch for symptom management at the end of life: <www.caresearch.com.au/caresearch/tabid/741/Default.aspx>.

It is time to think about all the cues that you have collected about this situation and to make inferences based on your analysis and interpretation of those cues.

Q   From what you know about Sally not eating and drinking, as well as your knowledge about palliative care, identify which of the following inferences is correct.

    a   Sally is experiencing terminal dehydration.

    b   Sally is not experiencing terminal dehydration.

(e) Predict

Now is the time to consider the consequences of your actions or inaction by predicting potential outcomes for your patient.

Q1   What could happen if Sally is given intravenous fluids? (Select the four that apply.)

    a   Sally's family would be more relaxed.

    b   Sally's breathing would become noisy from the excessive respiratory secretions.

    c   Sally's peripheral oedema will increase.

    d   Sally could develop pulmonary oedema.

    e   Sally could become hypoxic.

Q2   What could happen if Sally is not given intravenous fluids? (Select the three that apply.)

    a   Sally's condition will gradually deteriorate over the next few days.

    b   Sally's breathing will be easier and not require any scopolamine and atropine to dry up her secretions.

c Sally's urinary incontinence will be less.

d Sally will be less oedematous.

e Sally could become hypoxic.

Hint: Read van der Riet et al. (2009) for more information.

4. IDENTIFY THE PROBLEM/ISSUE

Identify the problem/ issue

At this stage, you bring together (synthesise) all of the facts you've collected and inferences you've made to identify definitive risk diagnoses for Sally.

Q Select from the following the *incorrect* nursing diagnoses for Sally at this time.

a Risk of aspiration related to oropharyngeal secretions and the provision of oral fluids

b Risk of abdominal discomfort related to accumulation of gas and fluids in the gastrointestinal tract and decreased peristalsis

c Risk of distress and discomfort associated with withholding fluids

d Risk of oral discomfort related to limited oral intake and poor oral care

e Risk of peripheral, cerebral or pulmonary oedema related to excess fluid intake

5. ESTABLISH GOALS

Establish goals

Before implementing any actions to improve this situation, it is important to clearly specify what you want to happen and when.

Q From the list below, choose the two most important *short-term* goals for Sally's management at this time.

a For Sally to be comfortable and treated with dignity

b For Sally to be hydrated with IV fluids

c To prevent dry mucous membranes and oral discomfort

Hint: Read Stein and McAlpine (2006) for more information.

6. TAKE ACTION

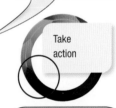

Take action

At this stage of the clinical reasoning cycle, you need to decide on your course of action to improve this situation. You should be alert to your role as patient advocate.

Q From the list below, choose the three *most immediate* actions you should take at this stage.

a Call the doctor and set up for the insertion of IV fluids.

b Explain to the family that IV fluids will not promote comfort for Sally. Her dying body has shut down and will not absorb intravenous fluids.

c Provide regular oral care, using moistening swabs with water (not glycerine swabs, as they dry mucous membranes), an oral gel or an oral spray.

d Explain to the family there has been a gradual decrease in food and fluid, and that, provided regular mouth care is given, Sally will not suffer the ill effects of terminal dehydration.

In person-centred care, you should refer to the patient and their family regarding their preferences for the use of music and aromatherapy. It is important that nurses do not push their own agenda and preferences.

7. EVALUATE

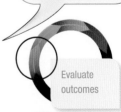

Evaluate outcomes

It is now 24 hours later. Sally's family have been keeping a bedside vigil. Her terminal restlessness has settled. You have been giving her gentle massages when you turn and sponge her. The use of aromatherapy (lavender) in a vaporiser, along with relaxation music, has helped to calm both Sally and her family.

8. REFLECT

Reflect on process and new learning

Caring for people who require palliative care can often be stressful and emotionally distressing. Your own fear of death and dying, and feelings of inadequacy in relation to the person's suffering, can add to feelings of distress. When caring for people who are dying, it is important that you have realistic expectations about the degree of support you can provide. It is also important that you know who you can access for support and advice.

Q1   What actions will you take in clinical practice as a result of your learning from this scenario?

Q2   Why are self-care strategies so important in palliative care nursing?

Q3   Who would you talk to if you felt distressed about a dying patient you have been caring for?

Q4   What self-care strategies could you use to assist you in caring for a dying patient?

Q5   What advice or support could you provide for a colleague who is caring for a dying patient?

> To find more information about the importance of self-care for your nursing career, go to PCC4U (2011).

> For the palliative care nurse, the death is not the completion of care. In many palliative care services, nurses will provide a bereavement service to the carers, the provision of support—supporting the expression of grief—and referral to bereavement counsellors or support networks if required.

EPILOGUE

Sally died peacefully two days after being admitted to the hospice. She was very calm and pain-free in the last two days of her life. A lavender infuser, low-level lighting and her favourite meditation music by 'Sacred Earth' created a peaceful environment. Sally's parents and her daughter, Olivia, were with her when she died and stayed with Sally for an hour longer to say their final farewell. They cried a lot and said how much they loved her. Sally's parents and Olivia chose not to assist in the final bathing of her, but they selected a dress they wanted Sally to wear. You sat with them for a while and gently held Olivia's hand.

Several months after Sally died, the hospice received a card from her mother to say how much they appreciated the care given to Sally. She spoke of the gentle massages given to Sally when she was restless, and how the time taken to communicate with and comfort the family will always be remembered. Sally's mother said that Olivia is living with them, and although she misses her mother very much she is a normal, active and happy teenager.

FURTHER READING

Cancer Council NSW. Available at <www.cancercouncil.com.au/>.

CareSearch (2011). *CareSearch: Palliative Care Knowledge Network*. Accessed March 2017 at <www.caresearch.com.au/Caresearch/Default.aspx>.

Elisabeth Kübler-Ross Foundation. Available at <www.ekrfoundation.org/>.

Palliative Care Curriculum for Undergraduates (PCC4U). (2011). *Teaching and Learning Hub: Palliative Care Learning Modules*. Accessed March 2017 at <www.caresearch.com.au/caresearch/pcc4u/tabid/1692/Default.aspx>.

REFERENCES

Adams, J. (2007). *Researching Complementary and Alternative Medicine*. Great Britain: Routledge.

Adams, J. (2006). An exploratory study of complementary and alternative medicine in hospital midwifery: Models of care and professional struggle. *Complementary Therapies in Clinical Practice, 12*(1), 40–47.

Amoah, C. (2011). The central importance of spirituality in palliative care. *International Journal of Palliative Care, 17*(9), 353–58.

Andrew, A. & Morgan, G. (2013). Constipation management in palliative care: Treatments and the potential of independent nurse prescribing. *International Journal of Palliative Care, 18*(1), 17–22.

Australian Bureau of Statistics (ABS). (2008). *4102.0—Australian Social Trends, 2008. 4102.0—Complementary Therapies*.

Australian Commission on Safety and Quality in Health Care (ACSQHC). (2016). *National Safety and Quality Health Service Standards Version 2*. Draft, Sydney, Australia.

Australian Institute of Health and Welfare (AIHW). (2010). *Australia's Health 2010*. Australia's Health No. 12. Cat. No. AUS122. Available at <www.aihw.gov.au/publications/ aus/ah08/ah08-c05.pdf>.

Baldacchino, D. (2008). Teaching on the spiritual dimension in care to undergraduate nursing students: The content and teaching methods. *Nurse Education Today, 28*, 550–62.

Bower, J. E., Crosswell, A. D., Stanton, A. L., Crespi, C. M., Winston, D., Arevalo, J., ... Patricia, A. (2015). Mindfulness meditation for younger breast cancer survivors: A randomized controlled trial. *Cancer, 121*(8), 1231–40. doi: 10.1002/cncr.29194

Cancer Insitute NSW. (2008). Cancer in NSW: Incidence and Mortality Report 2008. Accessed May 2017 at <www.cancerinstitute.org.au/how-we-help/reports-and-publications/cancer-in-nsw-incidence-and-mortality-2008>.

Droney, J., Ross, J., Gretton, S., Welsh, K., Sato, H. & Riley, J. (2008). Constipation in cancer patients on morphine. *Support Care Cancer, 16*(5), 453–59.

Dumitrescu, R. G. & Cotarla, I. (2005). Understanding breast cancer risk—Where do we stand in 2005? *Journal of Cellular and Molecular Medicine, 9*, 208–21.

Elisabeth Kübler-Ross Foundation. (2012). *Five Stages of Grief*. Accessed March 2017 at <www.ekrfoundation.org/five-stages-of-grief/>.

Ernst, E., Pittler, M. H. & Wider, B. (2006). *The Desktop Guide to Complementary and Alternative Medicine: An Evidence-Based Approach* (2nd edn). Philadelphia, USA: Mosby Elsevier.

Gallagher, L., Lagman, R. & Walsh, D. (2006). The clinical effects of music therapy in palliative medicine. *Support Care Cancer, 14*(8), 859–66.

Henneghan, A. & Harrison, T. (2015). Complementary and alternative medicine therapies as symptom management strategies for the late effects of breast cancer treatment. *Journal of Holistic Nursing, 33*(1), 84–97.

Higgins, I., van der Riet, P., Sneesby, L. & Good, P. (2014). Nutrition and hydration in dying patients: The perceptions of acute care nurses. *Journal of Clinical Nursing, 23*(17–18), 2609–17. doi: 10.1111/jocn.12478.

Kittelson, S., Eli, M. & Pennypacker, L. (2015). Palliative care symptom management. *Critical Care Nursing Clinics of North America, 27*, 315–39.

Kotsirilos, V., Vitetta, L. & Sali, A. (2011). *A Guide to Evidenced-Based Integrative and Complementary Medicine*. Sydney: Elsevier.

Larzelere, M., Campbell, J. & Robertson, M. (2010). Complementary and alternative medicine usage for behavioral health indications. *Primary Care, 37*(2), 213–36.

Lui, R., Chang, A., Reddy, S., Hecht, F. & Chao, M. (2016). Improving patient-centred care: A cross-sectional survey of prior use and interest in complementary and integrative health approaches among hospitalised oncology patients. *The Journal of Alternative and Complementary Medicine, 22*(2), 160–65.

Mansky, P. & Wallerstedy, D. (2006). Complementary medicine in palliative care and cancer symptom management. *Cancer Journal, 12*(5), 425–31.

Mason, D. (2014). Holism and embodiment in nursing. *Holistic Nursing Practice*, January–February, 55–64.

McCabe, P. (2005). Complementary and alternative medicine in Australia: A contemporary overview. *Complementary Therapies in Clinical Practice, 11*(1), 28–31.

McDonald, A., Burjan, E. & Martin, S. (2006). Yoga for patients and carers in a palliative care setting. *International Journal of Palliative Nursing, 12*, 219–23.

National Prescribing Service (NPS). (2010). *Complementary and Alternative Medicines*. Accessed June 2010 at <www.nps.org.au>.

Nursing and Midwifery Board of Australia (NMBA). (2016). *Registered Nurse Standards for Practice.* Retrieved from <http://nursingmidwiferyboard.gov.au/Codes-Guidelines-Statements/Professional-standards.aspx>.

O'Callaghan, V. (2011). *Patients' Perceptions of Complementary and Alternative Medicine*. Accessed September 2011 at <www.cancerforum.org.au/Issues/2011/March/Forum/Patients_perceptions_complementary_alternative.htm>.

Oechsle, K., Wais, M., Vehling, S., Bokemeyer, C. & Mehnert, A. (2014). Relationship between symptom burden, distress, and sense of dignity in terminally ill cancer patients. *Journal of Pain and Symptom Management, 48*(3), 313–21.

Palliative Care Australia. (2011). *About Palliative Care Australia*. Accessed September 2011 at <www.palliativecare.org.au/Default.aspx?tabid=1115>.

Palliative Care Australia. (2005). *Standards for Providing Quality Palliative Care for All Australians*. Accessed March 2017 at <http://palliativecare.org.au/wp-content/uploads/2015/07/Standards-for-providing-quality-palliative-care-for-all-Australians.pdf>.

Palliative Care Curriculum for Undergraduates (PCC4U). (2011). *Teaching and Learning Hub: Palliative Care Learning Modules*. Accessed September 2011 at <www.caresearch.com.au/caresearch/pcc4u/tabid/1692/Default.aspx>.

Palliative Care Outcomes Collaboration. (2011). *Symptom Assessment Scale*. Accessed December 2016 at <http://ahsri.uow.edu.au/content/groups/public/@web/@chsd/@pcoc/documents/doc/uow115384.pdf>.

Proulx, K. & Jacelon, C. (2004). Dying with dignity: The good patient versus the good death. *American Journal Hospice Palliative Care, 21*(2), 116–20.

Reid, R., Steel, A., Wardle, J., Trubody, A. & Adams, J. (2016). Complementary medicine used by the Australian population: A critical mixed studies systematic review of utilisation perceptions. *BMC Complementary and Alternative Medicine, 16*, 176. doi: 0.1186/s12906-016-1143-8

Sears, S., Kraus, S., Carlough, K. & Treat, E. (2011). Perceived benefits and doubts of participants in a weekly meditation study. *Mindfulness, 2*(3), 167–74. doi: 10.1007/s12671-011-0055-4

Sheppard-Hanger, S. & Hanger, N. (2015). The importance of safety when using aromatherapy. *International Journal of Childbirth Education, 30*(1), 42–47.

Smith, G. (2009). The need for complementary and alternative medicine familiarisation in undergraduate nurse education. *Journal of Clinical Nursing, 18*, 2113–15.

Smyth, T. & Allen, S. (2011). Nurses' experiences assessing the spirituality of terminally ill patients in acute clinical practice. *International Journal of Palliative Care, 17*(7), 337–43.

Stein, K. & McAlpine, C. (2006). The role of the nurse as advocate in ethically difficult care situations with dying patients. *Journal of Hospice and Palliative Nursing, 8*(5), 259–69.

Stephensen, P. & Berry, D. (2015). Describing spirituality at the end of life. *Western Journal of Nursing Research, 37*(9), 1229–47.

Tovey, P., Chatwin, J. & Broom, A. (2007). *Traditional Complementary and Alternative Medicine and Cancer Care*. London: Routledge.

van der Riet, P. J. (2011). Complementary therapies in health care. *Nursing & Health Sciences, 13*(1), 4–8. doi: 10.1111/j.1442-2018.2011.00587.x

van der Riet, P., Brooks, D. & Ashby, M. (2006). Nutrition and hydration at the end of life: Pilot study of a palliative care experience. *Journal of Law and Medicine, 14*, 182–98.

van der Riet, P., Francis, L. & Levett-Jones, T. (2011). Complementary therapies in healthcare: Design, implementation and evaluation of an elective course for undergraduate students. *Nurse Education in Practice, 11*, 146–52.

van der Riet, P., Good, P., Higgins, I. & Sneesby, L. (2009). Difficult clinical situations. *Journal of Clinical Nursing, 18*(14), 2104–11.

Walton, J. & Sullivan, N. (2004). Men of prayer: Spirituality of men with prostate cancer: A grounded theory study. *Journal of Holistic Nursing, 22*, 133.

World Health Organization (WHO). (2011). *Cancer: Palliative Care*. Accessed September 2011 at <www.who.int/cancer/palliative/en/>.

Wright, S. G. (2005). *Reflections on Spirituality and Health*. London: Whurr Publishers Ltd.

Yazdanimehr, R., Omidi, A., Sadat, Z. & Akbari, H. (2016). The effect of mindfulness integrated cognitive behaviour therapy on depression and anxiety among pregnant women: A randomised clinical trial. *Journal of Caring Sciences, 5*(3), 195–204.

CHAPTER 17

CARING FOR A PERSON WHO IS REFUSING TREATMENT

LORINDA PALMER

LEARNING OUTCOMES

Completion of the activities in this chapter will enable you to:

○ engage in the process of ethical reasoning to explore a complex ethical dilemma

○ examine the relationship between clinical reasoning and ethical reasoning

○ identify the nature and complexity of the ethical and legal dilemmas associated with refusal of potentially life-saving treatments

○ explain how advance care directives (ACDs) and the concepts of futile and burdensome treatment can inform decisions to withdraw or withhold treatment

○ assess the balance of benefits and harm associated with refusal of cardiopulmonary resuscitation (CPR)

○ assess how conflicting personal values may affect clinical decision making

○ consider how intuition, experience, emotion and context may affect the process of ethical reasoning

○ assess how actual and perceived loci of power and authority may affect the process of decisions to withhold CPR

○ identify the specific areas of legislation, case law, health department/ministry policies and hospital guidelines that are applicable to the refusal of CPR (and other potentially life-saving treatments) in the different states of Australia.

INTRODUCTION

This book would not be complete without a chapter illustrating the ethical dilemmas that nurses may encounter when caring for a person who does not wish to be 'rescued'. Mr George McAllister, who you will meet in the following pages, is one such person.

'Failure to rescue' can happen when nurses miss vital cues and fail to detect patient deterioration. But sometimes cues that patients are trying to refuse treatment might also be missed, misinterpreted or overlooked. Not all attempts at 'rescue' are appropriate, particularly if the treatment is futile and burdensome, not in the person's best interests, or not in accordance with their wishes.

However, the process of determining what is in a person's best interests and what accords with their wishes can be fraught with difficulties. Good communication skills are needed, as well as a willingness to engage in an examination of values—one's own as well as other people's, including the patient, their relatives and other members of the interprofessional team. Another complication is that, while many hospitals have clear protocols for how to respond when a patient's condition deteriorates, clear procedures do not always exist for when a patient wants to refuse treatment, particularly a potentially life-saving treatment such as cardio-pulmonary resuscitation (CPR).

The complex nature of these decisions means that they need to include both technical and ethical elements, that is, discussion of broader issues, such as the limits of technology, the uncertainty of outcomes, whether CPR should be offered at all, as well as death and dying (Hayes, 2013). These are difficult conversations to have, and there is evidence that health professionals are often reluctant to become involved in complex ethical matters, as decisions to withdraw or withhold life-saving treatment often are (Resuscitation Council UK, 2012). This situation is compounded by the lack of legal clarity, although this is perhaps less of an issue in jurisdictions where legislation addressing the refusal of life-saving treatment has been enacted. New South Wales is not one of those jurisdictions, so the legal situation there relies on common law cases and their interpretation in NSW Ministry of Health guidelines and hospital policies (Forrester & Griffiths, 2014). Refusal cues may also be overlooked if clinicians feel compelled to do everything possible to try to 'save' someone; and in many ways (in both myth and reality), performing CPR is one of the classic 'rescue' missions.

Whatever the reasons, decisions to withhold potentially life-saving treatments—not to rescue—are among the most frequent and

KEY CONCEPTS

ethical reasoning
ethical dilemma
advance care directive
futile and burdensome
    treatment
CPR decision-making
withdrawal of treatment
withholding treatment
end-of-life care

SUGGESTED READINGS

M.-J. Johnstone. (2015). *Bioethics: A Nursing Perspective* (6th edn). Sydney: Elsevier. Chapter 9: Ethical issues in end-of-life care

K. Forrester & D. Griffiths. (2014). *Essentials of Law for Health Professionals* (4th edn). Sydney: Elsevier. Chapter 8: Refusal of treatment

I. Kerridge, M. Lowe & C. Stewart. (2013). *Ethics and Law for the Health Professions* (4th edn). Sydney: Federation Press. Chapter 18: CPR and no-CPR orders

difficult moral problems that nurses encounter in practice (Adams et al., 2011). They require excellent clinical reasoning and decision-making capability, and a sound understanding of the relevant legislation and case law. This chapter explores how the clinical reasoning cycle can be used to assist in the ethical reasoning process associated with a situation involving the withholding of CPR.

Questions and answers in this chapter

Ethical dilemmas such as the ones explored in this chapter rarely have unequivocally correct answers. For this reason, the answers provided on the Pearson website to the questions asked in this chapter are not intended to be definitive. Instead, they are provided to promote reflection and discussion, and they also suggest avenues for further reading and learning.

SCENARIO 17.1 — The night before Christmas ...

SETTING THE SCENE

Access this AIHW website to find out more about the incidence, prevalence, morbidity and mortality risks associated with the four conditions that George either has had or may have: myocardial infarction, prostate cancer, stroke and type 2 diabetes. <www.aihw. gov.au/risk-factors-diseases-and-death/>.

It is late in the evening on Christmas Eve on a busy cardiology unit, about an hour before handover and change of shift, when notification comes of a new admission. He is Mr George McAllister, a 78-year-old man who had surgery that day at another hospital but is being transferred because he needs specialist cardiac care. He has had a post-surgical myocardial infarction following a radical prostatectomy. He has a bladder irrigation in-situ, a history of type 2 diabetes and a right-sided hemiplegia from a stroke five years ago.

George arrives just before the shift ends, so there isn't time to do much more than settle him in, ensure he is comfortable and pain-free, check whether he has any medications due, assess his vital signs and check that his bladder irrigation is patent.

George feels exhausted by his traumatic day—major surgery and the knowledge that he might have prostate cancer, as well as chest pain, a heart attack, a late-evening transfer to a different hospital, the pain from surgery and the discomfort caused by his urethral catheter.

In just a few hours it will be Christmas Day.

VALUES

Review the information on this NSW Ministry of Health website about advance care planning and how people can make their wishes known: <www.health. nsw.gov.au/patients/acp/ pages/default.aspx>.

Clinical decisions about treatment cannot be separated from the whole person. Up until this point, the health professionals involved in George's care have been focused on diagnosing, treating and, if possible, curing his medical conditions. But all of these things have a deep impact on George's life and his ability to live it in a way that is satisfying and meaningful to him. That is, George's values and perceptions of his quality of life, which up until now have not been a significant factor in his care, are about to become so. Thus far, he has accepted, in a fairly unquestioning way, advice about what surgeries, tests and treatments he should have. But things have now gotten to the point where he wants to reconsider the course he is on.

Thinking about this overnight, George decides that, if something happens and he has another heart attack, he does not want to be 'jumped on' and revived. He has known for quite some time that he doesn't want to be 'kept alive on machines', and he feels that now would be a good time to make that known. He is not sure what to say specifically or who to say it to, but he is sure that the nurses will know. He determines to ask someone about it in the morning. The young male nurse who settled him in said he would be back for the morning shift. George thought that he seemed really nice and very assured, and that he would be the right person to talk to.

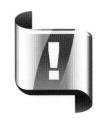

Something to think about …

George's personal values underpin his beliefs and guide his decisions. The nurse caring for George is guided by the values of his profession, which are expressed in the NMBA's Code of Ethics for Nurses in Australia *(2008a) and the* Registered Nurse Standards for Practice *(2016): <www.nursingmidwiferyboard.gov.au/ Codes-Guidelines-Statements/Professional-standards.aspx>.*

Review these professional codes and standards, and identify which values and standards are most relevant in this situation?

PERSON-CENTRED CARE—WHO IS GEORGE?

In order to understand why George might feel this way about his situation, it is necessary to know much more about him than just the results of his tests and scans. In common with many of his generation, who lived through the depression and the Second World War, George has worked hard all his life, and values independence and thrift. He has been married twice; his first wife is now deceased; his second marriage did not work out, resulting in divorce several years ago, and he has no contact with his ex-wife. His only daughter died over five years ago from cancer. Apart from his sister and her extended family, George has no close relatives. He tries to keep up an active social life and interests, and up until five years ago when he had the stroke he was very physically active. But the disability arising from the stroke has been a huge blow, from which he has not recovered. He has always been very particular about his appearance and his physical ability, and the loss of these has been steadily eroding his confidence and happiness. He has had counselling and psychological support but none of it has helped much and, for George, life entails a daily struggle to cope and deep wounds to his psyche that have never healed.

More than anything, George fears having another stroke or illness that renders him even more unable to function than he already is. Stroke survivorship has taught him harsh lessons about the nature of quality of life after stroke that perhaps only those who have lived through it—or care for those who do—can fully appreciate. He does not want to end his remaining years in a nursing home, or be dependent on full-time care. He has seen this happen to some of his relatives and friends, and he is determined that this will not happen to him.

Mostly, what George wants is that, when the time comes for him to die, he retains the same fierce independence, pride and dignity that have been so integral to his character for his entire life. He is not sure whether that time is now, but somehow it feels as though it might be. George is not afraid of dying. He has lived a good life and takes great comfort from his memories. What he is terribly afraid of now is losing control over his mind, body and life for whatever remaining time that he has.

> *This information about George is mostly unknown to the health professionals who have been caring for him. One reason is that few health assessments entail asking patients about their values, beliefs or wishes regarding the limits to continued treatment, such as CPR. Read* The value of taking an 'ethics history' *by Sayers et al. (2001) for a discussion on what this might entail: <www.jstor.org/stable/27718658>.*

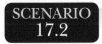

SCENARIO 17.2 Christmas morning

CHANGING THE SCENE

Next morning George is happy to see Greg, the nurse who looked after him the evening before, walk back into his room and greet him. Today George will find the right time to tell Greg about the decision he made the night before. Not just yet, though, because breakfast is arriving and there is quite a bit of festive cheer being bandied about. People are coming in and out of the four-bed room, and Greg looks a bit busy with other patients in the room; but soon, when the moment is right …

Eventually, the moment does arise and George tells Greg that he 'doesn't want any heroics' if he has another heart attack or stroke. Greg is surprised, because not many patients come out and say things so directly and he wasn't expecting this. But after a short conversation, he tells George that the best thing to do is to wait until a bit later in the morning when Dr Jones, George's cardiologist, does his rounds and the matter can be discussed with him.

It is now 1030 hours and George has been in the unit for just over 14 hours. Dr Jones has come to see him to assess his condition and options for treatment. The bedside visit is quite short and is focused on George's physical problems, particularly the tests and medications relating to his heart attack. George feels a bit intimidated. Dr Jones looks busy and the room is still quite noisy and full of people, and so George doesn't raise the issue of not wanting CPR. As Dr Jones leaves the room, George whispers a reminder to Greg to go after him and tell him about his decision. Greg catches up to Dr Jones at the desk as he is writing in George's notes and tells him what George has said to him earlier; how he feels about not having CPR. Dr Jones thinks for a moment and replies, 'We'll talk about that later after his pathology results [tests for prostate cancer] come back.' He closes the chart and walks away.

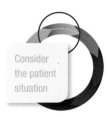

Consider
the patient
situation

1. CONSIDER THE PATIENT SITUATION

What should Greg do in this situation? He has a number of options, but finding the best—or least worst—will not be easy. He is having a very busy shift and, on top of that, it is Christmas Day. Should he seek advice from someone; if so, from whom? And what should he tell George now? Should he go after Dr Jones immediately and ask him to come back and talk to George? Should he just do as he was told and wait? What if George arrests in the meantime? Should Greg do CPR even though he now knows that George does not want it and has specifically refused it? Is that refusal legally valid?

Greg has spent only a few hours with George and does not know him very well. Could he be depressed? He has had a terribly stressful 24 hours. Is he in the right frame of mind to be making a decision like this? On the other hand, everyone has accepted that his frame of mind is perfectly okay to consent to continuing treatment, so why should it be questioned only when he wants to refuse it?

The dilemma Greg is facing here is not uncommon. There are a number of complex and conflicting issues and, before deciding what to do next, Greg needs to carefully think through the ethical and legal aspects of the situation. This is the process of ethical reasoning and decision making. The aim of this process is to try to identify what could be done, what should be done, what actually will be done and why.

Jewell (2000, cited in Henderson, 2005, p. 190) poses an interesting question; that is, is a moral person 'one who feels strongly about moral issues, one who understands moral issues or one who acts ethically when dealing with other[s]'?

Let's now work through the clinical reasoning cycle, with a focus on the ethical and legal dimensions of the situation, to see if you can identify what should be done, and what you actually would do if you were the nurse caring for George.

According to the clinical reasoning cycle, the first stage involves carefully considering the patient. Contextual reality may have a considerable impact at this stage. George's late arrival on Christmas Eve has the potential to be a distraction. Matters that are not urgent or life threatening, like advance directives and discussions about no-CPR decisions, can safely be left until after Christmas ... can't they?

Another factor is the sheer complexity and difficulty of the ethical problems that arise in healthcare. Ethical dilemmas, by their very nature, are often difficult and messy, and may involve conflict and take time to address and resolve. It requires a particular state of mind to 'see' the ethical dimensions of clinical situations and a deliberate act of will to go beyond the surface 'routine' of clinical practice to try to address the ethical complexities of the situation. Epstein (2006, p.115) calls the ability to do this 'mindful practice [in] the tacit ethics of the moment'. How the moral agent views these issues will have a significant impact on the way this situation unfolds, and on the outcome.

Therefore, the first stage of the clinical reasoning cycle, 'considering the patient's situation', should ideally focus as much on George as a person as on George having a number of serious and potentially life-threatening medical conditions. Will those caring for George consider his values and perspectives just as important as his diagnosis? Getting that balance right is extremely difficult and requires a high degree of willingness to listen to the points of view of others, as well as insight into one's own.

2. COLLECT CUES/INFORMATION

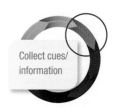

Collect cues/
information

(a) Review current information

There is a great deal that Greg does not know about George, especially the things that lie beneath the reasons for his decision to refuse CPR. One short conversation without privacy was not enough. George did appear to be very certain though, and what was also apparent was his trust in Greg and that he would know what to do.

On the other hand, Greg does not feel confident that George's refusal was sufficiently informed and not unduly influenced by his distressing experiences of the previous day. Greg wants to act in George's best interests, but it is not clear at the moment exactly what those are. Greg is very aware of the need for information to inform decisions, but he is also uncomfortable with Dr Jones' view that George cannot refuse CPR until he has a clearer diagnosis. Greg needs more information too, not only from George, but also about the wider ethical and legal ramifications of the situation.

(b) Gather new information

Nurses are familiar with conducting health assessments and taking patient histories, but such histories rarely involve deliberately eliciting information about a patient's values and treatment preferences, particularly concerning things like CPR. One of the ways of doing this is through an ethics history, in which information about George's understanding of his current situation, his values and wishes and the reasons for them, family relationships and other crucial but as yet unknown issues could be directly and explicitly explored. Sayers et al. (2001, p. 115) suggest some questions that could be useful in taking an ethics history, for example:

> *Very occasionally patients have what is called a cardiac arrest. This means their heart stops beating. Usually we try to restart it using artificial respiration, drugs and sometimes an electric shock. Usually doctors decide what to do, but some patients prefer to decide [this] for themselves.*
>
> *Would you like to make this decision?*
> *Would you like us, or a family member, to decide?*
> *Do you need more information before answering?*
> *Some people make advance directives or living wills. Have you heard of this? If so, are there any such directives that you would want us to know about?*

Greg also needs to know what processes should be followed for George's refusal of CPR to be recognised in law. There is variation between the states in regard to legislation and case law, so nurses need to be aware of the relevant polices and guidelines in their jurisdiction.

Consider the following questions:

Q1 Do you think that nurses should be involved in making CPR decisions, or is this outside their scope of practice? Explain.

Q2 The NSW Health (2005) guideline on *Using Advance Care Directives* (p. 4) lists six barriers to advance care planning. What are they?

Q3 The *Using Advance Care Directives* guideline identifies (on pp. 6 and 7) a number of best practice recommendations pertaining to advance care directives. Which ones are most relevant to George's situation?

Q4 What does the law say about the need for refusal of treatment decisions to be informed?

In Victoria, patients can fill out a refusal of treatment certificate (see Office of the Public Advocate Victoria, n.d.). In NSW, where advance directives are used, the following policies are relevant:

1 Using Advance Directives

2 End-of-Life Care and Decision Making

3 Using Resuscitation Plans in End-of-Life Decisions

Identify what laws and policies apply in your state.

(c) Recall knowledge

The knowledge of ethics and law that each individual nurse has will depend on their education, experience and professional ethos. While most nurses have had ethics content as part of their undergraduate education, one study found that many nurses (74 per cent) feel that they need more continuing ethics education in the workplace (Johnstone, Da Costa & Turale, 2004). One effect that ethics education has been found to have is to make it more likely that the nurse will encounter ethical issues in their practice. This is believed

The website, Respecting Patient Choices (supported by the Department of Health) has excellent state-based information and resources on advanced care planning: <www.respectingpatientchoices.org.au/>.

to be because they become increasingly likely to 'see' the ethical dimensions of practice; in other words, their perceptions fundamentally change as a result of such education. But being more attuned and aware of the ethical dimensions of practice is just the first step. To practise effectively, nurses also need to be able to correctly apply that knowledge to the situation at hand. This can be difficult, because the details of each case are frequently quite distinctive in their nuances and content, and clinicians have to make inferences to determine how the generalities of codes, or the specifics of different law cases, apply.

The NMBA's *Code of Ethics for Nurses in Australia* (2008a) should be well known to all nurses practising in Australia. Greg is aware that the Code of Ethics values quality nursing care, informed decision making, and respect and kindness. These value statements are quite broad and Greg has to translate them into the specifics of this situation. For example, this might entail:

- knowing what the benefits and risks of CPR actually are for George in this situation
- knowing how to assess whether George has made an informed refusal
- knowing how to ensure that George's values, beliefs and wishes are both elicited and respected
- knowing which actions are consistent with these value statements and which are not.

Greg is also aware that the NMBA's *Code of Professional Conduct* (2008b) requires him to practise in accordance with current laws. Some of the specific aspects of law that apply to this situation, and that Greg will need to know about, include:

- knowing what George's legal rights are in relation to refusing CPR
- knowing how best to inform George of these rights
- knowing his own legal responsibilities in either instigating or withholding CPR in the absence of a clearly documented no-CPR decision.

Consider the following questions.

Q1 Assuming that George does have decision-specific capacity, does he have the legal right to refuse CPR?

Q2 What might the potential legal consequences be of instigating CPR in the current situation (i.e. knowing George has refused it, but in the absence of any documentation)?

The epidemiology of in-hospital cardiac arrest

A famous study of the depiction of CPR in movies and television found that it was shown to be successful over 75% of the time, many times greater than happens in reality (Diemet et al., 1996; Portnova et al., 2015). For more details on the epidemiology of CPR, go to <www.ncbi.nlm.nih.gov/pubmed/23470471>.

Studies of the morbidity and mortality of in-hospital cardiac arrest show some interesting findings, some of which may surprise you. For example, post-arrest survival-to-discharge rates have not improved very much over the past 40 years, despite changes in technology and practice (Alabi & Haines, 2009). Conversely, patients and the general public considerably overestimate their chances of surviving a cardiac arrest. A study by Kaldjian et al. (2009) found that patients think the probability of surviving a cardiac arrest is 60 per cent, whereas actual rates are closer to 17–20 per cent. This figure may be even lower, depending on a number of factors such as age, co-morbidities and peri-arrest variables (such as time taken to initiate CPR). There are also other risks that many people may not be aware of, such as surviving with permanent neurological damage, and/or needing nursing home care rather than being able to be discharged home.

This doesn't mean that we should not be doing CPR. What it does mean is that the potential benefits and risks should be carefully and realistically considered for each patient's situation. In George's case, since he was so fearful of losing any more of his physical and mental capability, the risks are particularly applicable.

Q   How does this information affect your assessment of whether CPR is in George's best interests?

3. PROCESS INFORMATION

The third stage of the clinical reasoning cycle relates to the processing of information.

(a) Interpret

Interpretation can be difficult when the information that you are working with is subjective and not in the form of quantifiable and objective data, such as that derived from physiological signs and symptoms.

This stage of interpretation will also be filtered through the person doing the interpreting, and we know that human beings are not value-neutral when they make interpretations. Each person has had past experiences, both personal and professional, of situations such as this. Each person has personal beliefs and opinions about such matters, perhaps informed by a religion or perhaps not. These past experiences and personal values will affect how Greg feels about what George is requesting. Some nurses may interpret what George is requesting as irrational, a product of fear or stress or depression, and call into question his capacity to make such a decision. Others may interpret his refusal of treatment as synonymous with a wish to die. Greg's interpretation of these complex factors will have a significant impact on the outcome. Another nurse may interpret things differently and come to a quite different conclusion. This is yet one more way in which George is vulnerable in this situation. He is, to a considerable extent, dependent not only on the way others see him but also on their preparedness to act (or not) based on their interpretations.

Read about some of the debates on how humans came to be moral, the sources of our moral views and differences, and how we make moral judgments at The Situationist website: <http://thesituationist. wordpress.com/2008/ 06/17/jonathan-haidt-on-the-situation-of-moral-reasoning/>.

According to the moral psychologist, Jonathan Haidt (2000), human beings do not make moral judgments judicially and reasonably; rather, they do so quickly and instinctively, relying on innate intuitions, emotions, and socially and culturally derived perceptions and values. For Haidt, reason comes into play only after we have already made a judgment, and it is used mainly to rationalise or justify the judgment to ourselves and to others. Haidt's challenging ideas provide a fascinating insight into the ways in which a reasoning process may be far less rational than we realise.

Consider the following questions.

Q1 This situation potentially involves a clash of differing values and moral views. We are now well aware of George's values, but those of Greg and Dr Jones are much less visible. How might they affect the situation?

Q2 What values do you hold that would influence your interpretation of the information that you have about this situation?

(b) Discriminate, (c) Relate, (d) Infer and (e) Match

These elements of the clinical reasoning cycle might involve Greg being able to:

- distinguish what is more important from that which is less so
- identify what is most relevant from that which is least relevant
- identify which aspects of his past experiences with similar situations might be helpful in this one
- identify how his emotions and feelings about what has happened might be influencing his reasoning.

All of these elements require careful consideration of nuanced and detailed information. Is it more important that George's wishes be respected or more important that his carers are sure that those wishes are informed? Is following the 'correct' process of refusing CPR more or less important than the outcome? Is it possible that processes that are intended to give rise to better ethical decisions may not in fact do so in some situations? Could this be one of those? These four elements—discriminating, relating, inferring and matching—all require experience and skill to engage in effectively. If this is the first time that Greg has encountered this kind of situation, his thinking, feelings and overall approach at this stage of the clinical reasoning cycle are likely to be very different from his approach if he is used to and comfortable dealing with complexity, nuance and ambiguity.

(f) Predict

Thinking ahead to predict the outcome of each possible option for decisions in this situation is not a straightforward undertaking. There are a bewildering number of possibilities. However, Greg may identify the following options:

a Explain to George what has happened.

b Ask George whether he would like the involvement and support of family and/or friends.

c Undertake a proper ethics history.

d Make a thorough and detailed documentation of the information elicited from the ethics history.

e   Explain to George how he can go about making a legally binding advance directive.

f   Call Dr Jones back and ask him to see George again.

g   Notify the immediate clinical supervisor about what has happened and ask for advice.

h   Do nothing except document George's request and Dr Jones' response.

i   Do nothing at all now; not mention anything to George about what has happened and leave it until the next shift or even later, and not document anything.

j   Various combinations of the above.

Options (a) to (g) will, to varying degrees, be time consuming. Even though it is Christmas morning, it is still very busy and Greg has four other patients to care for. So it is possible that this will also be a factor in determining what happens next, even though this may not be explicitly acknowledged.

Apart from the time factor, there is also the question of how both Dr Jones and George might respond. Options (a) to (f) all require some degree and form of moral agency or advocacy from Greg, on George's behalf. Seal (2007), in a study of nurses and advocacy in advance care planning, found that up to 49 per cent of nurses felt powerless to advocate for their patients when issues of end-of-life care, or making decisions to withdraw or withhold treatment, were concerned. However, with the involvement of an institutionally supported intervention, the Respecting Patient Choices Program, this dropped to 19 per cent.

This suggests that even if Greg decides he should pursue options (e) and/or (f) he might feel he does not have the power to do so. Greg may feel that he lacks institutional or collegial support for any decision he might make that involves advocating for George, and his perception of the consequences of doing this may be a significant concern at this point.

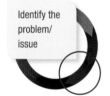

4. IDENTIFY THE ETHICAL PROBLEM/ISSUE

The core problem here is the question of who is responsible for making a no-CPR decision, and how that decision should be discussed, formally recognised and followed through. George thinks it is his decision. Unfortunately, he has little real understanding of the legal and procedural complexity that lies behind his request not to have CPR.

Dr Jones thinks it is his decision. He believes that he has both the expertise and the ultimate authority. The procedural need for formal documentation of some kind makes it unclear what should happen now, and if and how such an authority might legitimately and usefully be challenged.

Greg is caught in the middle, but if George has a cardiac arrest, then it will become Greg's decision. The moral problem for Greg is three-fold: First, can he find a way for George's refusal of treatment to be formally acknowledged? Second, can he make it happen in time? And, finally, what will he do if he can't?

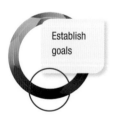

5. ESTABLISH GOALS

The people involved in this situation have different goals arising from their different values and perspectives about what is most important. Dr Jones values a clear diagnosis and that is his goal. His perception of George's best interest is to make a CPR decision based on having that information. George feels that he doesn't need that information. His decision about CPR isn't predicated on knowing if he has prostate cancer or not; it is about not wanting to live with a quality of life any less than he has now. These positions are fundamentally different.

The question is, whose goals (and values) come first? Nurses and doctors should and do put patients first, but it is possible (as we have seen) to have a different perspective about what that entails. In this situation, Greg's goal might well be to try to bridge the gap between George and Dr Jones, to make each aware of the other's position, and to try to resolve the situation in a collegial way that reflects the principles and goals of a best practice advance-care planning process.

There is something else that might be worth considering here. The Greek philosopher Aristotle wrote a great deal about the human virtues that lead to making good moral decisions. He believed that humans of good character or virtue would act rightly and make correct decisions, and that we should, throughout our lives, work consciously and deliberately to develop these character traits. For Aristotle, 'goodness' included traits such as kindness and generosity. He wrote in *Nichomachean Ethics*, '... we do not act rightly because we have virtue or excellence, but we rather have those because we have acted rightly. We are what we repeatedly do.'

Habits of thought and practice might be highly influential at this stage of the process. They may even determine the outcome. It is also possible that certain decisions and actions may be able to be definitely excluded as being the antithesis of 'goodness' and 'virtue'. Examples of such behaviours would include lying to George (even by omission) or avoiding him until the shift is over, behaviours that arise from self-centred rather than person-centred goals.

6. TAKE ACTION

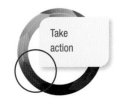

It turns out that Greg's time for thinking about the situation and taking action is cut short. What happens next is something he hasn't really believed could happen, even though he knows it is a possibility.

George's condition has been stable since his transfer and he's had no further chest pain. He begs Greg to allow him to take a shower on a commode chair, because he hates bed baths and doesn't want to have one on Christmas Day. So Greg takes him to the shower on a commode chair and is with him when George has a cardiac arrest.

Greg then has to make yet another decision about what to do, and this time there is no time for thinking. So he pushes the emergency buzzer, turns off the shower, eases George from the commode to the floor and starts CPR. The team arrives with the crash cart and George is carried naked from the bathroom to the corridor just outside, where an attempt to resuscitate him continues in full public view, with just a towel over his groin in a meagre attempt to preserve his modesty.

As someone else takes over doing chest compressions, the realisation hits Greg that what is happening is precisely what George has been trying to avoid.

After a prolonged resuscitation, George is taken to the Coronary Care Unit (CCU) and Greg is left to wonder if he has done the right thing, and what, if anything, he could have done differently.

7. EVALUATE

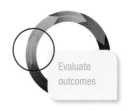

As Greg is thinking about what has happened and is wrestling with feelings of guilt, a call comes from the CCU. George's sister is there and wants to talk to him. Greg is a little apprehensive, but it turns out that she wants to talk about the documentation he wrote in the notes earlier, in which he explained in detail the results of his conversations with George. She has found out about it because the CCU staff wanted to confirm the information with her. George's sister tells Greg how thankful she is that Greg has done this, and has taken the trouble to get to know George. She tells Greg that George has told her several times that, when his time comes, he wants to go quickly and calmly. George's sister goes on to say that George has not regained consciousness and that his life support is about to be turned off. She then asks if Greg would like to be there when it is.

Greg agrees; so he, the last person to know George, is there with George's sister, who knows him best, to say goodbye at the end.

8. REFLECT

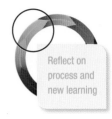

Reflecting on the whole situation afterwards, Greg realised that he could have done some things differently. He should have known that George was quite likely to have another cardiac arrest, and he should have factored that eventuality more into his thinking. But he also realised that, even knowing about the possibility, he hadn't really believed the cardiac arrest would happen when it did.

Greg felt sad and conflicted, knowing that George had an awful death, so lacking in the dignity that characterised his life, but also that without the CPR attempt his sister would not have had the opportunity to see him and say goodbye. So there had been both good and bad in what had happened. Greg knew, though, that he could never tell George's sister the reality of George's resuscitation, naked on the floor, in full view of almost the whole ward. So instead he gave a silent apology to George for not being able to protect him from that.

He wouldn't ever forget George, and if something like this happened again, Greg knew what he would do differently. He now knew that, whatever the time of day or year, patients' requests for refusing treatment have to be decisively followed up then and there. He knew now that he should have asked Dr Jones to go back and speak to George, instead of saying nothing as the doctor walked away. He also realised that the ward needed clearer guidelines on what the nurses should do in situations like this, so that outcomes would be less up to the vagaries of chance.

It is a hopeful signal for change that the need for better end-of-life care planning has been recognised and acted upon by the Australian Commission on Safety and Quality in Health Care. The draft NSQHS Standards include a Comprehensive Care standard which aims to address gaps in quality and safety in specific conditions, such as the failure to 'work in partnership with patients' and to 'determine their preferences for care' (ACSQHC, 2016, pp. 36–41). The future prospects for comprehensive end-of-life care planning for patients like George are now much improved.

Reflect on your learning from this scenario and consider the following questions:

Q1   What are three of the most important things that you have learnt from this scenario?

Q2   Identify the full range of specific nursing actions that may have prevented George from having CPR against his wishes.

Q3   Considering your answer to the above, what would you have done in this situation and why?

Q4   If what you would do is different from what you think you should do, explain why this is the case.

Q5   What specific further knowledge do you think you need in order to be able to practise ethically and legally in situations involving refusal of treatment?

FURTHER READING

Australian Commission on Safety and Quality in Health Care (ACSQHC). (2016). *End-of-Life Care.* Available at <www.safetyandquality.gov.au/our-work/end-of-life-care-in-acute-hospitals>.

Relevant legislation and case law:

Anderson v St Francis–St George Hospital: <http://findarticles.com/p/articles/mi_qa3689/is_199803/ai_n8807845/>.

Brightwater Care Group Inc. v Rossiter: <www.supremecourt.wa.gov.au/publications/pdf/proceedings.pdf>.

Hunter and New England Area Health Service v A: <www.austlii.edu.au/>.

Medical Treatment Act 1988 (Vic): <www.austlii.edu.au/au/legis/vic/consol_act/mta1988168/>.

REFERENCES

Adams, J. A., Bailey, D. E., Anderson, R. A. & Docherty, S. L. (2011). Nursing roles and strategies in end-of-life decision making in acute care: A systematic review of the literature. *Nursing Research and Practice*. doi: 10.1155/2011/527834

Alabi, T. O. & Haines, C. A. (2009). Predicting survival from in-hospital CPR. *Clinical Geriatrics, 17*(12), 34–36.

Aristotle. (n.d.). *Nichomachean Ethics*. Available at <http://classics.mit.edu/Aristotle/nicomachaen.html>.

Australian Commission on Safety and Quality in Health Care (ACSQHC). (2016). *National Safety and Quality Health Service Standards Version 2*. Draft, Sydney, Australia.

Diem, S. J., Lanton, J. D. & Tulsky, J. A. (1996). Cardiopulmonary resuscitation on television— Miracles and misinformation. *New England Journal of Medicine, 334*, 1578–82. doi: 10.1056/NEJM199606133342406

Epstein, R. M. (2006). Mindful practice and the tacit ethics of the moment. In W. Shelton (Ed.), *Advances in Bioethics*. New York: Emerald.

Forrester, K. & Griffiths, D. (2014). *Essentials of Law for Health Professionals* (4th edn). Sydney: Elsevier.

Haidt, J. (2000). The emotional dog and its rational tail: A social intuitionist approach to moral judgment. *Psychological Review, 108*, 814–34.

Hayes, B. (2013). Clinical model for ethical cardiopulmonary resuscitation decision making. *Internal Medicine Journal, 43*(1), 77–83. doi: 10.1111/j.1445-5994.2012.02841.x

Henderson, L. (2005). Combining moral philosophy and moral reasoning: The PAVE moral reasoning strategy. *International Education Journal, 6*(2), 184–93.

Johnstone, M., Da Costa, C. & Turale, S. (2004). Registered and enrolled nurses' experiences of ethical issues in nursing practice. *Australian Journal of Advanced Nursing, 22*(1), 24–30.

Kaldjian, L. C., Erekson, Z. D., Haberle, T. H., Curtis, A. E., Shinkunas, L. A., Cannon, K. T. & Forman-Hoffman, V. L. (2009). Code status discussions and goals of care among hospitalised adults. *Journal of Medical Ethics, 35*(6), 338–42.

Nursing and Midwifery Board of Australia (NMBA). (2016). *Registered Nurse Standards for Practice*. Retrieved from <www.nursingmidwiferyboard.gov.au/Codes-Guidelines-Statements/Professional-standards.aspx>.

Nursing and Midwifery Board of Australia (NMBA). (2008a). *Code of Ethics for Nurses in Australia*. Australian Nursing and Midwifery Council/Australian College of Nursing/Australian Nursing Federation. Retrieved from <www.nursingmidwiferyboard.gov.au/Codes-Guidelines-Statements/CodesGuidelines.aspx#competencystandards>.

Nursing and Midwifery Board of Australia (NMBA). (2008b). *Code of Professional Conduct for Nurses in Australia*. Australian Nursing and Midwifery Council/Australian College of Nursing/Australian Nursing Federation. Retrieved from <www.nursingmidwiferyboard.gov.au/Codes-Guidelines-Statements/Codes-Guidelines.aspx#competencystandards>.

NSW Health. (2005). *Using Advance Care Directives*. Accessed April 2017 at <www1.health.nsw.gov.au/pds/ActivePDSDocuments/GL2005_056.pdf>.

Office of the Public Advocate Victoria. (n.d.). *Refusal of Medical Treatment*. Available at <www.publicadvocate.vic.gov.au/medical-consent/refusal-of-treatment>.

Portnova, J., Irvine, K., Yi, J. Y. & Enguidanos, S. (2015). It isn't like this on TV: Revisiting CPR survival rates depicted on popular TV shows. *Resuscitation, 96*, 148–50. doi: 10.1016/j.resuscitation.2015.08.002

Resuscitation Council UK. (2012). *Emergency Care and CPR Decision-Making*. Available at <www.resus.org.uk/statements/emergency-care-and-cpr-decision-making>.

Sayers, G. M., Barratt, D., Gothard, C., Onnie, C., Perera, S. & Schulman, D. (2001). The value of taking an 'ethics history'. *Journal of Medical Ethics, 27*, 114–17.

Seal, M. (2007). Patient advocacy and advance care planning in the acute hospital setting. *Australian Journal of Advanced Nursing, 24*(4), 29–36.

GLOSSARY

acquired brain injury	Any injury or damage that occurs to the brain after birth.
acute pain	A severe pain episode lasting from a few seconds to six months duration that may occur due to trauma, surgery or a medical condition.
advanced directive	A document by which a person makes provision for healthcare decisions in the event that, in the future, he/she becomes unable to make those decisions.
adverse drug event	A harmful or unintended reaction or symptom from an administered medication.
aetiology	The cause or origin of a disease or abnormal condition.
altered level of consciousness	Any level of consciousness other than normal rousability and responsiveness.
analyse	Separation into components: the breaking down of the whole into its parts (deductive reasoning).
anchoring	The tendency to lock onto salient features in the patient's presentation too early in the clinical reasoning process, and failing to adjust this initial impression in light of later information.
anxiety	Feelings of apprehension, uneasiness, tension and restlessness, often precipitated by different or unfamiliar experiences.
arrhythmias	Abnormal heart rhythms or beats.
ascertainment bias	When a nurse's thinking is shaped by prior assumptions and preconceptions, e.g. ageism, stigmatism and stereotyping.
asthma	A respiratory condition that causes airways to become inflamed, swell and narrow; along with extra production of mucus, breathing becomes difficult.
autoimmune disease	A condition where the immune system responds abnormally and attacks healthy cells within the body.
blood component therapy	Transfusion of one or a number of components of whole blood, e.g. packed red cells or platelets.
cardiac arrest	An emergency situation where a person's cardiac output and effective circulation suddenly ceases.
cerebral palsy	A group of permanent disorders of development, movement and posture caused by non-progressive disturbances to the developing brain during pregnancy or soon after birth.
chest pain	A physical symptom requiring immediate evaluation, diagnosis and treatment. May be symptomatic of a cardiac complication, or could be musculoskeletal, gastrointestinal or psychogenic.
chronic	Persisting for a long time, either recurring frequently or continuing for the rest of a person's life.
clinical reasoning	The process by which nurses (and other clinicians) collect cues, process the information, come to an understanding of a patient problem or situation, plan and implement interventions, evaluate outcomes, and reflect on and learn from the process.

cognitive decline	A gradual reduction in the speed at which individuals acquire information as they age.
community-acquired pneumonia	Pneumonia (acute infection of the lungs) that has developed in the community, outside of a healthcare setting.
co-morbidity	Two or more diseases experienced at the one time that are connected with each other via pathogenetic mechanisms.
complementary therapies	A group of diverse medical and healthcare systems, practices and products that are not generally considered to be part of conventional medicine.
confirmation bias	The tendency to look for confirming evidence to support a nursing diagnosis rather than look for disconfirming evidence to refute it.
critical thinking	A complex collection of cognitive skills and affective habits of the mind.
cues	Identifiable physiological or psychosocial changes experienced by the patient, perceived through history or assessment and understood in relation to a specific body of knowledge and philosophical beliefs. Cues also include the context of care and the surrounding clinical situation.
cultural safety	Effective person-centred healthcare of an individual and/or their family as determined by their cultural background and traditional wishes.
data	A piece or pieces of information about health status.
dehydration	Extreme loss of fluid from cellular tissues in the body as a result of illness or lack of fluid intake.
delirium	An acute reversible clinical syndrome of cognitive function, characterised by an acute decline that impairs cognitive and physical function.
dementia	An umbrella term that is used to describe a gradual, progressive, irreversible deterioration of cerebral function, which results in disturbance of many higher cortical functions, including memory, thinking and judgment.
depression	A mood disorder that causes a persistent feeling of sadness and loss of interest, and that can affect how a person feels, thinks and behaves.
deterioration	Gradual decline or worsening of a condition.
diabetes	A term covering a complex group of dangerous diseases that result in an imbalance of blood glucose levels. The three key types of diabetes include type 1 (insulin in pancreas is destroyed by the immune system); type 2 (pancreas does not produce enough insulin, or the insulin produced is not effective); and gestational diabetes (occurs during pregnancy, usually disappearing after birth of baby).
diabetic ketoacidosis	A highly dangerous complication of diabetes that may occur when the body is profoundly deficient in insulin with symptoms of hyperglycaemia, ketosis, acidosis and dehydration.
diagnostic momentum	When a label attached to a patient starts as a possibility but gathers increasing momentum until it is seen as definite and other possibilities are excluded.
disability	A physical or mental condition that limits a person's movements, senses or activities.
discharge planning	Activities that facilitate continuity of care during a person's transfer from one healthcare setting to another, or to home. It is a multi-disciplinary process involving doctors, nurses, social workers and possibly other healthcare professionals.

discriminate	To use good judgment, note or observe a difference accurately, distinguish relevant from irrelevant information, recognise inconsistencies, narrow down information to what is most important and recognise gaps in cues collected.
dying with dignity	Death that occurs in accordance with the wishes and values of a patient.
electrolyte imbalance	An imbalance of electrolytes in the body, such as sodium, potassium, magnesium or calcium.
ethical dilemma	Situations in which there is a choice to be made between two options, neither of which resolves the situation in an ethically acceptable fashion.
ethical reasoning	The ability to identify, assess and develop ethical arguments from a variety of ethical positions.
evaluate	To make a judgment about the worth or value of something.
'failure to rescue'	Mortality of patients who experience a hospital-acquired complication.
family-centred care	Healthcare delivery centred around a partnership with a child's family and/or significant others.
fundamental attribution error	The tendency to be judgmental and blame patients for their illnesses rather than examine the circumstances that may have been responsible.
goals	A desired outcome and a guidepost to the selection of nursing interventions.
haemotological diseases	Diseases or disorders affecting the blood.
healthcare transition	The coordination and continuity of healthcare during a movement from one healthcare setting to another or to home, and/or between healthcare providers during the course of a chronic or acute illness.
heart failure	When the heart is not able to effectively maintain blood flow to ensure sufficient circulation. Sometimes referred to as chronic or congestive heart failure.
holistic healthcare	Comprehensive healthcare that takes into consideration a person's physical, emotional, social, economic and spiritual needs.
hyperglycaemia	An abnormally high blood glucose level.
hypervolaemia	An abnormally high level of fluid in the circulating blood volume—or fluid volume deficit.
hypoglycaemia	An abnormally low blood glucose level.
hypovolaemia	An abnormally low level of fluid in the circulating blood volume.
hypoxia	When an inadequate amount of oxygen is reaching tissues in parts of the body.
inconsistency	Something that contradicts something else or that is not in keeping with it; not regular or predictable.
infer	To make deductions or form opinions that follow logically by interpreting subjective and objective data; to consider alternatives and consequences.
interpret	Analyse data to come to an understanding; to explain or tell the meaning of; to present in understandable terms.
ischaemia	A restriction or lack of blood supply to tissues in the body causing inadequate oxygen levels, sometimes leading to tissue necrosis.
kidney disease	A disease where renal function is impaired, either acutely or chronically, sometimes requiring dialysis.
match	Information or cues that correspond to each other or cluster together naturally.

medication error	A preventable incident where an incorrect medication is administered which may lead to patient harm or inappropriate use.
medication safety	A model that aims to prevent medication errors occurring.
mental state examination	A clinical assessment tool used in mental health assessment that provides a methodical way to observe and record an individual's thoughts, emotions, behaviour and demeanour.
mild cognitive impairment	A syndrome characterised by cognitive decline that is different from normal ageing and does not meet the criteria for mild dementia.
multi-disciplinary healthcare team	When healthcare professionals from a range of disciplines with different but complementary skills, knowledge and experience work together to deliver comprehensive care aimed at providing the best possible outcome for the physical and psychosocial needs of a patient and their carers.
multimodal pain management	A combination of two or more analgesic medications or techniques acting on different mechanisms to provide optimal pain relief whilst using less opioids.
multimorbidity	Two or more diseases appearing randomly without any connection to each other through pathogenetic mechanisms.
multisystem autoimmune disease	An autoimmune disease that impacts multiple organs.
neurological deterioration	Gradual decline or worsening of the neurological state, which may appear as a decline in sensory and motor responses.
nursing diagnosis	A patient problem that becomes apparent following a thorough and systematic interpretation of subjective and objective data.
outcome	A measurable change in a client's status in response to nursing care.
overconfidence bias	Believing we know more than we do, reflecting a tendency to act on incomplete information, intuition or hunches.
oxygenation	The process of oxygen diffusing from the alveolus to the pulmonary capillary.
pain management plan	An agreement made between the medical officer and patient to use medication and/or alternative therapies in an effort to meet pain management goals.
pain myths	A well-known but false idea or belief about pain and/or pain management.
palliative care	An approach that improves the quality of life of people facing a life-limiting illness, through the prevention and relief of suffering by identification, assessment and treatment of pain and other physical, psychosocial and spiritual problems.
persistent (chronic) pain	Pain that continues past a 'normal' healing time of around three months.
person-centred care	A holistic approach to the planning and delivery of healthcare that is grounded in a philosophy of personhood. It is a way of practising that acknowledges and respects each individual's autonomy, personal beliefs, values, needs and desires.
predict	To envisage or foresee something that may happen.
pre-emptive pain management	Analgesia that is initiated before surgery in order to prevent the establishment of central sensitisation evoked by the incisional and inflammatory injuries occurring during surgery and in the early post-operative period. Also refers to all analgesic strategies that aim to prevent rather than treat pain after it has manifested.
premature closure	The tendency to accept a nursing diagnosis without sufficient evidence and before it has been fully verified.

psychosis	A state of mind where there is a disconnect with reality.
psych-out error	When clinical reasoning errors occur in people with mental illness, and co-morbid conditions are overlooked or minimalised. A variant is when medical conditions (e.g. hypoxia, delirium, electrolyte imbalance or head injuries) are misdiagnosed as psychiatric conditions.
raised intracranial pressure	A rise in pressure of the cerebrospinal fluid surrounding the brain and spinal cord, due to either an increase in fluid volume or swelling of the brain.
rapid response	A system whereby a team of healthcare professionals (sometimes referred to as a medical emergency team) immediately responds to a call for a patient who is exhibiting signs of serious clinical deterioration.
recall	To remember or recollect a past situation or piece of knowledge.
recovery model	A model that supports an individual's recovery from mental illness.
reflection	A critical review of practice with a view to refinement, improvement or change; the process of looking back and the careful consideration of an experience; to explore the understanding of what one did and why and the impact it has on themselves and others.
rehabilitation	The process of restoring an individual's health and mental or physical abilities to the pre-operative or pre-injury level through guided therapy.
relate	To connect or link; to discover new relationships or patterns; to cluster cues together to identify relationships between them.
'rescue'	The ability to recognise deteriorating patients and to intervene appropriately.
respiratory distress	A life-threatening condition involving breathing difficulties due to narrowed airways or when alveoli fill with fluid.
risk nursing diagnosis	A clinical judgment about a potential problem where the presence of risk factors indicates that a problem may develop unless nurses intervene appropriately.
sepsis	A potentially life-threatening infection—often of the blood.
septic shock	A serious medical condition that occurs when sepsis, which is organ injury or damage in response to infection, leads to dangerously low blood pressure and abnormalities in cellular metabolism. It can cause multiple organ failure and death.
stigma	A mark, blemish or sign of disgrace, shame or dishonour.
stroke	Brain damage from an interruption to the blood supply. Two types of stroke include haemorrhagic (bleeding in the brain) and ischaemic (blocked artery). A transient ischaemic attack (TIA) may also occur, which is when the blood supply is interrupted, but for a short time only.
substance use	A condition in which the use of one or more substances leads to a clinically significant impairment or distress. It refers to a cluster of cognitive, behavioural and physiological symptoms indicating that the individual continues using the substance despite significant substance-related problems.
synthesis	The putting together of parts into the whole (inductive reasoning); the integration of new knowledge with previous knowledge, to form a 'new whole'.
terminal dehydration	A type of isotonic fluid imbalance that occurs at the end of life, which can lead to feelings of euphoria and an increasing level of comfort during the dying process.

terminal restlessness   A particularly distressing form of delirium that sometimes occurs in dying patients characterised by spiritual, emotional or physical restlessness, anxiety, agitation and cognitive failure.

transfusion reactions   Adverse signs or symptoms that appear or occur during, or up to 24 hours after, infusion of transfused product.

unpacking principle   Failure to collect and unpack all relevant cues, and consider differential diagnoses, resulting in significant possibilities being missed.

INDEX